OXFORD MEDICAL PUBLICATIONS

The Making of the Nervous System

THE MAKING
OF THE NERVOUS
SYSTEM

EDITED BY

J. G. PARNAVELAS
University College London

C. D. STERN
University of Oxford

AND

R. V. STIRLING
National Institute for Medical Research, London

OXFORD NEW YORK TOKYO
OXFORD UNIVERSITY PRESS
1988

Oxford University Press, Walton Street, Oxford OX2 6DP

Oxford   New York   Toronto
Delhi   Bombay   Calcutta   Madras   Karachi
Petaling Jaya   Singapore   Hong Kong   Tokyo
Nairobi   Dar es Salaam   Cape Town
Melbourne   Auckland

and associated companies in
Beirut   Berlin   Ibadan   Nicosia

Oxford is a trade mark of Oxford University Press

Published in the United States
by Oxford University Press, New York

British Library Cataloguing in Publication Data
The Making of the nervous system.
(Oxford medical publications).
1. Developmental neurology
I. Parnavelas, J.G.   II. Stern, C.D.
III. Stirling, R.V.
591.1'88   QP363.5
ISBN 0-19-854224-0

Library of Congress Cataloging in Publication Data
The Making of the nervous system.
(Oxford medical publications)
Based on a conference held at Wye College, Kent, in June 1986.
Bibliography: p.
Including index.
1. Nervous system—Growth—Congresses.   2. Developmen-
tal neurology—Congresses.   I. Parnavelas, J. G. (John G.)
II. Stern, C. D. (Claudio D.)
III. Stirling, R. V. (R. Victoria)   IV. Series. [DNLM:
1. Central Nervous System—growth & development—
congresses.   2. Neurobiology—congresses. WL 300 M235 1986]
QP363.5.M35   1988   591.1'88   87-18658
ISBN 0-19-854224-0

Set and Printed in Great Britain by
The Alden Press, Oxford

Preface

The mechanisms that play roles in the making of the nervous system (and, indeed, of the whole animal) are remarkably diverse. While many of them are still mysterious, a number of powerful techniques have recently become available which may help elucidate them.

The availability of these new techniques carries an intrinsic danger: their indiscriminate application can give rise to a plethora of facts and figures without a clear sense of direction. For example, the recent application of molecular biology to developmental neurobiology has led to a proliferation of reports of messenger RNAs that are expressed in some portion or other of the nervous system. However, these findings have yet to add to our understanding of how the development of the nervous system is controlled. In other words, knowledge is more than the sum of the facts. Occasionally, however, a discovery is made that is able to bring many facts together. As Hermann Bondi has put it: 'at times we make discoveries that sharply reduce the knowledge that we have, and it is discoveries of this kind that are indeed the seminal point in science. It is they that are the real roots of progress and lead to the jumps in understanding'. In attempting to synthesize our knowledge of the processes that shape the nervous system, neurobiologists inevitably choose particular model systems, which, they argue, are representative of all others, and which, by virtue of their simplicity in one or another respect, are preferable to anyone else's model system. To quote Hermann Bondi once more, 'the search for simplicity is a powerful driving force, but it does not necessarily get us there'. One problem is that it is not so easy to establish where 'there' is.

It is surprising, perhaps, to find that we still need to be reminded of some of the basic problems to be addressed in developmental neurobiology. After attending a rather confused lecture on the development of the nervous system in 1983, we decided that it was high time to put together a conference, perhaps a book, in which we would attempt to identify some of these problems. The conference took place in June 1986 at Wye College, in Kent.

This book does not aim to be a comprehensive survey of the events that take place during the development of the nervous system, nor does it provide solutions to the unanswered questions in developmental neurobiology. Rather, we have tried to bring together the thoughts of some workers confronted with similar problems of differing complexity in different animals, to warn the student of neurobiology about some of the pitfalls that lie on the path, to inform him about the current state of the art, and to remind him of the questions that remain to be addressed. In order to aid the student in this quest and to give more coherence to the book, we have grouped the chapters into five parts, each of which is preceded by a short introduction designed to present each major area. A short list of recommended reading relating to these sections will be found at the back of the book. The references in this list are compiled to help the student to understand some of the basic concepts used in this book.

Oxford and London   J.G.P.
October 1986   C.D.S.
                                                             R.V.S.

Acknowledgements

We are especially grateful to The Brain Association for their support, which ensured the success of the Wye meeting. Thanks are also due to the following for financial contributions to the meeting: Arnold R. Horwell Ltd., Millipore (UK) Ltd., Stag Instruments Ltd., Anachem, Raymond A. Lamb, Imperial Chemical Industries plc., Sigma Chemical Co. Ltd., Merck, Sharpe & Dohme Ltd., Parke Davis & Co. Ltd., The Royal Society, The Wellcome Trust, The British Council, IBRO, and Centre for Neuroscience. We are deeply indebted to Mrs Chris Richards for her invaluable assistance before, during, and after the meeting, to Mr James Cope for his help during the conference, and to Miss Eva Franke for her assistance during the preparation of the manuscripts for publication. For allowing us to reproduce those figures that had already been published elsewhere, we owe our gratitude to the Copyright Clearance Centre, to the editors of the journals and books where they appeared and, in some cases, to the authors of the original sources. We are also grateful to Mrs Georgina Ferry for her coverage of the conference on behalf of BBC Radio 4, and to *Nature* for publishing a report on the meeting. We thank those who gave up their time repeatedly to comment on chapters and editorial sections, in particular Drs. J. Adam and R. J. Keynes. We are greatly indebted to the Staff of Oxford University Press for their support and help during all the stages of the publication of this book. Finally, we are grateful to the authors for complying promptly and without hesitation to our multiple, and often unreasonable, requests.

Contents

List of contributors

JONATHAN P. BACON, School of Biological Sciences, University of Sussex, Falmer, Brighton BN1 9QG, UK.

MARTIN BERRY, Department of Anatomy, U.M.D.S., Guy's Hospital Medical School, London SE1 9RT, UK.

SUSANNA BLACKSHAW, Department of Physiology, University of Glasgow, Glasgow G12 8QQ, UK.

MARIANNE BRONNER-FRASER, Department of Developmental and Cell Biology, and The Developmental Biology Center, University of California, Irvine, CA 92717, USA.

PAUL R. CARNEY, Neuroscience Program, Department of Developmental Genetics, School of Medicine, Case Western Reserve University, Cleveland, Ohio 44106, USA.

MARION E. CAVANAGH, Department of Anatomy and Embryology, University College London, Gower Street, London WC1E 6BT, UK.

SUSANNAH CHANG, Max-Planck-Institut für Entwicklungsbiologie, Spemannstrasse 35, D-7400 Tübingen, Federal Republic of Germany.

RICHARD DURBIN, MRC Laboratory of Molecular Biology, Hills Road, Cambridge CB2 2QH, UK.

JAMES W. FAWCETT, The Salk Institute for Biological Studies and the Clayton Foundation for Research, California Division, P.O. Box 85800, San Diego, California 92138, USA. (Present address: University Laboratory of Physiology, University of Cambridge, Downing Street, Cambridge CB2 3DY, UK.)

SCOTT E. FRASER, Department of Physiology and Biophysics, and The Developmental Biology Center, University of California, Irvine, CA 92717, USA.

JOHN FREDIEU, Neuroscience Program, Department of Developmental Genetics, School of Medicine, Case Western Reserve University, Cleveland, Ohio 44106, USA.

R. W. GUILLERY, Department of Human Anatomy, University of Oxford, South Parks Road, Oxford OX1 3QX, UK.

STEPHEN P. HUNT, MRC Molecular Neurobiology Unit, Medical Research Council Centre, Hills Road, Cambridge CB2 2QH, UK.

GIORGIO M. INNOCENTI, Institut d'Anatomie, Rue de Bugnon 9, 1005 Lausanne, Switzerland.

MARCUS JACOBSON, Department of Anatomy, University of Utah School of Medicine, Salt Lake City, Utah 84132, USA.

JOSEF P. KAPFHAMMER, Max-Planck-Institut für Entwicklungsbiologie, Spemannstrasse 35, D-7400 Tübingen, Federal Republic of Germany.

ROGER J. KEYNES, Department of Anatomy, University of Cambridge, Downing Street, Cambridge CB2 3DY, UK.

JEFF W. LICHTMAN, Department of Anatomy and Neurobiology, Washington University School of Medicine, 660 South Euclid Avenue, St. Louis, Missouri 63110, USA.

RONALD M. LINDSAY, Sandoz Institute for Medical Research, 5 Gower Place, London WC1E 6BN, UK.

ANDREW G. S. LUMSDEN, Department of Anatomy, U.M.D.S., Guy's Hospital Medical School, London SE1 9RT, UK.

ANDREW MATUS, Friedrich-Miescher Institute, P.O. Box 2543, 4002 Basel, Switzerland.

ROBERT H. MILLER, Medical Research Council Neurobiology programme, Department of Zoology, University College London, Gower Street, London WC1E 6BT, UK.

NANCY A. O'ROURKE, Department of Physiology and Biophysics, and The Developmental Biology Center, University of California, Irvine, CA 92717, USA.

JOHN G. PARNAVELAS, Department of Anatomy and Embryology, University College London, Gower Street, London WC1E 6BT, UK.

MICHAEL R. POSTON, Neuroscience Program, Department of Developmental Genetics, School of Medicine, Case Western Reserve University, Cleveland, Ohio 44106, USA.

JOHNATHAN A. RAPER, Max-Planck-Institut für Entwicklungsbiologie, Spemannstrasse 35, D-7400 Tübingen, Federal Republic of Germany.

FRITZ G. RATHJEN, Max-Planck-Institut für Entwicklungsbiologie, Spemannstrasse 35, D-7400 Tübingen, Federal Republic of Germany.

MARTIN SADLER, Department of Anatomy, U.M.D.S., Guy's Hospital Medical School, London SE1 9RT, UK.

JOHN T. SCHMIDT, Department of Biological Sciences and Neurobiology Research Center, State University of New York at Albany, 1400 Washington Avenue, Albany, New York 12222, USA.

JERRY SILVER, Neuroscience Program, Department of Developmental Genetics, School of Medicine, Case Western Reserve University, Cleveland, Ohio 44106, USA.

CLAUDIO D. STERN, Department of Human Anatomy, University of Oxford, South Parks Road, Oxford OX1 3QX, UK.

R. VICTORIA STIRLING, National Institute for Medical Research, The Ridgeway, Mill Hill, London NW7 1AA, UK.

CLAUDIA A. O. STUERMER, Friedrich-Miescher-Laboratorium der Max-Planck-Gesellschaft, Spemannstrasse 37–39, D-7400 Tübingen, Federal Republic of Germany.

DENNIS SUMMERBELL, National Institute for Medical Research, The Ridgeway, Mill Hill, London NW7 1AA, UK.

ANNE WARNER, Department of Anatomy and Embryology, University College London, Gower Street, London WC1E 6BT, UK.

RICHARD WETTS, Department of Physiology and Biophysics, and The Developmental Biology Center, University of California, Irvine, CA 92717, USA.

. . . so much concerning the several classes of Idols, and their equipage: all of which must be renounced and put away with a fixed and solemn determination, and the understanding thoroughly freed and cleansed.

Francis Bacon

PART I

Generating cell diversity

Introduction

In the formation of its nervous system, the organism must ensure that all the necessary cell types are available and that they are put together appropriately in space. There are two broad strategies that organisms might use: one is to generate cell diversity first, independently of any pattern, and then to assemble the different cells into a pattern; the other is to arrange groups of uncommitted cells into a gross pattern first, and then to generate diversity by cell interactions in different regions of the pattern. Each of these strategies has advantages and disadvantages for the embryo, and it is not yet known to what extent each plays a role during normal development.

If cell diversity is generated independently of the pattern ('mosaic' development; for definitions of classical embryological terms, see Slack 1983), cells should be allocated to different fates in the correct proportions. This is easy to achieve if cell fates are assigned entirely on the basis of the mitotic history of the cells (their 'lineage'). However, one has to explain the ability of a cell, tissue, or embryo to participate in generating normal organization after experimental interference ('embryonic regulation'). If cells are already committed to their fates, regulation has to be explained by interactive processes such as cell sorting.

The mechanisms that assign cells to different fates can be investigated by combining three approaches: by studying cell lineages in the normal embryo, by experimental interference (such as transplantation or ablation of individual identified cells), and by searching for the appearance of cell-type-specific determinants.

Organisms are amenable to the study of cell lineages if they allow some tracer to be introduced into individual, identified cells in the embryo. The markers may be genetic, such as mutant genes which may be introduced by various techniques (for example, using viral vectors or by genetic recombination) into individual cells, or they may be enzymes (such as horseradish peroxidase) or fluorescent tracers. The disadvantage of non-genetic markers is that they may become diluted by cell division and growth. Genetic markers have come into their own in organisms in which many genetic mutations are available; in particular, this approach has been exploited in the fruitfly, *Drosophila*. While the epidermal lineages in *Drosophila* are reasonably well understood, little is known yet about the lineage of neural cells. This is because the deep-lying nervous system of these organisms is more difficult to screen than the epidermis in assays that involve a large number of individuals.

The following chapters review our knowledge of the mechanisms that allocate cells to different fates in the nervous systems of three organisms: the nematode, the leech, and the frog. Since planning this volume, elegant studies of the cell lineage of the nervous system in the zebrafish embryo have been conducted, and the reader is referred to the original publications.

1

Determination of cell type in the ventral nervous system of the nematode *Caenorhabditis elegans*

RICHARD DURBIN

In the formation of a nervous system a large number of distinct neuronal types must be produced. In this chapter I will consider the problem of determination of cell type in an invertebrate nervous system. In general, cell determination may be influenced both by the ancestry of the cell and by its environment. To study the interactions between these intrinsic and extrinsic factors inside individual cells it is necessary either to study a very homogeneous population of cells or, ideally, to study single cells. The latter possibility is available in some of the simpler invertebrates whose nervous systems are highly reproducible from one animal to the next at a cellular level.

The animal for which the studies of development and anatomy have been brought together at the finest level of detail is the nematode, *Caenorhabditis elegans*, which is a small roundworm about 1 mm in length. In this chapter I intend to summarize our current knowledge about how neuronal cell types are determined in *C. elegans* by focusing on the development of one part of its nervous system, the ventral nerve cord. The cell types in the ventral cord provide examples of most of the principle patterns of determination that have been observed.

There are two features in particular that make *C. elegans* a powerful developmental model system. The first is that because of its transparency and small number of cells (959 somatic cells) it is possible to follow directly individual cells throughout development by light microscopy. By this means it has been discovered that all the cell positions and divisions outside the germ line are essentially invariant between individuals. Therefore the cell lineage tree, which contains the complete pattern of cell division from the zygote to all the final differentiated cells, is also essentially invariant, and so it has been possible to provide a complete description of the lineage (Sulston and Horvitz 1977; Kimble and Hirsh 1979; Sulston, Schierenberg, White and Thomson 1983). The second advantageous feature is the original reason for its selection as a model organism: it is particularly suitable for genetic analysis (Brenner 1974). Many mutants have been isolated that affect development, and the use of genetic techniques has allowed us to probe into the mechanisms that execute observed patterns of development.

The neuronal development of *C. elegans* has been reviewed previously by Sulston (1983) and by Chalfie (1984). Less complete data on the role of lineage in neuronal development are also available for several other invertebrate species, each of which has its own advantageous features as a model system. The early lineages in the leech are discussed by Blackshaw (this volume, Chapter 2). In the fruit-fly, *Drosophila*, the techniques of molecular genetics are revealing the mechanisms involved in subdividing the embryo into, and distinguishing between, ectodermal compartments (Scott and O'Farrell 1986). These compartments are lineally segregated subregions of the embryo that give rise to the repeated epidemal segments and their associated neuronal ganglia. In the grasshopper, whose nervous system shows similarities to that of *Drosophila* (Thomas, Bastiani, Bate and Goodman 1984), the determination of neuroblasts and their division patterns (Bate 1976; Doe and Goodman 1985) can be linked up with studies on process outgrowth from the resulting neurons (Bastiani, Doe, Helfand and Goodman 1985; see also Bacon this volume, Chapter 13).

THE NERVOUS SYSTEM OF *C. ELEGANS*

All 302 neurons in *C. elegans* are individually and reproducibly identifiable from animal to animal. Hence it has been possible to reconstruct the typical anatomy and synaptic connectivity of each neuron from electron micrographs of serially sectioned worms (White, Southgate, Thomson and Brenner 1976, 1986).

The main part of the nervous system lies on the inner surface of the hypodermis, which is the outer layer of cells lying under the external cuticle. There is also a miniature, almost independent nervous system in the pharynx, a muscular throat which pumps food into the intestine (Albertson and Thomson 1976). Neuronal cell bodies are mostly located in ganglia in the head or tail, or, in the case of body motoneurons, in the ventral cord. The neuropil essentially consists of bundles of parallel nerve fibres that run either longitudinally along the animal or circumferentially around it, as does the nerve ring, which is the main centre of synaptic activity (Fig 1.1).

The ventral nerve cord runs along the ventral midline and is the largest longitudinal nerve bundle. It contains the motor circuitry for controlling most of the body musculature together with about 20 interneuron processes that run between the nerve ring in the head and several smaller ganglia in the tail (White *et al.* 1976). The motor circuitry consists of 75 motoneurons and five pairs of interneurons that synapse onto them.

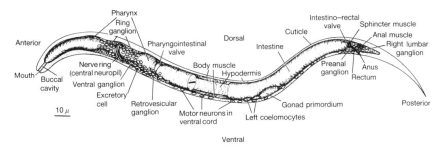

Fig. 1.1. General anatomy of the newly hatched juvenile. Labelled cell types and tissues include those that are discussed in the text [reproduced from Sulston *et al.* (1983) by kind permission of Academic Press, New York].

CELL TYPES IN THE VENTRAL CORD

The 75 ventral cord motoneurons can be assigned to eight different classes, DA, DB, DD, VA, VB, VC, VD, and AS, on the basis of their process morphology and synaptic connectivity. Each class has between seven and thirteen members that are distributed along the length of the cord and numbered from anterior to posterior, e.g. DA1 to DA9. One of these classes, VC, is sex specific and innervates vulval muscles in the hermaphrodite. It is replaced in the male by two different classes that are derived from the same precursor cells as the hermaphrodite VC neurons. The members of each of the other classes have consecutive non-overlapping regions of neuromuscular output, so that in any one region there is one cell of each class that is active. The boundaries of activity of motoneurons within one class in general bear no simple relation to those of another class. As will become apparent later, some of the motoneurons arise from a repeated developmental unit, but there does not appear to be an overall repeated framework for developmental control, as in truly segmented animals such as *Drosophila* or the leech.

C. *elegans* development can be split into two phases: embryonic development, during which a viable worm is created from a fertilized egg, and post-embryonic development, during which various additional structures are generated as the worm grows in size via four moults. The DA, DB, and DD classes are made during embryogenesis, while the VA, VB, VC, VD, and AS classes are post-embryonic.

GERM LAYER FORMATION

Classically, neuronal cells are considered to be produced together with epidermal tissue types by the ectoderm, which is the outermost of the three germ layers that are established by the process of gastrulation. This early restriction of tissue-type potential is universal to all higher animals and is presumably fundamental to their development, although, as we shall see below, it is sometimes not strictly maintained.

In nematode eggs it was seen early on that the germ layers are formed semi-clonally (reviewed in Chitwood and Chitwood 1974). The initial single zygotic cell, P_0, proceeds through a series of unequal divisions, producing the founder cells, AB, E, MS, C, and D, and the germ line precursor P_4 (Fig. 1.2). In general, each founder cell generates a clone of identical-looking cells through a series of equal and synchronous divisions, the doubling time being different and characteristic for each clone, although in fact the grand-daughters of each of MS and C split into two groups and the AB lineage desynchronizes rapidly. When gastrulation takes place the E cells enter the body first and go to form the gut, which constitutes the endoderm. They are followed by P_4, together with the mesodermal precursors, the MS, D, and half the C cells, which produce muscle, coelomocytes, and the somatic gonad. Most of the remaining cells, i.e. the AB descendants and the second half of the C progeny, form the ectoderm, an external monolayer of cells that generates almost all the neurons, neuronal support cells, and hypodermis. However, a number of AB derivatives enter the body at the front of the embryo at the end of gastrulation and join some of the MS descendents to form a distinct ball of cells that becomes the pharynx.

The initial conception that germ layer formation is an early stage in absolute tissue-type restriction, e.g. that ectoderm could not produce muscle, was found to be incorrect (Oppenheimer 1940). For instance, in the chick the neural crest, which is an ectodermal derivative, makes contributions to striated muscle, which is classically a mesodermal cell type (Le Douarin 1980). There are similar exceptions in *C. elegans*; four muscle cells are produced by

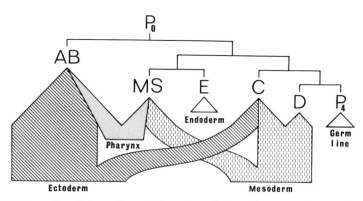

Fig. 1.2. Generation of the embryonic founder cells from the zygote, P_0, together with an indication of their contributions to the various germ layers.

the ectoderm (they are AB derivatives) and four glial cells by the mesoderm (from MS). Interestingly both cases involve penetration of another germ layer by the exceptional cells: the AB muscles are formed from a group of cells at the back of the animal that invaginates to contact the gut and form the rectum, while the MS glial cells are formed where some MS muscles push forward through AB derivatives into the front of the head (Sulston *et al.* 1983). As regards the pharynx, which contains muscle, neurons, gland cells, and specialized structural cells, all generated from both AB and MS precursors, there is even uncertainty as to which germ layer it should be assigned to.

In summary, almost all the neuronal cells come from the AB-derived ectoderm, but there are also two that are derived from the C-derived ectoderm, several pharyngeal neurons from both AB and MS, and four glial cells from the mesoderm, also from MS. There is further general localization within the ectoderm: neuronal precursors lie mainly ventral and anterior, and are separated from hypodermis, most of which starts as a dorsal patch of contiguous cells that spreads out over the rest of the embryo at the beginning of the final morphogenesis.

DETERMINATION OF INDIVIDUAL CELL TYPES

After establishing a general pool of neuronal precursor cells, the next major problem is to generate distinctions between cells so that they can differentiate into the identified neuron types. Insight into how this is done can be obtained by considering classes of equivalent cells, such as the ventral cord motoneuron classes. Such equivalent cells are termed analogues, while cells that come from corresponding developmental, particularly lineal, origins are termed homologues. We shall see that many neural analogues are also lineal homologues, suggesting that lineage is important in specifying cell type. However, there are also examples of both non-homologous analogues, i.e. equivalent cells with different origins, and non-analogous homologues, cells with corresponding lineal positions that adopt different fates. Such cells might be candidates for having been determined by external interactions with neighbouring unrelated cells. Below I discuss first the spatial and lineal patterns that give rise to the ventral cord motoneuron cell types, and second the evidence for and against intercellular interactions as a determining factor at various stages of development.

Lineal derivation of cell types

One simple way to generate a class of neurons would be to make them all as a clone from a single determined precursor. There is some weak evidence for such a scheme amongst the embryonic motoneurons, which differentiate from the apparently homogeneous ventral ectoderm of the post-gastrulation embryo. Figure 1.3 shows the positions and recent lineages of the precursors of all the embryonic motoneurons just before they divide and overt terminal differentiation begins. The DD neurons arise as two clonal groups, one on each side of the animal. Sisters of DA neurons tend to be DA neurons (6 out of 9), and in two of the three cases where this is not so the sister either becomes a DA-like post-embryonic motoneuron (Y, sister of DA7) or divides to give a DA-like head motoneuron and another cell (SABVR, niece of DA1). However, except in one case, the parents of DA neurons are not closely related, although some are related to DD precursors, suggesting a possible tendency towards clonal generation of motoneurons.

However, no other neuronal classes in the animal show even this degree of clonal derivation. For instance, the DB neurons are very distantly related to

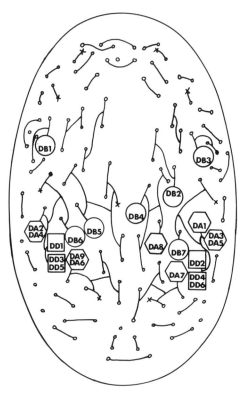

Fig. 1.3. The ventral ectoderm of the embryo prior to morphogenesis, showing the precursors of the embryonic ventral cord motoneurons. Cells undergoing programmed cell death are indicated by crosses, and other cells by small circles. Most ectodermal cells at this stage will divide just once more. Recent lineages are shown by linking sister cells, and are taken back several generations for the motoneuron precursors [adapted from Sulston *et al.* (1983) by kind permission of Academic Press, New York].

each other; one has to go back five generations to find a common ancestor for even the most closely related pair. They are also widely scattered over the ventral surface of the post-gastrulation embryo, so it is unlikely that they are specified as a regional group.

An alternative lineal origin for a class of cells might be that analogous cells could come from the homologous position in terminal lineages that are not themselves closely related. In fact, the DB cells fit this pattern partially, since all but one of them are posterior daughters of posterior daughters, and many other neuronal cell classes fit it completely, although most of them contain only two or four symmetrically placed cells. The relevance of the principle to embryonic development is best seen in the establishment of bilateral symmetry.

Left/right symmetry

It is immediately clear from Fig. 1.3 that left/right symmetry is an important principle in organizing neuronal cell fate, even for cells such as the ventral cord neurons which will eventually lie in a row along the ventral midline and show no mirror symmetry. Apart from the central two lines of precursor cells which produce mainly unpaired cells, e.g. DB4, both the ultimate fates of cells and the recent lineages that have created them are remarkably symmetrical.

However, this symmetry is not a continuous feature of embryonic development. The early lineages and cell positions are highly asymmetrical. It is only as gastrulation progresses that bilateral symmetry is established in the ectoderm; if one traces back the lineage trees from Fig. 1.3 one gets back to a set of cell pairs that produce homologous lineages, with analogous terminal cell types, but which are not themselves related homologously, i.e. they do not bear the same lineal relation amongst themselves on the left-hand side as they do on the right-hand side (Fig. 1.4).

Post-embryonic sublineages

The principle of producing analogous cell types from homologous terminal lineages is seen particularly clearly in the generation of several sets of post-embryonic neurons, including the post-embryonic ventral cord neurons, which are produced by a row of 13 neuroblasts on the ventral side of the larva, W and P1.a to P12.a. P1.a to P12.a are the anterior daughters of the embryonic ventral hypodermal cells, P1 to P12. Each of the neuroblasts gives rise to five cells by the same division pattern and, in general, each of the five cells differentiates into one of the five post-embryonic motoneuron types, VA, VB, VC, AS and VD (see Fig. 1.5). Such a spatially repeated division and differentiation pattern has been called a sublineage (Sternberg and Horvitz 1981).

Although there is a canonical differentiation pattern, many of the neuroblasts produce variant patterns; only six of the thirteen sublineages produce the full complement of five neurons (Fig. 1.5). The most common

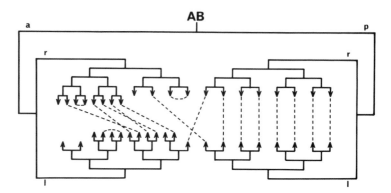

Fig. 1.4. Origin of bilateral symmetry within the AB lineage. Precursors that generate similar terminal lineages producing bilaterally symmetrical cell types are connected by dotted lines [reproduced from Sulston (1983) by kind permission of Cold Spring Harbor Press, New York].

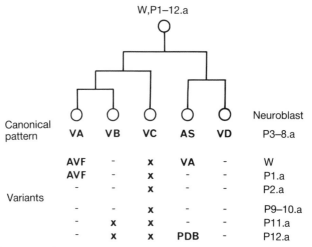

	VA	VB	VC	AS	VD	Neuroblast
Canonical pattern	VA	VB	VC	AS	VD	P3–8.a
	AVF	-	x	VA	-	W
	AVF	-	x	-	-	P1.a
	-	-	x	-	-	P2.a
Variants	-	-	x	-	-	P9–10.a
	-	x	x	-	-	P11.a
	-	x	x	PDB	-	P12.a

Fig. 1.5. The post-embryonic ventral cord motoneuron sublineage in the hermaphrodite, with the canonical assignment of cell types and the variant assignments produced by the anterior and posterior neuroblasts. In the male the cell in the VC position divides once in the P3 to P11.a sublineages and dies in the W and P1.a sublineages.

alternative fate of a cell is to die rather than to differentiate. This happens in the VC position in W, P1.a, P2.a, and P9 to P12.a and in the VB position in P11.a and P12.a. It seems that there is an underlying plan which is seen in its raw form in the middle of the body, but which is adapted to meet local needs at the two ends of the cord. This view is supported by the identification of genetic mutants that revert some of the alternative fates to the underlying pattern. For example, in animals mutant for the gene *mab-5* the deaths at the VB positions at the back of the cord do not take place. The extra cells have been seen in electron microscope reconstructions to have motoneuron properties, although the posterior neuropil is somewhat disorganized (Kenyon 1986). Mutants in *mab-5* show other abnormalities in the back of the animal, most of which can be interpreted as removing posterior specific post-embryonic specialization.

Cell death   The cell deaths that take place in the ventral cord follow a very typical course (Robertson and Thomson 1982). Similar deaths are seen in the embryo (as indicated in Fig. 1.3) and in other post-embryonic lineages, usually neuronal; 17 per cent of the embryonic cells die this way. Death occurs soon after the cell is born (30 minutes to one hour), before any overt alternative differentiation has taken place. It is therefore unlikely that it is due to functional competition between neurons as seen in vertebrates (Cowan, Fawcett, O'Leary and Stanfield 1984). Instead, it seems to be a form of preprogrammed suicide, whose purpose is presumably to remove an unwanted cell. Some cases seem to be used to create diversity in a repeated sublineage, as in the ventral cord, but in others there is no apparent reason for the cell to have been born. This suggests either that the extra divisions are necessary for correct determination and differentiation, or that the deaths might be evolutionary fossils, removing once-used cells that are no longer needed.

The proposal that there is a standard suicide mechanism is supported by the identification of two genes, *ced-3* and *ced-4*, that are required for all such deaths (Ellis and Horvitz 1986). In mutants for these genes many of the undead cells appear to differentiate into identifiable cell types; in particular, an electron microscope reconstruction of the posterior ventral nerve cord of a *ced-3* mutant showed extra motoneurons that probably correspond to the extra VB and VC cells (White and Southgate, unpub. obs.). None of the undead cells has been seen to divide, suggesting that programmed cell death is not used to prevent continued proliferation.

Production of a variant cell type   Apart from variation due to cell death there are four cases where a Pn.a descendant differentiates into a neuron but of a different cell type from that expected (Fig. 1.5). The front two VA homologues become the AVF interneurons, which send processes forward into the ring and back along the whole length of the ventral cord. The other two cases both affect AS homologues; the front AS homologue becomes a VA cell (recall that both the front VA cells had been replaced by AVF cells), and the back AS homologue becomes PDB, which is a unique neuron. The AS-to-VA switch can be seen as only a partial switch, since VA neurons receive the same types of synaptic input that AS cells do, except for missing a single chemical synapse characteristic of AS cells, although they are distinguishable on the basis of

Another is that a complex interaction may take place between a set of cells in such a way that any one cell is non-essential.

Replacement regulation   An example of replacement regulation after laser ablation involves the anteriormost ventral cord neuroblast, W. W migrates onto the ventral midline from the right as its homologue G2 migrates in from the left, in a similar fashion to the Pn cells discussed above, but earlier. If G2 is ablated then the cell that would have become W replaces G2 and no W is made. If W is ablated then it is not replaced (Sulston *et al.* 1983). This is a typical result; there is a primary fate, in this case G2, a secondary fate, in this case W, and a pair of cells that appear to have equivalent potential. Normally the two cells fill the two different fates, but if either cell is ablated then the primary fate is filled and not the secondary one. The known cases where replacement regulation takes place all follow this type of plan. In particular they involve a group of cells in analogous positions and of similar appearance, known as an equivalence group (Kimble, Sulston, and White 1979), and the replacement is always due to a switch in fate; there is never an extra cell made to fill the gap.

Almost all the equivalence groups that have been discovered so far contain post-embryonic blast cells. Amongst them, not surprisingly, are many of the groups of cells that show natural indeterminacy. For instance, if the ventral cord precursor P1 is killed, then P2.a generates an AVF cell rather than a VA cell (White and Sulston, pers. comm.). It is interesting that the capacity for regulation seems to be limited to blast cells and is lost in their descendants. This has not been shown in the ventral cord, but there is a similar series of neuronal sublineages produced on the male posterior lateral hypodermis (they generate the ray sensilla) that is susceptible to regulation at the blast cell level, but has resisted extensive attempts to show regulation when cells within the sublineage are killed (Sulston and White 1980). Similar results have been obtained recently in ablation experiments on the developing grasshopper nervous system, which have indicated that neuroblast formation and assignment is regulative but that cell generation by a neuroblast is not (Doe and Goodman 1985).

Interactions without replacement   There are only a few cases where ablation of a cell has led to large-scale morphological change in structures produced by other cells. A good example is in the post-embryonic development of the hermaphrodite vulva, where the participating hypodermal divisions are absolutely dependent on the presence of a gonadal cell, the anchor cell (Kimble 1981). In contrast, a set of mid-embryonic ablations of neuronal precursors showed neither replacement nor extensive morphological disruption, although some animals did die due to the failure of their incomplete hypodermis to enclose the embryo (Sulston *et al.* 1983).

However, there is more evidence for interactions playing a part in establishing the correct morphology of differentiated cell types, especially in the nervous system. In the same set of mid-embryonic ablations described above the fine structure of the head sensilla was scored, and in most cases additional processes from either neurons or their support cells had gone astray. More recently, the parent cells of two particular ventral cord interneurons have been ablated, in each case disrupting the normal pattern of process growth from other nerve cells (Durbin, unpub. obs.). These interactions during differentiation may not be unexpected, but they indicate that there is substantial capacity for specific intercellular interaction between cells whose determination seems largely intrinsic.

Genetics and intercellular interaction

Many mutants have been isolated that are altered in the numbers and positions of cells, including nerve cells, generated during development (e.g. Sulston and Horvitz 1981; reviews include Sternberg and Horvitz 1984; Hedgecock 1985; Greenwald, 1985a). The most interesting of these result in changes of the fate of specific cells, so that they behave like other cells elsewhere in the body. An example is provided by mutations in the *mab-5* gene that were discussed earlier as affecting several posterior-specific features of post-embryonic development. Genes defined by such mutations are candidates for control genes (Garcia-Bellido 1975; Greenwald 1985a), which act as switches to turn developmental pathways on or off.

Many known genes with these properties are thought to determine decisions that are normally influenced by extracellular inductions. For instance, the multivulva and vulvaless genes described by Ferguson and Horvitz (1985) act at the same determination step as the wild-type induction of the vulva by the anchor cell. Similarly the homoeotic genes of *Drosophila*, which act to distinguish different body regions from each other, are thought to set up their expression patterns from external positional information, possibly indirectly via the segmentation genes (Scott and O'Farrell 1986).

Why might switch genes be more common for decisions established by extracellular induction? Whenever a whole developmental decision can be triggered by the binary state of a single signal then any gene whose product is required solely for the establishment or transduction of that signal will behave as a switch gene. This is likely to arise in the case of a simple external induction, where one might expect a specific signalling factor and receptor, together with possibly less specific internal factors that cause release of the signal and respond to its reception. In contrast, although we know very little about intrinsic differentiation mechanisms, presumably a large number of different factors could influence the asymmetrical segregation of developmental potential in a cell division. Possible examples are factors involved in the physical control of the mitotic spindle, or the localization of cytoplasmic components. If these factors interact in a complex fashion then damage to any one might result in general problems rather than in a developmental switch. It is therefore not necessary in the case of an internal decision to postulate gene products whose absence would result in a clean switch of fate, although it is possible for them to exist, and indeed there are some genes for which mutations cause an apparently intrinsic switch, such as *unc-86*.

One particular switch gene seems likely to be involved in communication between cells. The *lin-12* gene acts at various different stages of development (mainly post-embryonic) in many different groups of cells, most of which are equivalence groups subject to replacement regulation (Greenwald, Sternberg and Horvitz 1983). For example, it affects the G2/W group considered earlier, which normally produces one G2 cell and one W cell. Instead *lin-12* dominant mutants produce two G2 cells, while *lin-12* null mutants produce two W cells. The *lin-12* gene has recently been cloned and sequenced. It encodes a polypeptide with marked similarity to a family of extracellular and cell surface proteins that includes epidermal growth factor precursor and the LDL receptor (Greenwald 1985*b*). Following this and other recent work on cloning developmentally important *C. elegans* genes, we can look forward to the direct study of the molecular mechanisms of cell determination.

CONCLUSIONS

C. elegans is clearly a species for which lineage-intrinsic determination is an important developmental mechanism. In the early embryo the lineal production of the founder cell clones appears partly to prespecify the fundamental events of gastrulation and germ layer formation. After gastrulation lineal homology of the left and right sides of the embryonic ectoderm is rapidly established and appears to be essentially imperturbable by ablation experiments (the only two exceptions being analogous to post-embryonic situations). Even in post-embryonic development, where a fair amount of regulation is demonstrable, all the interactions seem to take place at the level of blast cell specification, while the terminal sublineages produced by the blast cells have been unaffected by ablations when these have been attempted.

The most pervasive feature of those parts of the lineage that create the nervous system is the principle of the sublineage. In contrast, clonal specification plays a minor part in the nervous system, although it is a common feature of mesodermal and endodermal lineages. The presence of sublineages suggests that there are developmental subprograms which can be triggered in unrelated cells. In some cases during post-embryonic development the triggering has been shown to be external by ablation experiments, but there is no reason why a sublineage should not be initiated by a cell-intrinsic mechanism. This seems likely in many cases, since often during development cell ablations fail to produce any major disruptions. Once a sublineage is initiated it seems to run autonomously, even when the decision to initiate was determined externally. Kenyon (1985) has discussed possible mechanisms for cell-intrinsic lineage determination.

It is important to recognize that determination does not necessarily have to take place by a progressive restriction of absolute potential. We have seen that in *C. elegans* both repeated sublineages and clones are subject to terminal variation away from the standard pattern, involving either partial or total transformation of a few final cell types, as indeed are the early germ layers themselves. A hypothetical alternative to the model of progressive restriction of potential is that propensities to become a particular type of cell are established during development by various means (e.g. internal subprogram, clonal descent, external induction) and that these propensities may in some cases be conflicting. When differentiation is triggered then the propensities present in any particular cell could interact and compete to determine the final cell type. Such a proposal indicates how the informational basis for determination could be set up throughout development, even in cases where true commitment takes place only very late.

Ultimately, cell determination may not always be separable from cell differentiation. *In vitro* studies on rat neural crest cells suggest that they can change cell type as a result of external factors after the start of differentiation (Doupe, Landis and Patterson 1985). It is clear that many specific cellular interactions must take place during differentiation, particularly in a spatially complex tissue such as the nervous system. In *C. elegans* ablations of nerve cell precursors in the late embryo have been seen to result in positional defects of other nerve processes (Durbin, unpub. obs.). Many genes have been identified on the basis of an uncoordinated phenotype (Brenner 1974), and mutants in some of them show defects in the nervous system, affecting either process guidance (Hedgecock, Culotti, Thomson and Perkins 1985; McIntire, pers. comm.) or synaptic specificity (White and Nawrocki, pers. comm.). Since these defects involve detailed behaviours, they may provide the best approach to studying the detailed interactions that must be important in the differentiation of complex cell types and may also be important for their correct final determination.

ACKNOWLEDGMENTS

I would like to thank T. Hyman, C. Kenyon, J. Priess, J. Sulston and J. White for discussions and comments on the manuscript.

REFERENCES

Albertson, D. G. and Thomson, J. N. (1976). The pharynx of *Caenorhabditis elegans*. *Phil. Trans. R. Soc. Lond. B* **275.** pp. 299–325.

Bacon, J. P. (1987). Transplantation of sensory neurons in the insect. In *The making of the nervous system* (eds. J. G. Parnavelas, C. D. Stern and R. V. Stirling), pp. 248–267. Oxford University Press, Oxford.

Bastiani, M. J., Doe, C. Q., Helfand, S. L. and Goodman, C. S. (1985). Neuronal specificity and growth cone guidance in grasshopper and *Drosophila* embryos. *Trends Neurosci.* **8**, pp. 257–66.

Bate, C. M. (1976). Embryogenesis of an insect nervous system I. A map of the thoracic and abdominal neuroblasts in *Locusta migratoria*. *J. Embryol. exp. Morphol.* **35**, pp. 107–23.

Blackshaw, S. (1987). Cell lineage and the development of identified neurons in the leech. In *The making of the nervous system* (eds. J. G. Parnavelas, C. D. Stern and R. V. Stirling), pp. 22–51. Oxford University Press, Oxford.

Brenner, S. (1974). The genetics of *Caenorhabditis elegans*. *Genetics* **77**, pp. 71–94.

Chalfie, M. (1984). Neuronal development in *Caenorhabditis elegans*. *Trends Neurosci.* **7**, pp. 197–202.

Chalfie, M., Horvitz, H. R. and Sulston, J. E. (1981). Mutations that lead to reiterations in the cell lineages of *C. elegans*. *Cell* **24**, pp. 59–69.

Chitwood, B. G. and Chitwood, M. B. (1974). *Introduction to nematology*. University Park Press, Baltimore, MD.

Cowan, W. M., Fawcett, J., O'Leary, D. and Stanfield, B. (1984). Regressive events in neurogenesis. *Science* **225**, pp. 1258–65.

Doe, C. Q. and Goodman, C. S. (1985). Early events in insect neurogenesis II. The role of cell interactions and cell lineage in the determination of neural precursor cells. *Dev. Biol.* **111**, pp. 206–19.

Doupe, A. J., Landis, S. C. and Patterson, P. H. (1985). Environmental influences in the development of neural crest derivatives: glucocorticoids, growth factors, and chromaffin cell plasticity. *J. Neurosci.* **5**, pp. 2119–42.

Ellis, H. M. and Horvitz, H. R. (1986). Genetic control of programmed cell death in the nematode *C. elegans*. *Cell* **44**, pp. 817–29.

Ferguson, E. L. and Horvitz, H. R. (1985). Identification and characterization of 22 genes that affect the vulval cell lineages of the nematode *Caenorhabditis elegans*. *Genetics* **110**, pp. 17–72.

Garcia-Bellido, A. (1975). Genetic control of wing disc development in *Drosophila*. In *Cell patterning, Ciba Foundation Symp.* **29**. pp. 161–82.

Greenwald, I. (1985a). The genetic analysis of cell lineage in *Caenorhabditis elegans*. *Phil. Trans. R. Soc. Lond. B* **312**, pp. 129–37.

Greenwald, I. (1985b). *lin-12*, a nematode homeotic gene, is homologous to a set of mammalian proteins that include epidermal growth factor. *Cell* **43**, pp. 583–90.

Greenwald, I. S., Sternberg, P. W. and Horvitz, H. R. (1983). The *lin-12* locus specifies cell fates in *Caenorhabditis elegans*. *Cell* **34**, pp. 435–44.

Hedgecock, E. (1985). Cell lineage mutants in the nematode *Caenorhabditis elegans*. *Trends Neurosci.* **8**, pp. 288–93.

Hedgecock, E. M., Culotti, J. G., Thomson, J. N. and Perkins, L. A. (1985). Axonal guidance mutants of *Caenorhabditis elegans* identified by filling sensory neurons with fluoroscein dyes. *Dev. Biol.* **111**, pp. 158–70.

Hodgkin, J., Horvitz, H. R. and Brenner, S. (1978). Nondisjunction mutants of the nematode *Caenorhabditis elegans*. *Genetics* **91**, pp. 67–94.

Kenyon, C. (1985). Cell lineage and the control of *Caenorhabditis elegans* development. *Phil. Trans. R. Soc. Lond. B* **312**, pp. 21–38.

Kenyon, C. (1986). *mab-5*, a gene involved in the development of the posterior body region of *C. elegans*. *Cell* **46**, pp. 477–87.

Kimble, J. (1981). Alterations in cell lineage following laser ablation of cells in the somatic gonad of *Caenorhabditis elegans*. *Dev. Biol.* **87**, pp. 286–300.

Kimble, J. and Hirsh, D. (1979). The postembryonic cell lineages of the hermaphrodite and male gonads in *Caenorhabditis elegans*. *Dev. Biol.* **70**, pp. 396–417.

Kimble, J., Sulston, J. E. and White, J. G. (1979). Regulative development in the post-embryonic lineages of *Caenorhabditis elegans*. In *Cell lineages, stem cells and cell determination, INSERM Symposium 10* (ed. N. Le Douarin), pp. 59–68. Elsevier/North Holland Biomedical Press, Amsterdam.

Le Douarin, N. (1980). Migration and differentiation of neural crest cells. In *Current topics in developmental biology, Vol. 16* (eds. A. A. Moscana and A. Monray), pp. 31–85. Academic Press, New York.

Oppenheimer, J. (1940). The non-specificity of the germ layers. *Q. rev. Biol.* **15**, 96–124.

Robertson, A. M. G.and Thomson, J. N. (1982) Morphology of programmed cell death in the ventral nerve cord of *Caenorhabditis elegans* larvae. *J. Embryol. exp. Morphol* **67**, pp. 89–100.

Scott, M. P. and O'Farrell, P. H. (1986). Spatial programming of gene expression in early *Drosophila* embryogenesis. *Ann. Rev. Cell Biol.* **2**, pp. 49–80.

Sternberg, P. W. and Horvitz, H. R. (1981). Gonadel lineages of the nematode *Panagrellus redivivus* and implications for evolution by the modification of cell lineage. *Dev. Biol.* **88**, pp. 147–66.

Sternberg, P. W. and Horvitz, H. R. (1984). The genetic control of cell lineage during nematode development. *Ann. Rev. Genet.* **18**, pp. 489–524.

Sulston, J. E. (1983). Neuronal cell lineages in the nematode *Caenorhabditis elegans*. *Cold Spring Harbor Symp. Quant. Biol.* **48**, pp. 433–52.

Sulston, J. E. and Horvitz, H. R. (1977). Post-embryonic cell lineages of the nematode *Caenorhabditis elegans*. *Dev. Biol.* **56**, pp. 110–56.

Sulston, J. E. and Horvitz, H. R. (1981). Abnormal cell lineages in mutants of the nematode *Caenorhabditis elegans*. *Dev. Biol.* **82**, pp. 41–55.

Sulston, J. E. and White, J. G. (1980). Regulation and cell autonomy during postembryonic development of *Caenorhabditis elegans*. *Dev. Biol.* **78**, pp. 577–97.

Sulston, J. E., Schierenberg, E., White, J. G. and Thomson, J. N. (1983). The embryonic cell lineage of the nematode *Caenorhabditis elegans*. *Dev. Biol.* **100**, pp. 64–119.

Thomas, J. B., Bastiani, M. J., Bate, C. M. and Goodman, C. S. (1984). From grasshopper to *Drosophila:* a common plan for neuronal development. *Nature* **310**, pp. 203–7.

White, J. G., Southgate, E., Thomson, J. N. and Brenner, S. (1976). The structure of the ventral nerve cord of *Caenorhaditis elegans*. *Phil. Trans. Roy. Soc. London Ser. B* **275**, pp. 327–48.

2

Cell lineage and the development of identified neurons in the leech

SUSANNA BLACKSHAW

The central nervous system of invertebrates usually occupies a ventral rather than a dorsal position both in the embryo and in the adult, and the adult nervous system is organized into a series of ganglia rather than into a brain and spinal cord. In leeches the adult ventral nerve cord contains around 15 000 cells and is composed of segmentally repeating units, the segmental ganglia, that are virtually identical to each other. Each contains about 400 bilaterally paired neurones, eight paired giant glial cells, and a few unpaired neurones (Fig. 2.1). Particular sensory, motor, and interneurons can be recognized from segment to segment and from animal to animal, and, in some cases, homologous neurons can be recognized across species (Muller, Nicholls, and Stent 1981). The peripheral nervous system is similarly stereotyped, though less well characterized. It consists of a bilaterally symmetrical and segmentally repeating system of four circumferential nerve trunks (AA, MA, PP, and DP) and their peripheral branches which contain the axons of CNS (central nervous system) neurons and the centrally directed axons of neurons situated in the periphery. Some of the peripheral neurons have been identified and their functions established (Kretz, Stent, and Kristan 1976; Friesen 1981; Blackshaw, Nicholls, and Parnas 1982a; Blackshaw, Mackay, and Thompson 1984; Thompson 1986; Blackshaw and Thompson 1986a, 1987; Elliot 1987; Blackshaw 1987).

The stereotyped arrangement of the nervous system and the relatively small number of cells mean that leeches offer us the possibility of studying the development of a nervous system in terms of individually recognizable cells. Leeches were in fact a focus of interest in the late 19th century, not only for anatomists of the adult CNS such as Retzius, Cajal, and Sanchez, but also for the pioneers of experimental embryology. On the basis of his observations in the light microscope on the early cleavage of a glossiphoniid leech egg, Whitman (1878) first stated the idea that each identified cell in the early embryo is developmentally distinct, and that each identified blastomere and the clone of its descendant cells plays a specific predestined role in later development.

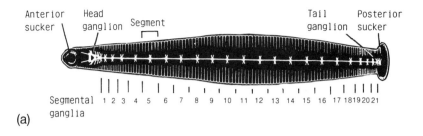

(a)

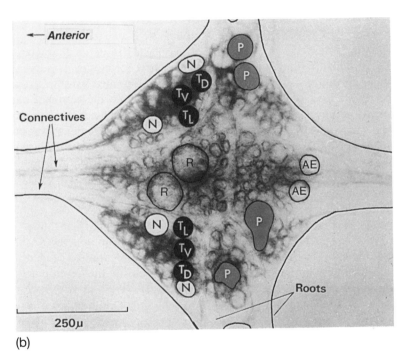

(b)

Fig. 2.1. (a) The medicinal leech, like other annelids, has both the body and the nervous system made up of very similar repeating units. Externally each segment is divided into annuli (five in the mid-body region). The ventral nerve cord consists of a chain of 21 segmental ganglia, with some concentration of ganglia at the head and tail ends. (b) Segmental ganglion viewed from the ventral aspect. Cells labelled include the T, P and N mechano–sensory cells which respond to touch, pressure, or noxious stimulation of the skin; the AE motoneurones which innervate the muscles responsible for raising the annuli into ridges; and the giant serotonin-containing Retzius cells (R). Individual touch cells innervate specific areas of ventral (T_V), lateral (T_L), or dorsal (T_d) skin. [Reproduced with modifications from Nicholls and Baylor (1968) by kind permission of the Americian Physiological Society, Bethesda, MD.]

Today, with the development of new techniques for cell lineage analysis and the detailed description of the cellular elements of the adult leech nervous system, it is possible to unravel certain rules for the development of this relatively simple nervous system. Thus the key decisions of early development seem to be made at a very early stage when there are relatively few cells in the embryo (Slack 1983). By labelling individually identified blastomeres with vital cell lineage tracers and following the fate of their descendent cells it has been shown that the orderly sequence of embryonic cleavages subdivides cell fates in a highly determinate pattern. A particular identified blastomere of the early embryo regularly gives rise to a particular part of the adult tissue, although the particular part contributed by a given teloblast comprises a variety of cell types. In the case of the nervous system each segmental ganglion of the adult is derived from five pairs of teloblasts through a characteristic pattern of cell divisions, and the developmental stereotypy is such that particular groups of neurons in each body segment, termed 'kinship' groups, can be traced back to particular primary blast cells in the germinal band. Although the lineage of identified neurons of the adult nervous system is highly determinate, in that a given neuron or glial cell invariably belongs to a particular kinship group, neurons within a kinship group are not obviously related in structure or function. Cell migration and cell death, which are features of development of the vertebrate nervous system, also shape the leech nervous system and it appears that regional differences in the architecture of the leech CNS arise only after the initial condensation of the ganglion rudiments. The stereotypy of the migration routes and of the final cell positioning suggests that mechanisms exist that constrain migrating cells to move along appropriate pathways. Studies of the differentiation of identified neurons of the adult nervous system show that, during the development of sensory fields, individual axons grow directly to their appropriate skin territories without initial overgrowth and subsequent elimination of excess processes. Selective loss of neural processes is, however, a feature of developing central arborisations.

SUMMARY OF EARLY DEVELOPMENT IN GLOSSIPHONIID LEECHES

Early development of glossiphoniid leeches has been described by several authors (Weisblat, Sawyer, and Stent 1978; Fernandez 1980; Fernandez and Stent 1980; Weisblat, Harper, Stent, and Sawyer 1980; Weisblat 1981; Fernandez and Olea 1982; and Stent, Weisblat, Blair, and Zackson 1982). A distinct feature of neural development in the leech is the formation during the first stages of development, via a series of well-defined cell divisions, of a germinal plate from which the ectoderm- and mesoderm-derived tissues of the adult arise. The initial cleavages follow the typical spiral pattern of the annelid phylum (Anderson 1973). The first three divisions divide the egg into eight blastomeres, four small micromeres at the animal pole marking the site of the future head, and four large yolky vegetal macromeres. Three of the macromeres (A, B, and C) cease dividing after producing only a few micromeres and eventually are incorporated into the gut. The D lineage plays a crucial role in development, as it does in other invertebrates such as molluscs, since all segmental tissues, including the nervous system, arise from it. Cleavages of the D macromere give rise by the end of embryonic stage 6 to five bilateral pairs of teloblasts (M, N, O/P, O/P, Q) of which four pairs (N, O/P, O/P, Q) are the precursors of the definitive ectoderm and the fifth pair (M) is the precursor of the mesoderm (Fig. 2.2).

During stage 7, each of the five pairs of teloblasts begins to carry out a series of highly unequal divisions, budding off, over the course of many hours, a series of several dozen smaller primary blast cells, which form a longitudinal row or bandlet. The five bandlets on either side of the midline merge to form a bilaterally symmetrical pair of prominent cell ridges, the right and left germinal bands, which overlie the macromeres. Each germinal band consists of a superficial layer of four ectodermal precursor bandlets designated n, o, p, q, and a deeper layer provided by the mesodermal precursor bandlet on each side, m. Within each bandlet, the first-born and developmentally oldest blast cells are located at the anterior end, and their progeny will contribute to the anterior most segments of the body. Progressively younger blast cells are located progressively more posteriorly in the bandlet, and will contribute their progeny to correspondingly more posterior segments. Any given developmental event such as formation of the ventral nerve cord occurs first in the anterior most segments and progressively later in the progressively more posterior segments.

A series of morphogenetic movements of the five bilateral pairs of bandlets occurs during stage 8. With ongoing production of primary blast cells the germinal bands lengthen and their mid-portions move circumferentially onto the future ventral surface. Gradually, left and right germinal bands meet and coalesce along the ventral midline, beginning at the head end and continuing rearward, like a zipper. As they coalesce, the germinal bands form the germinal plate which straddles the ventral midline. In the course of formation and circumferential movement the blast cells change their positions; the medio–lateral order of the bandlets becomes inverted so that the left and right n ectodermal bandlets come to lie together along the future ventral midline of the embryo. The midline position of the two n bandlets lead early embryologists to propose that the nervous system arises entirely from their progeny, an idea which could not be tested because cells within the germinal plate were too numerous and too small for their fates to be followed precisely with the techniques then available, and which was subsequently shown to be wrong. During stage 9 the germinal plate lengthens, broadens, and thickens due to a progressive increase in the number of cells in all the bandlets, and expands

paired connectives and the unpaired midline *Faivres* nerve of the adult nervous system. The definitive anatomy is largely established at stage 10 of embryogenesis. By that point there has been a secondary fusion of the four most anterior segments and of the seven most posterior segments. The 21 intervening segments show relatively little variation in structure.

BODY WALL MUSCLES AS ANATOMICAL LANDMARKS

The M teloblasts are the first to cease forming teloblasts at mid-stage 8 and, as previously mentioned, segmentation is first seen in the mesodermal tissue derived from the m bandlet. By the time formation of the 32 ganglia primordia is complete, formation of the 32 blocks of mesodermal tissue has been completed for several hours. In each hemisegment of the stage-9 germinal plate, individual identified muscle fibres differentiate in a stereotyped order and in stereotyped positions (Stuart, Thompson, Weisblat, and Kramer 1982; Torrence and Stuart 1986). Layers of outer circular and inner longitudinal muscle fibres differentiate deep to the definitive epidermis and nervous system which now form the surface of the germinal plate. The first circular muscle fibre ('primary circular'; Torrence and Stuart 1986) to differentiate in each hemisegment spans the distance from the ventral midline to the lateral margin of the germinal plate. It marks the position of the future cleft between ganglia and defines the anterior edge of the segment. Deep to the circular muscle a layer of longitudinal fibres differentiates. The primary circular and deep longitudinal muscle fibres can be visualized by labelling with a monoclonal antibody to leech muscle, Lan 3–14 (Zipser and McKay 1981; Stuart *et al.* 1982) before the ganglia become morphologically distinct. When the ganglia first appear each occupies the rectangular space bounded by two successive primary circular fibres and the right and left deep longitudinal fibres. Thus the muscle fibres outline the presumptive ganglion territory in each segment, within which the neural precursors of the ganglionic rudiment are to coalesce.

ORIGIN OF THE VENTRAL NERVE CORD AS DETERMINED BY LINEAGE TRACING TECHNIQUES

To establish the line of descent of the constituent cells of the leech nervous system, Whitman's (1878) lineage studies have been extended and refined by the introduction of novel tracer techniques by Weisblat, Stent, and colleagues. These techniques were first used to derive a fate map of the early leech embryo (Weisblat *et al.* 1978) and have subsequently been used for lineage analysis in frogs (Hirose and Jacobson 1979), mice (Balakier and Pedersen 1982), tunicates (Nishida and Satoh 1983) and the zebrafish (Kimmel and Warga 1986). In these techniques a tracer molecule such as horseradish peroxidase (Weisblat *et al.* 1978) or a fluorescent compound that does not require a histochemical reaction (Weisblat, Zackson, Blair, and Young 1980; Gimlich and Braun 1985) are micro-injected into an identified cell of the early embryo. The tracer is subsequently inherited by all the progeny of the injected cell. The embryo is allowed to develop to a chosen end-point when the distribution of the labelled cells is mapped.

Use of the lineage tracer technique has shown that the leech nervous system is derived from all five teloblasts (Weisblat, Harper, *et al.* 1980; Weisblat, Kim, and Stent 1984) and therefore has several embryonic sources, in contrast to the single source proposed for it on the basis of direct observations (Whitman 1878; Schleip 1936). For the experiments, horseradish peroxidase (HRP) was injected into each identified blastomere in turn in a stage-6 or -7 embryo (see Fig. 2.2) and the resulting distribution of HRP-labelled cells was then examined in the late embryo (stage 10). In this way it was shown that each of the four paired ectodermal teloblasts, N, O/P, O/P, Q, gives rise to a topographically characteristic set of neurons in the ganglia and body wall and in addition a characteristic territory of non-neuronal cells in the epidermis, whereas the mesodermal M teloblast gives rise to the longitudinal, circular, and oblique muscle fibres of the body wall as well as to the longitudinal muscle fibres in the nerve cord and to a few presumptive neurons within the ganglion. Thus the nervous system and epidermis of the leech have a common ectodermal origin in accord with general embryological principles. The relative circumferential position of each teloblast's epidermal contribution to the embryonic body wall corresponds to the relative position of its blast cell bandlet in the germinal plate: the n bandlet and its very few epidermal descendants lie nearest to the ventral midline; the q bandlet lies furthest from the ventral midline and its epidermal descendants are destined for the dorsal body wall; and the o and p bandlets lie between the n and q bandlets and their epidermal descendants are destined for the ventro–lateral body wall.

Of the four ectodermal teloblasts, the N teloblast contributes most cells to the ipsilateral segmental ganglion (about 90 N-derived cells per half-ganglion) as well as a few cells outside the ganglion in the body wall. The O-pattern contribution to the hemiganglion consists of about 60 cells (Fig. 2.3). There is also a substantial extraganglionic contribution to the ipsilateral body wall. The P pattern contributes about a dozen cells to the half-ganglion and also, like the O pattern, a substantial contribution to the ipsilateral body wall outside the ganglion. Of the four ectodermal teloblasts, the Q with the most lateral blast cell bandlet in the germinal plate makes the smallest contribution: about ten cells to the ipsilateral half-ganglion. The principal contribution of the Q teloblast is the epidermis of the future dorsal body wall.

Following injection of an M teloblast, labelled cells are distributed throughout the ipsilateral body wall in stage-10 embryos. The most prominent

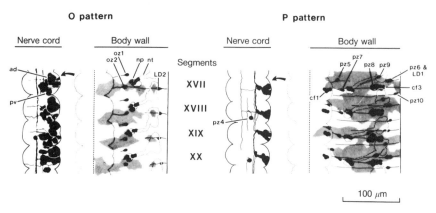

Fig. 2.3. *Camera lucida* tracings of HRP-labelled O and P descendant patterns in a series of four consecutive mid-body segments. Labelled cell bodies and axons are shown in black, with the shaded regions representing labelled portions of the squamous epidermis. The ventral nerve cord is shown separately, and its location relative to the body wall is marked by a dotted outline. The nephridia are also shown by a dotted outline on the right side of each segment. Note that the labelled tissues lie on only one side of the midline (dotted line), and that—with the exception of the P-derived neuron pz4—the pattern of labelled tissues is repeated in every segment. The 32 body segments are numbered from head to tail, with the unfused abdominal segments designated: V–XXV.ad, antero–dorsal cell cluster; pv, postero–ventral cell cluster; nt, nephridial tubule; np, nephridiopore; cf1 and cf3, cell florets 1 and 3; peripheral neurons as in the text. [Reproduced from Shankland and Weisblat (1984) by kind permission of Academic Press, New York.]

of these labelled cells are the longitudinal, circular, and oblique muscle fibres of the body wall, as well as the nephridia. Thus, again in accord with general embryological principles, muscles, nephridia, and connective tissue of the leech are of common mesodermal provenance. HRP-injection of an M teloblast also results in the labelling of a few cells within the nerve cord, which on morphological grounds appear to be interneurons—an unusual example of nervous tissue of mesodermal origin (Weisblat *et al.* 1984).

These experiments have shown that development of the leech is highly stereotyped, in the sense that particular identifiable blastomere of the early embryo regularly gives rise to a particular part of the adult, although the particular part contributed by a given teloblast comprises a variety of cell types. In the case of the nervous system, this developmental stereotypy is such that a particular group of neurones in each body segment can be traced back to a particular primary blast cell in the germinal band. Within each half-ganglion, therefore, the cells fall into five kinship groups according to their teloblasts of origin. Each kinship group has a characteristic cell number and a unique distribution in the segment as a whole and within the segmental ganglion in particular. Since the identified neurons and glia of the adult ganglion are themselves stereotypically located (Muller, Nicholls, and Stent 1981), it can be inferred that each kinship group normally comprises a particular set of neurons and that in leech development neuronal cell lineage is highly determinate.

THE TELEOLOGICAL SIGNIFICANCE OF THE TELOBLAST-DERIVED KINSHIP GROUPS

The existence of the teloblast-derived kinship groups raises the question of whether neurons related by lineage share common functional or morphological properties that distinguish them from members of other kinship groups. To answer this question, identified CNS neurons and glia in *Haementaria ghilianii* were traced to particular M, N, O, P, and Q kinship groups (Kramer and Weisblat 1985). In these experiments it was necessary to be able to identify individual neurons and, in the same preparation, assay for the presence or absence of lineage tracer (Fig. 2.4). A teloblast was injected with the fluorescent rhodamine peptide tracer (RDP) in an early stage-7 embryo and the embryo was dissected at stage 10 or 11, by which time individual neurons have differentiated and are identifiable. If RDP fluorescence was seen to be localized within a putative mechano–sensory neuron the identity of the neuron was confirmed by intracellular recording and Lucifer-yellow dye injection (Kuwada and Kramer 1983). These experiments showed that the lineage of identified neurons is highly determinate in that a given neuron or glial cell was invariably found to belong to a particular kinship group. Thus, of the mechano–sensory neurons, the touch (T) and nociceptive (N) neurons belong to the N kinship group, the pressure-sensitive neuron innervating ventral skin (P_V) to the P kinship group, and the pressure-sensitive neuron innervating dorsal skin (P_D) to the O kinship group. The giant glial cells (Kuffler and Potter, 1964) arise from all four ectodermal teloblasts. Conversely, neurons within a kinship group are not obviously related in structure or function: the N kinship group includes a variety of neuronal types— sensory, motor and interneurons. So far no neuronal characteristic unique to the N kinship group has emerged. Thus in leech development the determinants of neuronal identity are not segregated in any obvious thematic way in the cleavages that give rise to the five bilateral pairs of teloblasts.

CELL MIGRATION IN LEECH GANGLIOGENESIS

Although the stereotyped pattern of cell divisions in leech embryogenesis causes many cells to arise near the site of their ultimate differentiation, some precursors of neurons and glia of the CNS do arise outside the presumptive

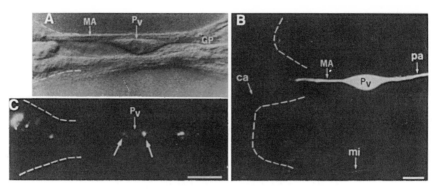

Fig. 2.4. Localization of lineage tracer within an identified neuron. (A) Differential interference contrast (Nomarski) photomicrograph of P_V mechano–sensory neuron cell body pulled outside the ganglion (whose boundaries are indicated by *dashed lines*) on the MA segmental nerve. Other cell bodies remained within the ganglion. GP: germinal plate. (B) Processes of the P_V cell in (A) revealed by intracellularly injected, fluorescent Lucifer-yellow dye. Morphology is unambiguously that of the P_V neuron: a peripheral axon (pa) in the ipsilateral MA nerve tract with an intersegmental central axon (ca) that exits the adjacent ganglia as minor field peripheral axons (mi). (C) Same areas as in (A) photographed to reveal fluorescent granules of the RDP lineage tracer, which had been injected into a generative P teloblast in this specimen. RDP granules located within the P_V cell body are indicated by arrows. Position of the PV cell body is apparent from its weak, uniform fluorescence that results from the injected Lucifer-yellow dye (i.e. Lucifer-induced red fluorescence). Note that Lucifer-yellow fluorescence is concentrated in the cell nucleus (at PV-labelled arrow), whereas RDP is excluded from the nucelus. (A) and (C) are at the same magnification. Scale bars: 20 μm. [Reproduced from Kramer and Weisblat (1985) by kind permission of the Society for Neuroscience, Bethesda, MD.]

domain of the ventral nerve cord (Weisblat *et al.* 1984) and therefore must migrate centripetally to enter the CNS (Torrence 1984; Stuart *et al.* 1982; Torrence and Stuart 1986). Early in stage 9 when the ganglion first appears, the germinal plate is still a flat strip of tissue about 300 μm wide and 40 μm thick (Fernandez and Stent 1982), extending longitudinally over the ventral surface of the embryo with structures at its lateral margins that are ultimately destined to lie along the dorsal midline of the future leech. Within the germinal plate the four pairs of ectodermal bandlets lie in a single layer arranged on either side of the embryo in the medio–lateral order, n, o, p, q. Each of the ectodermal blast cells has divided several times so that the bandlets are more than one cell wide in transverse section (Fig. 2.5). The mesodermal blast cells have also divided a number of times and have given rise to an essentially solid mass of mesodermal tissue.

At the beginning of gangliogenesis, the presumptive ganglion territory occupies somewhat less than half of the width of the germinal plate and, on each side, corresponds to a region of the embryo initially occupied by the n

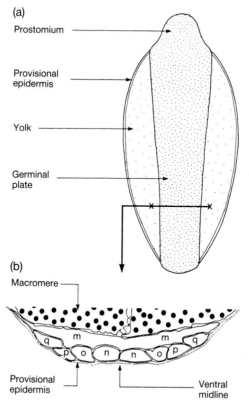

(a)

Prostomium

Provisional epidermis

Yolk

Germinal plate

(b)

Macromere

q m   m q
p o n   n o p

Provisional epidermis

Ventral midline

Fig. 2.5. The anatomy of the germinal plate of *Theromyzon rude*. (a) View of the ventral surface of an early-stage-9 embryo. Anterior is uppermost. The germinal plate (dense stippling) extends longitudinally over the ventral surface on either side of the midline. The interior of the embryo is occupied by large yolky cells, the macromeres, and the surface is covered by the provisional epidermis. (b) Diagrammatic transverse section along the line X–X in (a) showing the positions of the eight ectodermal (right and left n, o, p and q) and two mesodermal (right and left m) bandlets. Because of cellular proliferation, bandlets are more than one cell wide in transverse section; thus the bandlet contours drawn here encompass more than one cell each (cf. Fig. 2.2). The large dots in the macromeres symbolize yolk granules. [Reproduced from Torrence and Stuart (1986) by kind permission of the Society of Neuroscience, Bethesda, MD.]

bandlet and about half of the width of the o bandlet. Neuroblasts and glioblasts that are destined for the CNS and are derived from the n and o bandlets arise predominantly within the presumptive ganglion territory and can be incorporated directly into the ganglion rudiment. The p and q bandlets, however, lie furthest from the ventral midline at the lateral margins of the germinal plate outside the presumptive ganglion territory and, although their principal contribution is to the ipsilateral lateral and dorsal body wall (Weisblat *et al.* 1984), both also contribute cells to the CNS.

To follow the central migration of neuroblasts and glioblasts derived from the p and q bandlets the distribution pattern of lineage tracer labelled cells belonging to p and q kinship groups was examined in a series of segments of embryos of *Theromyzon rude* during embryo stage 9 (Fig. 2.6). (Since any

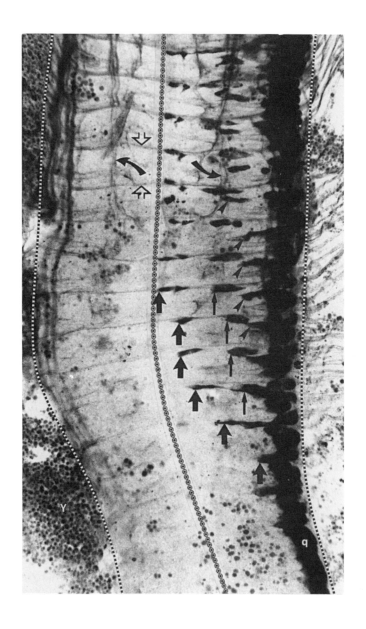

given developmental event occurs first in the anterior most segment and progressively later in progressively more posterior segments, each embryo provides an orderly and finely graded series of developmental substages in which the embryo's longitudinal axis is equivalent to a developmental time axis from which sequential developmental events may be inferred.) These experiments show that the neuroblasts and glioblasts that belong to p and q ectodermal kinship groups and are destined for the CNS migrate from their bandlet of origin along stereotyped pathways to reach their definitive locations in and near the ganglion rudiment. For example, migrating cells in the q kinship group first appear as a medially directed protrusion from the q bandlet. This consists initially of only three or four cells which move medially immediately posterior to the primary circular muscle fibre (see p. 28) along the path that will later be taken by the AA segmental nerve. The leading two cells separate from the trailing cells and enter the ganglion rudiment. One settles at the intersection of the ventral midline and the anterior margin of the segment. This is the *glioblast*, which will give rise to the glia of the ipsilateral connective nerve. The other is a neuron that settles just lateral to the connective glioblast

---

Fig. 2.6. Centripetal migration of neural precursor cells from the q bandlet toward the central nervous system. Approximately 16 segments of the germinal plate of a stage-9 embryo of *Theromyzon rude* are shown. Anterior is up. The left and right margins of the germinal plate are indicated by dashed lines and the ventral midline by the dotted line. The left (apparent right) q bandlet was labelled with rhodamine-dextran-amine cell lineage tracer by injection of its precursor, the Q teloblast, and is seen extending along the margin of the germinal plate. In addition, developing circular and longitudinal muscle fibres were stained by indirect immunofluorescence using a mouse monoclonal antibody directed against leech muscles and a fluorescein-conjugated second antibody. Circular muscle fibres appear as dark horizontal lines and longitudinal muscles as dark vertical lines. The micrograph was printed as a negative image, so that the fluorescent labels appear dark against a light background. The presumptive domain of each segmental ganglion is outlined by particular identified circular (hollow arrows) and longitudinal (curved arrows) muscle fibres. The rostro–caudal gradient of developmental age that is characteristic of leech embryos allows the events of cell migration to be followed in progression from the less developed, posterior segments at the bottom of the micrograph to the more developed, anterior segments at the top of the micrograph. In each segment small groups of neural precursor cells migrate from the labelled q bandlet toward the ventral midline (from right to left in the figure) along stereotyped routes. In the posteriormost segments shown here migration is just beginning. From the initial protrusion of cells from the q bandlet, two cells in each segment move quickly to the ventral midline (large straight arrows), and a larger group of cells migrates slightly later along the same path (small straight arrows). A third group of cells in each segment leaves the q bandlet later still, and migrates along a second, more posterior path. In the anteriormost segments shown here many of the migrating neuroblasts are only just entering the ganglionic primordium. (Photograph courtesy of Dr S. Torrence.)

and immediately begins to extend ipsilateral neurites anteriorly and posteriorly in the forming longitudinal fibre tracts. The trailing groups of cells follow the same pathway into the ganglion rudiment but pause at the lateral margin where the cells proliferate. The progeny subsequently move deep into the ganglion rudiment and most settle near the earlier arrived neuron. A few remain outside the ganglion rudiment and contribute to the cluster of peripheral neurons found along the MA nerve in the adult (Rude 1969). Another small group of cells migrates medially along a second mid-segmental pathway roughly half-way between successive primary circular muscle fibres—this route corresponds to the path later taken by the MA segmental nerve (which is also the route taken by the migrating cells from the p kinship group)—and stop when they reach the ganglion. They also contribute to the MA cluster of peripheral neurons.

Thus cell migration, which is a feature of development of the vertebrate nervous system, also shapes the leech nervous system. Centrifugal as well as centripetal migrations occur. For example, peripheral neurons derived from the n kinship group arise within the presumptive ganglion territory and must migrate laterally to reach their characteristic positions in the periphery (Weisblat *et al.* 1978). The stereotypy of the migration routes and of the final cell positioning suggests that mechanisms exist that constrain migrating cells to move along appropriate pathways. A variety of cell types including the muscle fibres, is present along the paths of the migrating neuroblasts and glioblasts and might provide guidance or positional clues.

SEGMENTAL DIFFERENCES IN THE ARCHITECTURE OF THE LEECH CNS: THE ROLE OF CELL DEATH AND CELL PROLIFERATION

In animals with a segmented nervous system, the ganglia of the ventral nerve cord often have considerably different cell numbers. In the grasshopper, for example, the thoracic ganglia have between 2000 and 3000 neurons, whereas the abdominal ganglia have around 500 (Bate 1976), and it has been suggested that this difference is principally the result of cell death. Despite the metamerically stereotyped architecture of the leech nervous system, significant regional differentiation of the adult leech nerve cord does exist. For instance, the four most anterior and seven most posterior segmental ganglia which arise as separate ganglion rudiments in the embryo are fused into compound suboesophageal and caudal ganglia in the adult (Mann 1962; Muller *et al.* 1981), and ganglia in the genital segments (5 and 6) contain more neurons than the typical mid-body ganglion (Zipser 1979; Macagno 1980). Certain cells associated with a particular function are found only in a restricted number of ganglia (Thompson and Stent 1976; Stent and Kristan

1981; Shafer and Calabrese 1981; Weeks 1982). No regional differences were seen, however, in any aspect of the cell migration that occurs during stage 9 of glossiphoniid embryos (Torrence and Stuart 1986), supporting the view that regional differences in the architecture of the leech CNS arise only after the initial condensation of the ganglionic rudiments.

A similar conclusion was reached by Stewart and Macagno (1984) for regional differentiation of the hirudinid leech *Haemopis marmorata* on the basis of comparative cell counts in ganglia of genital and non-genital segments. Counts of cell populations in *Haemopis* embryos from ten days of development when the 32 metameres are clearly visible, up to hatching, show that all ganglia behave equally in early development, and up to day 20 of embryogenesis there is no detectable difference between sex and non-sex segmental ganglia. However, over this period the mean number of cells per ganglion decreases significantly and pyknotic cells are seen within the ganglia indicating that cell death is one of the ways in which cell number is adjusted in the leech CNS. The first signs of sex segmental differences appear just before hatching when the number of neurons in ganglia 5 and 6 begins to increase. This increase continues post-embryonically over several months until the adult number of between 600 and 700 neurons is reached (Stewart, Spergel, and Macagno 1986). Thus the segmental differences in size of neuronal populations in *Haemopis* are due to selective cell addition. In another annelid, the earthworm *Pheretima communissima*, there is a three- to four-fold increase in the number of neurons in the reproductive segments from hatching to sexual maturity (Ogawa, 1939). The capacity to add nerve cells post-embryonically could be a general property of annelid central nervous systems, and in this respect the annelid CNS may differ from that of grasshoppers, where some segment-specific differences appear at the earliest stages of neurogenesis (Doe and Goodman 1985), although for the most part a stereotyped segmental complement of neural cells arises in each ganglion and is subsequently remodelled by segment-specific patterns of cell death and differentiation (Goodman 1982).

SEGMENT-SPECIFIC DIFFERENCES IN IDENTIFIED NEURONS: THE POSSIBLE ROLE OF TARGET INTERACTIONS

Regional differences occur in the adult nervous system in the branching architecture of homologous neurons in different segments. For example, sensory and motoneurons at head and tail ends of the cord arborize over more ganglia than their counterparts in the mid-body ganglia (Yau 1976a; Gillon and Wallace 1984; Johansen, Hockfield, and McKay 1984). Some differences may be the consequence of the secondary fusion of ganglia during embryogenesis to form the head and tail 'brains' (see p. 27); other differences are found between the free segmental ganglia. The large serotoninergic Retzius cells in segments 5 and 6 differ from Retzius cells in all the other segmental ganglia in their central arborization and synaptic relations, as well as in their peripheral projections. In standard mid-body ganglia the peripheral axons of Retzius cells innervate skin mucus glands and body wall muscles (Yaksta-Sauerland and Coggeshall 1973). By contrast, in segments 5 and 6 they do not innervate the body wall but instead innervate the male and female reproductive organs found only in these segments. The differences in the morphology of Retzius cells in segments 5 and 6 apparently arise only after their growth cones contact the developing reproductive tissue. At this time the cells stop expanding neurites into the body wall and intersegmental connectives and appear rather to devote their entire peripheral innervation to the developing male and female reproductive organs, suggesting that an interaction with the target may be important in the development of segment-specific differences (Mason, Glover, and Kristan 1984; Jellies, Loer, and Kristan 1985; Loer, Jellies, and Kristan 1985). The ability to ablate or transplant tissue in early leech embryos should make it possible to test such ideas.

DIFFERENTIATION OF NEURONS STUDIED WITH TECHNIQUES THAT LABEL GROUPS OF CELLS: THE EXPRESSION OF ANTIGENS BY EMBRYONIC NEURONS

Some of the monoclonal antibodies raised against adult leech nervous systems (Zipser and McKay 1981) label identified cells or small groups of cells, showing that there are individual molecular signatures in the adult nervous system. For example, the antibody Lan 3–2 is specific in adult *Haemopis* for the two pairs of nociceptive neuron cell bodies within the ganglion which respond to noxious stimulation of the skin and gut (Nicholls and Baylor 1968; Blackshaw *et al.* 1982*a*) and for a subset of axon fascicles in the connectives. (In the related species *Hirudo* and *Helobdella*, Lan 3–2 cross-reacts only with axon fascicles and not with central N cell bodies.) The grouped subset of axons stained by Lan 3–2 are symmetrically located in the centro–lateral part of left and right connectives and maintain their stereotyped location along the entire length of the ventral nerve cord in all animals of the same species and frequently in animals of different species (see Fig. 2.6; McKay, Hockfield, Johansen, Thompson, and Frederiksen 1983). Lan 3–2 binds to all of the axons within particular fascicles delineated by glial cell processes, as does a second antibody, Lan 4–2, which binds to a different, overlapping set of axons, raising the possibility that there might be molecular markers for each fascicle in the connectives. In electron micrographs of antibody-stained adult nervous systems the Lan 3–2 and Lan 4–2 staining is associated with the perimeter of stained axons rather than with the axoplasm showing that these antibodies bind to surface antigens (Fig. 2.7). On immunoblots of proteins extracted from the leech nervous system, Lan 4–2 binds to a high-molecular-weight antigen of 130 Kd which co-migrates with the band of antigens of high molecular size (90 Kd to 130 Kd) recognized by the antibody Lan 3–2. The antigens recognized by both Lan 3–2 and Lan 4–2 are protease-sensitive and both have been shown by lectin-binding experiments to be glycosylated (McKay *et al.* 1983; Flanagan, Flaster, MacInnes, and Zipser 1986).

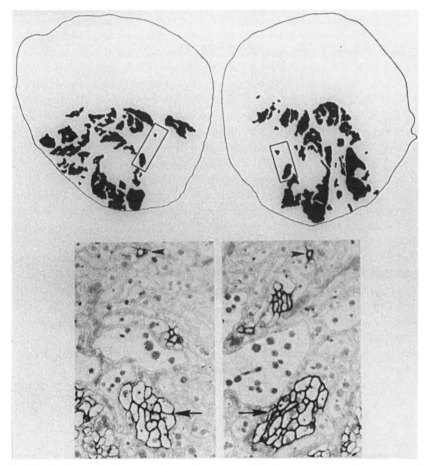

Fig. 2.7. Antibody binding to subsets of axons: distribution of axon bundles in the left and right connectives identified by Lan 3–2 are shown. The boxes marked in the diagram are shown in the inset electron micrographs. [Reproduced from McKay *et al.* (1983) by kind permission of the American Association for the Advancement of Science, Washington, DC.]

The mechanisms underlying the grouping and path-finding of axons are largely unknown. Most proposals invoke specific molecular markers (Sperry 1963). The fact that the axon surface can carry specific markers that distinguish axons in a given fascicle from axons in neighbouring fascicles suggests a possible role of the surface antigens in the formation of fascicles. Experiments in which the developmental appearance of the Lan 3–2 antigen has been studied in leech embryos show that this family of protease-sensitive, glycosylated antigens are differentially expressed by some neurons from the earliest stages of axon outgrowth. In the embryos of two species of leech, *Haemopis marmorata* and *Helobdella triserialis*, the antigen is seen first in the peripheral nervous system in groups of cells associated with the segmental sensilla along the central annulus of each segment on the dorsal body wall (McKay *et al.* 1983; Johansen, Thompson, Stewart, and McKay 1985; Stewart, Macagno, and Zipser 1985). Only a few neurons in each sensillum are stained and they are associated with a 5–10 μm cilium making it likely that they correspond to uniciliate primary sensory neurons thought to be involved in water-movement detection in adult leeches (Friesen 1981). The axons carrying these specific antigens grow into the CNS from the cell bodies in the periphery, so forming distinct fibre bundles with the processes of more proximally located groups of neurons. They arborize within the CNS and send processes rostrally and caudally to form antigenically positive bundles of axons in the connectives at early stages of development. The antibody Lan 3–6 (Zipser and McKay 1981) also labels cells in segmental sensilla in *Haemopis* embryos but a different population of ciliated cells from those labelled with Lan 3–2, indicating that the different kinds of ciliated cells in a sensillum possess different antigenic markers. Lan 3–6 also labels previously undescribed ciliated peripheral neurons of unknown modality located in the epidermis of the other annuli (Fig. 2.8). Peripheral neurons label first in the middle annulus of each segment, beginning at the head end of the embryo and progressing rostro–caudally, and label last in the most anterior and posterior annuli of each segment. Thus there are two kinds of temporal organization in the developing leech body wall: an overall rostro–caudal sequence, which is also apparent in other tissues, and a local ordering from the middle annulus towards the anterior and posterior boundaries of each segment.

DEVELOPMENT OF SENSORY FIELDS: PRIMARY AXON OUTGROWTH AND THE FORMATION OF RECEPTIVE FIELDS BY IDENTIFIED MECHANO–SENSORY NEURONS

In the vertebrate nervous system the outgrowth of populations of axons from identified sensory and motor pools has been shown to be highly selective from

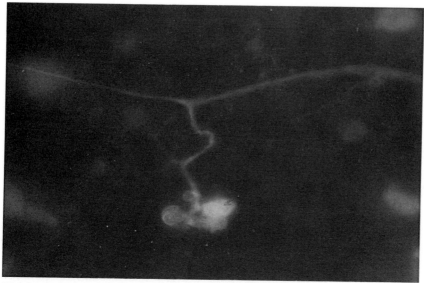

Fig. 2.8. Peripheral neurons in a 20-day *Hirudo* embryo labelled with *lan 3–6* (antibody kindly supplied by Dr B. Zipser).

the beginning, suggesting that neurons have identities prior to innervation and choose specific pathways to find their targets (Landmesser and Morris 1975; Landmesser 1978; Lance-Jones and Landmesser 1980; Scott 1982). In the leech nervous system, with its relatively small number of neurons, it is possible to study in the embryo the behaviour of single axons as they establish their territories. The striking feature of the innervation of skin by mechano–sensory neurons in adult leeches is its orderliness. In each of the 21 segmental ganglia along the along the length of a leech, individual touch (T), pressure (P), or nociceptive (N) cells innervate the same specific areas of skin. For example, there are six T sensory cells in each ganglion, symmetrically arranged in pairs, and each of the three cells on one side innervates a discrete area of either dorsal, lateral, or ventral skin (Nicholls and Baylor 1968). Within their particular body wall territories, touch cell axons branch profusely and the endings of the axons form specialized mechano–receptors (Fig. 2.9). An individual T cell may have as many as a thousand terminals distributed throughout its receptive field (Blackshaw 1981). The other types of mechano–sensory cells, the pressure (P) and nociceptive (N) neurons, also innervate specific territories in the skin. They have different peripheral axon branching patterns, terminals with a different morphology (Blackshaw, Nicholls, and Parnas 1982*a*), and their receptive fields overlap those of T cells but have different boundaries.

For touch and pressure cells the specificity of skin innervation is carried further in that each cutaneous branch of the axon innervates a specific part of

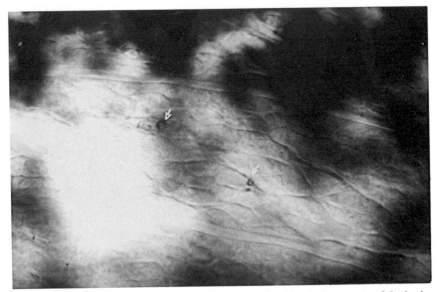

Fig. 2.9. Touch mechano–sensory cell endings visualized in whole mounts of the body wall after injection of horse-radish peroxidase into their cell bodies in the ganglion. Nomarski photograph of the surface of the ventral skin showing the profiles of the skin epithelial cells and two adjacent terminals (arrows) of the T cell innervating the ventral skin and lying between the epithelial cells at the skin surface.

the cell's field. Major fields are innervated by large calibre axon branches in the nerve roots of the cell's own ganglion. In addition, there are fine calibre axon branches in the connectives to adjacent ganglia which innervate accessory fields in adjacent body segments (Fig. 2.10). The boundaries between the subfields are quite distinct and usually correspond to annular margins (Yau 1976*b*; Kramer and Goldman 1981). Thus the innervation pattern of a single neuron and its numerous branches appears like a patchwork quilt with individual branches innervating a discrete territory in the skin with no overlap by other branches of the same cell.

Although different branches of the same cell do not overlap, the fields of homologous T cells in neighbouring ganglia overlap extensively along the length of a leech. There is also a small amount of overlap dorso–ventrally between the fields of touch cells within a ganglion. Thus innervation of a patch of skin by a touch cell does not preclude the presence of other touch cells, or of pressure or nociceptive cells.

The precise way in which the skin is innervated in the leech makes it possible to ask particular questions about the way in which the sensory fields are established during embryogenesis. For example: How does a neuron recognize and acquire its territory and what limits its spread? Do neurons innervate initially only the appropriate territory of skin or do they also innervate

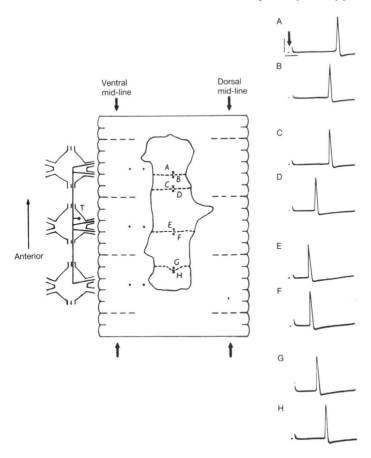

Fig. 2.10. Subfields of a touch cell that innervated lateral skin. Each subfield was innervated by a separate branch of the cell passing through either a root of its ganglion or that of an adjacent ganglion. Adjacent subfields had negligible overlap with each other, as indicated by discrete jumps in the time delay of intracellularly recorded action potentials (records on the right) when a mechanical stimulus was moved across the boundary between two adjoining subfields. Vertical calibration: 20 mV; horizontal calibration: 10 msec. Arrow indicates the time when the mechanical stimulus was applied. [Reproduced from Yau (1976*b*) by kind permission of the Physiological Society.]

inappropriate skin territory from which their axons later withdraw? Why is it that a touch cell will innervate territory occupied by another touch cell or by a pressure or a nociceptive neuron but will not invade the territory of another branch of its own axon? Are receptive subfields non-overlapping because during development the different peripheral branches of the same axon avoid each other or compete for a place on their common target?

Innervation of skin by identified pressure-sensitive neurons in embryos of the glossiphoniid leech *Haementaria ghilianii* has been followed from the time of initial outgrowth of the axons by injecting Lucifer-yellow intracellularly at successive developmental stages until the receptive field has achieved its adult configuration (Kuwada and Kramer 1983). Each segmental ganglion in *Haementaria* contains two pairs of pressure cells, each of which innervates a specific area of dorsal or ventral skin in adult leeches. During embryogenesis the ventral germinal plate near the ganglion is the target of the P_V neuron and the more distal germinal plate the target of the P_d neuron. These experiments show that P neurons send their first or 'primary' peripheral axons directly to their separate targets and begin to innervate them at approximately the same time. Thus the P_D neuron shows an early preference in embryogenesis for dorsal skin, growing across ventral germinal plate directly to dorsal germinal plate despite an opportunity to innervate ventral germinal plate, the target of the P_V neuron. The specificity of the P neuron is therefore not accounted for by temporal differences in the outgrowth of the primary axons, as has been shown for the formation of appropriate neuronal connections in the developing arthropod visual system (Anderson 1978; Macagno 1978). The smaller secondary subfields develop later from secondary and intersegmental axons. These axons too grow directly to their appropriate skin territories, and their arborization expands until the adult receptive field pattern is established late in embryogenesis. They do not appear initially to overgrow and later to trim down to the normal boundaries of the receptive field.

Not only do the neurons grow directly to target territory, but they arborize in that territory in a highly stereotyped way as if the peripheral axons were growing along predetermined pathways (Kramer and Kuwada 1983). The primary axon branch grows out circumferentially, perpendicular to the long axis of the embryo, along that area of the germinal plate from which will arise the central annulus of the segmental skin. First-order longitudinal branches emerge at characteristic locations around the circumference and grow anteriorly and posteriorly along the length of the leech. As these grow longitudinally, second-order annular branches emerge circumferentially along the central portions of the future skin annuli (Fig. 2.11). This consistently rectilinear pattern appears to match the grid-like arrangement of muscle fibres in the body wall (see pp. 28 and 35–6) whose development precedes the outgrowth of the primary axon. It has been suggested that as well as guiding migrating neuroblasts and glioblasts earlier in development, the muscles might delineate the peripheral pathways of differentiating CNS neurons.

A striking feature of the arborization within the receptive fields is that throughout embryogenesis, as in the adult leech, separate axon branches of the same neuron are virtually non-overlapping, in marked contrast to the extensive contact and overlap between axon branches of homologous P neurons. It appears that the sharp boundaries between the major and minor

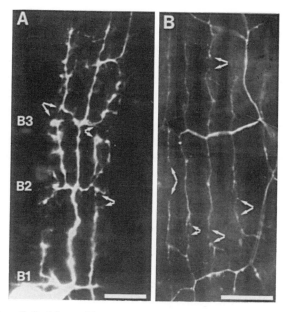

Fig. 2.11. Growth-limiting self-encounters of P_V neuron axons as seen among peripheral axons of Lucifer-yellow-filled P_V neurons photographed in whole mount. (A) The major field axons at stage 10(2/5). Laterally directed second-order annular branches from B1 and B2 branches encounter the B2 and B3 branches, respectively (at arrows). These axons are spatially separated, but focusing through the preparation revealed apparent filopodial contacts between the encountering branches; filopodia projecting from ends of axons are blurred in the photograph. (B) Encounter of fourth-order circular branches in a neuron in the mid-body at stage-11 (2/20). Circular branches growing from neighbouring third-order longitudinal branches along the same circumferential path encounter each other at arrows (that point to ends of axons) and are separated. Blurred filopodia are visible between the ends of some pairs of circular branches. The thick, faintly fluorescent circumferential stripe beneath each row of circular branches is an autofluorescent circular muscle fibre. Calibration: 50 μm. [Reproduced from Kramer and Kuwada (1983) by kind permission of the Society for Neuroscience, Bethesda, MD.]

subfields are established because the major and minor field axons of the same neuron stop growing towards each other when they meet. Thus each axon branch excludes the other from the territory it already occupies. Kramer and Kuwada (1983) suggest that the peripheral axon arborization is constrained by a process of neuronal self-avoidance. This idea has been tested directly by delaying or surgically preventing the outgrowth of minor or major field axon branches (Kramer and Stent 1985). Interference with the outgrowth of a minor field axon results in the spread of the major field axon branch into the territory normally occupied by the absent or delayed branch, and vice versa.

This non-overlap of isoneuronal processes, which is so apparent in the leech mechano–sensory neurons, may be a general phenomenon of neuronal development. Whatever the underlying mechanism, one consequence of self-avoidance by isoneuronal processes in the development of receptive fields could be to ensure optimal coverage of target territory. Other neurons with similar two-dimensional fields of processes are the alpha cells of the retina and the cerebellar Purkinje cells. The mutual territorial exclusion obtains only for isoneuronal branches and consequently is likely to be a different mechanism to that underlying heteroneuronal exclusion found in adult leeches between axon branches of homologous mechano–sensory neurons maintaining receptive fields in adjacent skin territories (Blackshaw *et al.* 1982*b*).

SELECTIVE LOSS OF NEURITES WITHIN THE CNS DURING DIFFERENTIATION OF IDENTIFIED NEURONS

Although initial overgrowth and subsequent elimination of excess processes does not appear to be a feature of the development of sensory fields in the peripheral nervous system, selective loss of neurites does occur during the differentiation of the central arborization of both motor and sensory neurons. A striking feature of developing motoneurons to annulus erector muscles (AE motoneurons) in *Hirudo* is the projection of processes, not normally seen in adult AE motoneurons, into the connectives of the ventral nerve cord. These '*extra*' central processes are present at eight days of development, by which time the motoneurons have already extended peripheral axons out of developing segmental nerve roots towards the annulus erector muscles in the adjacent body wall. The central processes continue to extend as the connectives between ganglia elongate during development, but over the subsequent six days they become gradually thinner, while the peripheral axons are increasing in calibre, and they continue to atrophy until the neurons attain the adult morphology between two and three weeks after hatching. By contrast, developing motoneurons in ganglia at the head and tail ends of the ventral cord retain extra processes. These continue to increase in calibre within the CNS as the cells grow and eventually send branches out of the roots of more rostral and caudal ganglia to innervate the peripheral musculature (Wallace 1984).

A selective loss of processes from the central arbor also occurs in mechan–sensory neurons over a similar developmental time-scale (Blackshaw, Parnas, and Thompson 1984). Individual adult mechano–sensory neurons have arborizations that span three segmental ganglia: they contact their post-synaptic cells via an array of fine branches within their own ganglion and they also project axon branches into anterior- and posterior-going connectives to neighbouring ganglia where they synapse and send branches to the periphery

(Yau 1976*b*). In adult neurons the axon branches in the connectives do not normally have collaterals but project directly from one ganglion to the next as single fibres of passage. By contrast, labelling of identified neurons with Lucifer yellow or horseradish peroxidase in embryonic and newly hatched *Hirudo* shows that both T and N cells have extra axon branches within the connectives. N cells have several additional fine axon branches arising both within the neuropil of the ganglion and as side branches of the main axon within the connectives, that typically run for hundreds of microns parallel to the main axon branch, whereas touch cell connective axons have numerous short secondary branches that arise in a tuft and end within a few microns.

ACKNOWLEDGEMENTS

Unpublished work by the author was supported by the SERC.

REFERENCES

Anderson, D. T. (1973). *Embryology and phylogeny in annelids and arthropods.* Pergamon Press, Oxford.

Anderson, H. (1978). Postembryonic development of the visual system of the locust *Schistocerca gregaria. J. Embryol. exp. Morphol.* **45**, pp. 55–83.

Balakier, H. and Pedersen, R. A. (1982). Allocation of cells to inner cell mass and trophectoderm lineages in preimplantation mouse embryos. *Dev. Biol.* **90**, pp. 352–62.

Bate, C. M. (1976). Embryogenesis of an insect nervous system. I. A map of the thoracic and abdominal neuroblasts in *Locusta migratoria. J. Embryol. exp. Morphol.* **35**, pp. 107–23.

Blackshaw, S. E. (1981). Morphology and distribution of touch cell terminals in the skin of the leech. *J. Physiol. (Lond.)* **320**, pp. 219–28.

Blackshaw, S. E. (1987). Organisation and development of the peripheral nervous system in annelids. In *Nervous systems in invertebrates* (ed. M. A. Ali) (in press). NATO-ASI Series, Plenum Press, New York.

Blackshaw, S. E. and Thompson, S. W. N. (1986). Hyperpolarising response to stretch in neurones innervating body wall muscle in the leech. *J. Physiol. (Lond.)* **371**, 58P.

Blackshaw, S. E. and Thompson, S. W. N. (1987). Hyperpolarising responses to stretch in sensory neurones innervating leech body wall muscle. *J. Physiol. (Lond.)* (in press).

Blackshaw, S. E., Mackay, D. A., and Thompson, S. W. N. (1984). The fine structure of a leech stretch receptor neurone and its efferent input. *J. Physiol. (Lond.)* **360**, 76P.

Blackshaw, S. E., Nicholls, J. G., and Parnas, I. (1982*a*). Physiological responses, receptive fields and terminal arborisations of nociceptive cells in the leech. *J. Physiol. (Lond.)* **326**, pp. 251–60.

Blackshaw, S. E., Nicholls, J. G., and Parnas I. (1982*b*). Expanded receptive fields of cutaneous mechanoreceptor cells following deletion of single neurones in the CNS of the leech. *J. Physiol. (Lond.)* **326,** pp. 261–68.

Blackshaw, S. E., Parnas, I., and Thompson, S. W. N. (1984). Changes in the central arborisation of primary afferent neurones during development of the leech nervous system. *J. Physiol. (Lond.)* **353,** 47P.

Doe, C. Q. and Goodman, C. S. (1985). Early events in insect neurogenesis. I. Development and segmental differences in the pattern of neuronal precursor cells. *Dev. Biol.* **111,** 193–205.

Elliot, E. J. (1987). Morphology of chemosensory organs required for feeding in the leech *Hirudo medicinalis*. *J. Morphol.* **192,** pp. 181–7.

Fernandez, J. (1980). Embryonic development of the glossiphoniid leech *Theromyzon rude*: characterization of developmental stages. *Dev. Biol.* **76,** 245–62.

Fernandez, J. and Olea, N. (1982). Embryonic development of glossiphoniid leeches. In *Developmental biology of freshwater invertebrates* (eds. F.W. Harrison and R.C. Cowden), pp. 317–61. Liss, New York.

Fernandez, J. and Stent, G. S. (1980). Embryonic development of the glossiphoniid leech *Theromyzon rude*: structure and development of the germinal bands. *Dev. Biol.* **78,** pp. 407–34.

Fernandez, J. and Stent, G. S. (1983). Embryonic development of the hirudiniid leech *Hirudo medicinalis*: structure, development and segmentation of the germinal plate. *J. Embryol. exp. Morphol.* **72,** pp. 71–96.

Flanagan, T., Flaster, M. S., MacInnes, J., and Zipser, B. (1986). Probing structural homologies in cell-specific glycoproteins in the leech CNS. *Brain Res.* **378,** pp. 152–8.

Friesen, W. O. (1981). Physiology of water motion detection in the medicinal leech. *J. exp. Biol.* **92,** 255–75.

Gillon, J. W. and Wallace, B. G. (1984). Segmental variation in the arborisation of identified neurones in the leech central nervous system. *J. Comp. Neurol.* **228,** pp. 142–8.

Gimlich, R. L. and Braun, J. (1985). Improved fluorescent compounds for tracing cell lineage. *Dev. Biol.* **109,** pp. 509–14.

Goodman, C. S. (1982). Embryonic development of identified neurones in the grasshopper. In *Neuronal development* (ed. N. C. Spitzer), pp. 171–212. Plenum Press, New York.

Hirose, G. and Jacobson, M. (1979). Clonal organization of the central nervous system of the frog. I. Clones stemming from individual blastomeres of the 16-cell and earlier stages. *Dev. Biol.* **71,** pp. 191–202.

Jellies, J., Loer, C. M., and Kristan, W. B. (1985). Morphogenesis of segment specific innervation patterns in an identified leech neuron. *Soc. Neurosci. Abstr.* **11,** p. 956.

Johansen, J., Hockfield, S., and McKay, R. D. G. (1984). Axonal projections of mechanosensory axons in the connectives and peripheral nerves of the leech *Haemopis marmorata*. *J. Comp. Neurol.* **226,** pp. 255–62.

Johansen, J., Thompson, I., Stewart, R. R., and McKay, R. D. G. (1985). Expression of surface antigens by the monoclonal antibody Lan 3–2 during embryonic development of the leech. *Brain Res* **343,** pp. 1–7.

Kimmel, C. B. and Warga, R. M. (1986). Tissue specific cell lineages originate in the gastrula of the zebrafish. *Science* **231,** pp. 365–8.

Kramer, A. P. and Goldman, J. R. (1981). The nervous system of the glossiphoniid leech *Haementeria ghilianii*. I. Identification of neurones. *J. Comp. Physiol. A* **144**, pp. 435–48.

Kramer, A. P. and Kuwada, J. Y. (1983). Formation of the receptive fields of leech mechanosensory neurons during embryonic development. *J. Neurosci.* **3**, pp. 2474–86.

Kramer, A. P. and Stent, G. S. (1985). Developmental arborisation of sensory neurons in the leech *Haementeria ghilianii*. II. Experimentally induced variations in the branching pattern. *J. Neurosci.* **5**, pp. 768–75.

Kramer, A. P. and Weisblat, D. A. (1985). Developmental neural kinship groups in the leech. *J. Neurosci.* **5**, pp. 388–407.

Kretz, J. R., Stent, G. S., and Kristan, W. B. (1976). Photosensory input pathways in the medicinal leech. *J. Comp. Physiol.* **106**, pp. 1–37.

Kuffler, S. W. and Potter, D. D. (1964). Glia in the leech nervous system: physiological properties and neuron-glia relationships. *J. Neurophysiol.* **27**, pp. 290–320.

Kuwada, J. Y. and Kramer, A. P. (1983). Embryonic development of the leech nervous system: primary axon outgrowth of identified neurons. *J. Neurosci.* **3**, pp. 2098–111.

Lance-Jones, C. and Landmesser, L. (1980). Motoneurone projection patterns in embryonic chick limbs following partial deletions of the spinal cord. *J. Physiol. (Lond.)* **302**, pp. 559–80.

Landmesser, L. (1978). The development of motor projection patterns in the chick hind limb. *J. Physiol. (Lond.)* **284**, pp. 391–414.

Landmesser, L. and Morris, D. G. (1975). The development of functional innervation in the hindlimb of the chick embryo. *J. Physiol. (Lond.)* **249**, pp. 310–26.

Loer, C. M., Jellies, J., and Kristan, W. B. (1985). The possible role of target interactions in the development of segment-specific differences of an identified neuron. *Soc. Neurosci. Abstr.* **11**, 957.

Macagno, E. R. (1978). A mechanism for the formation of synaptic connections in the arthropod visual system. *Nature* **275**, pp. 318–20.

Macagno, E. R. (1980). Number and distribution of neurones in leech segmental ganglia. *J. Comp. Neurol.* **190**, pp. 283–302.

Mann, K. H. (1962). *Leeches (Hirudinea)*. Pergamon Press, New York.

Mason, A. J. R., Glover, J. C., and Kristan, W. B. (1984). Embryonic development of segmentally specialised serotonergic neurones in the leech *Hirudo medicinalis*. *Soc. Neurosci. Abstr.* **10**, p. 1033.

McKay, R. D. G., Hockfield, S., Johansen, J., Thompson, I., and Frederiksen, K. (1983). Surface molecules identify groups of growing axons. *Science* **222**, pp. 788–94.

Muller, K. J., Nicholls, J. G., and Stent, G. S. (1981). Neurobiology of the leech. Cold Spring Harbor Publications, New York.

Nicholls, J. G. and Baylor, D. A. (1968). Specific modalities and receptive fields of sensory neurones in the CNS of the leech. *J. Neurophysiol.* **31**, pp. 740–56.

Nishida, H. and Staoh, N. (1983). Cell lineage analysis in ascidian embryos by intracellular injection of a tracer enzyme. I. Up to the 8 cell stage. *Dev. Biol.* **99**, pp. 382–94.

Ogawa, F. (1939). The nervous system of earthworm *Pheretima communissima* in different ages. *Sci. Rep. Tokohu Univ.* **13**, pp. 395–488.

Rude, S. (1969). Monoamine containing neurons in the central nervous system and peripheral nerves of the leech, *Hirudo medicinalis*. *J. Comp. Neurol.* **136**, pp. 349–71.

Schliep, W. (1936). Ontogenie der Hirudineen. In *Klassen und Ordnungen des Tierreichs* (ed. H. G. Bronn), vol. 4, div. III, book 4, part 2, pp. 1–121. Akad. Verlagsgesellschaft, Leipzig.

Scott, S. A. (1982). The development of the segmental pattern of skin sensory innervation in the embryonic chick hindlimb. *J. Physiol. (Lond.)* **303**, pp. 203–20.

Shafer, M. R. and Calabrese, R. L. (1981). Similarities and differences in the structure of segmentally homologous neurons that control the hearts in the leech, *Hirudo medicinalis. Cell Tissue Res.* **214**, pp. 137–53.

Shankland, M. and Weisblat, D. A. (1984). Stepwise commitment of blast cell fates during the positional specification of the O and P cell lines in the leech embryo. *Dev. Biol.* **106**, pp. 326–42.

Slack, J. M. W. (1983). *From egg to embryo.* Cambridge University Press, Cambridge.

Sperry, R. W. (1963). Chemoaffinity in the orderly growth of nerve fiber patterns and connections. *Proc Natl. Acad. Sci. USA* **50**, pp. 703–10.

Stent, G. S. and Kristan, W. B. (1981). Neural circuits generating rhythmic movements. In *Neurobiology of the leech* (eds. K. J. Muller, J. G. Nicholls, and G. S. Stent), pp. 113–46. Cold Spring Harbor Publications, New York.

Stent, G. S., Weisblat, D. A., Blair, S. S., and Zackson, S. L. (1982). Cell lineage in the development of the leech nervous system. In *Neuronal development.* (ed. N. Spitzer), pp. 1–44. Plenum Press, New York.

Stewart, R. R. and Macagno, E. (1984). The development of segmental differences in cell number in the CNS of the leech. *Soc. Neurosci. Abstr.* **10**, p. 512.

Stewart, R. R., Macagno, E., and Zipser, B. (1985). The embryonic development of peripheral neurons in the body wall of the leech, *Haemopis marmorata. Brain Res.* **332**, 150–7.

Stewart, R. R., Spergel, D., and Macagno, E. R. (1986). Segmental differentiation in the leech nervous system: the genesis of cell number in the segmental ganglia of *Haemopis marmorata. Proc. Natl. Acad. Sci. USA* **83**, pp. 2746–50.

Stuart, D. K., Thompson, I., Weisblat, D. A., and Kramer, A. P. (1982). Antibody staining of embryonic leech muscle, blast cell migration and neuronal pathway formation. *Soc. Neurosci. Abstr.* **8**, p. 15.

Thompson, S. W. N. (1986). Morphological and physiological studies of a stretch receptor neurone in the leech *Hirudo medicinalis.* PhD thesis, University of Glasgow, Glasgow, UK.

Thompson, W. and Stent, G. S. (1976). Neuronal control of heartbeat in the medicinal leech. II. Intersegmental coordination of heart motoneuron activity by heart interneurons. *J. Comp. Physiol.* **111**, pp. 281–307.

Torrence, S. A. (1984). Neuroblast migration in leech embryos. *Soc. Neurosci. Abstr.* **10**, p. 512.

Torrence, S. A. and Stuart, D. K. (1986). Gangliogenesis in leech embryos: migration of neural precursor cells. *J. Neurosci* **6**, pp. 2736–46.

Wallace, B. G. (1984). Selective loss of neurites during differentiation of cells in the leech central nervous system. *J. Comp. Neurol.* **228**, pp. 149–53.

Weeks, J. C. (1982). Synaptic basis of swim initiation in the leech. II. Pattern generating neuron (cell 208) which mediates motor effects of swim-initiating neurons. *J. Comp. Physiol.* **148**, pp. 265–79.

Weisblat, D. A. (1981). Development of the nervous system. In *Neurobiology of the leech* (eds. K. J. Muller, J. G. Nicholls, and G. S. Stent), pp. 173–96. Cold Spring Harbor Publications, New York.

Weisblat, D. A., Kim, S. Y., and Stent, G. S. (1984). Embryonic origins of cells in the leech *Helobdella triserialis*. *Dev. Biol.* **104**, pp. 65–85.

Weisblat, D. A., Sawyer, R., and Stent, G. S. (1978). Cell lineage analysis by intracellular injection of a tracer enzyme. *Science* **202**, pp. 1295–8.

Weisblat, D. A., Harper, G., Stent, G. S., and Sawyer, R. T. (1980). Embryonic cell lineages in the nervous system of the glossiphoniid leech *Helobdella triserialis*. *Dev. Biol.* **76**, pp. 58–78.

Weisblat, D. A., Zackson, S. S., Blair, S. S., and Young, J. D. (1980). Cell lineage analysis by intracellular injection of fluorescent tracers. *Science* **209**, pp. 1538–41.

Whitman, C. O. (1878). The embryology of *Clepsine*. *Q.J. Micros, Sci.* **18**, pp. 215–315.

Yaksta-Sauerland, B. A. and Coggeshall, R. E. (1973). Neuromuscular junctions in the leech. *J. Comp. Neurol.* **151**, pp. 85–99.

Yau, K. W. (1976a). Physiological properties and receptive fields of mechanosensory neurones in the head ganglion of the leech: comparison with homologous cells in segmental ganglia. *J. Physiol. (Lond.)* **263**, pp. 489–512.

Yau, K. W. (1976b). Receptive fields, geometry and conduction block of sensory neurones in the CNS of the leech. *J. Physiol. (Lond.)* **262**, pp. 513–38.

Zackson, S. L. (1982). Cell clones and segmentation in leech development. *Cell* **31**, pp. 761–70.

Zackson, S. L. (1984). Cell lineage, cell–cell interactions, and segment formation in the ectoderm of a glossiphoniid leech embryo. *Dev. Biol.* **104**, pp. 143–60.

Zipser, B. (1979). Identifiable neurons controlling penile eversion in the leech. *J. Neurophysiol.* **42**, pp. 455–64.

Zipser, B. and McKay, R. G. (1981). Monoclonal antibodies distinguish identifiable neurones in the leech. *Nature* **289**, pp. 549–54.

3

Vital-dye analyses of neural development and connectivity

RICHARD WETTS, NANCY A. O'ROURKE,
AND SCOTT E. FRASER

The nervous system is created by many dynamic processes, starting with the initial determination of the neural precursors and ending with the final patterning of neural connections. The cells divide, migrate, change their appearance (differentiate), and elongate processes far from their somas. It is necessary to study these changes directly in order to understand the mechanisms of development. Observation of dynamic behaviour, however, presents a challenge, since it requires a practical way of identifying a cell (or group of cells) in different animals at different stages. In an ideal experiment, an identified group of cells could be followed in the same animal over several stages of development. It is also advantageous to be able to visualize the projection patterns of the identified cells. Recent experiments are more frequently overcoming these obstacles in a satisfying way with fascinating implications for neural development.

In some invertebrate systems (leech, grasshopper, nematode), the following of identified cells is a relatively minor task. The regular positions and small numbers (at least at early stages) of developing neurons have permitted straightforward analyses of the developmental history of single cells. In the extreme example of the nematode *C. elegans*, the lineage and position of each cell that contributes to the nervous system have been directly followed by light microscopy in the intact animal through the use of Nomarski optics (Sulston and Horvitz 1977; Sulston, Schierenberg, White, and Thomas 1983). The small size of the organism allowed projection patterns of each neuron to be elucidated 'simply' by reconstruction of electron micrographs of serial sections (White 1985). With few exceptions (the Mauthner cell and the Rohon–Beard cells), however, this type of analysis is not possible in vertebrates for three reasons: (a) there is a much larger number of cells with less noticeable spatial organization; (b) the individual cells usually cannot be observed directly; and (c) there are a large number of progenitors (which are not uniquely identifiable) initiating lineages which appear to be less rigidly regulated. To study the mechanisms of vertebrate neural development in a practical way, it is necessary to be able easily to observe a small group of the cells of interest. Until recently, examination of the developing nervous system have been limited to studies in which a capricious technique such as the Golgi stain is used to visualize a random subset of neurons. By examining different animals, fixed and stained at various stages, a likely sequence of the development of individual cells can be cautiously reconstructed. In the past, alternative methods have employed vital dyes that might leak from cell to cell, or interspecific chimerae which may introduce artefacts arising from slight species incompatibility.

In response to the need for a cell-autonomous cell lineage tracer, Stent and his co-workers (Weisblat, Sawyer, and Stent 1978) micro-injected the enzyme horseradish peroxidase (HRP) into individual cells of a leech embryo and identified the descendants of the injected cells by use of sensitive histochemistry specific for HRP. HRP has the additional advantage of being transported anterogradely down the axons of the developing neurons thus revealing their connection patterns. Therefore the same experiment yields results both about the lineage of the nervous system and about its developing connectivity. These techniques, adapted for use in *Xenopus* by Jacobson and co-workers, permitted a fate map of the early frog embryo to be created (cf. Hirose and Jacobson 1979) and allowed the pathways of early developing spinal neurons to be traced (Moody and Jacobson 1983; Jacobson and Huang 1985. The major limitation of the HRP technique is that the tissue must be fixed and processed before the cells can be imaged. An ideal lineage tracer would be one that could be observed in the cells as they develop, thereby allowing developmental phenomena to be monitored directly in individual live animals.

Fluorescent dextrans, which have recently been introduced as lineage tracers, come closest to this ideal (Gimlich and Braun 1985). These dyes serve well as cell-autonomous lineage tracers because they can be injected easily into a cell, but they are too large and too highly charged to escape through either cell junctions or cell membranes. The fluorescence allows observation of the labelled tissue *in vivo*. Lysinated derivatives of the fluorescent dextrans have free amino groups, rendering them fixable and so allowing them to be observed in fixed and sectioned tissues. In addition, for reasons yet to be understood, some batches of the dye remain diffusible in neuronal cell bodies and fill both the axon and the dendrites. Hence these dyes, which were originally designed for lineage studies, also serve as invaluable tools for studying issues of axon outgrowth and patterns of connectivity (cf. Eisen, Myers, and Westerfield 1986; O'Rourke and Fraser 1986a, 1986b).

The availability of fluorescent dextrans as intracellular vital dyes has ushered in exciting new classes of experiments in vertebrate neurogenesis. After direct injection of the dye into blastomeres of fish embryos, the descendants can be followed over time in these optically transparent animals. With this procedure, Kimmel and Warga (1986) have demonstrated both a dramatic amount of cell mixing and the variety of lineages among the cells that contribute to the nervous system. This cell mixing during early fish development has been used advantageously to follow the developing morphology of individual motoneurons. A single blastomere was injected and then, later, when a labelled motoneuron ended up fortuitously among unlabelled cells, it could be examined in detail since it was relatively unobscured by other labelled cells (Eisen *et al.* 1986). In another approach, a defined, coherent group of cells can be studied in detail. An entire embryo is injected with the dye at the one- or two-cell stage, resulting in an embryo with all of its cells labelled. Classical embryological techniques are then used to graft cells from the labelled animal into an unlabelled host (Gimlich and Gerhart 1984; Dale, Smith and Slack 1985; O'Rourke and Fraser 1986*a*, 1986*b*).

Here we will describe two different applications of the fluorescent dextrans as vital dyes in investigations of neurogenesis in the frog, *Xenopus*. First, we will present studies that use direct micro-injection of the dye to follow the descendants of the early blastomeres of *Xenopus*. Such work can address several issues, including the fate map of the embryo, the intermixing of the clone with other cells, and the presence of lineage restriction boundaries. Second, we will describe experiments in which groups of labelled eye-bud cells are grafted to an unlabelled host, thereby permitting the experimenter to follow the early establishment of topography in the *Xenopus* retinotectal projection.

CELL LINEAGE AND MIXING IN FROG EMBRYOS

The lineages of cells which give rise to the nervous system and the mechanisms that determine their fates are far from known, as evidenced by the recent questioning (Jacobson 1982) and reconfirmation (Gimlich and Cooke 1983; Smith and Slack 1983; Jacobson 1984) of the role of a grafted dorsal lip in organizing a second neural axis. In addressing further issues of neural development, amphibian embryos are ideally suited for lineage studies with the fluorescent dextran dyes. Cleavage stage *Xenopus* embryos have large cells which can be pressure-injected with dye. Up to the 64-cell stage, each blastomere is uniquely identifiable due to its position relative to the natural pigmentation of the egg. A micropipette (tip diameter approximately 2 μm), filled at the tip with lysinated fluorescein dextran (LFD) or lysinated rhodamine dextran (LRD), is inserted into the target blastomere under a dissecting microscope, and pulses of air pressure are used to inject 5–10 nl of the dye into the cell. After injection, the embryos continue development in a simple saline solution. Importantly, the total volume of amphibian embryos does not increase for the first few days of life, thereby avoiding any dilution of injected dye. The health of the injected animal and the position of some of the labelled cells can be followed with an epifluorescence microscope. However, since the yolk granules contained within the early amphibian embryo scatter the fluorescence from any but the surface cells, conventional histological techniques must be used to follow all of the injected cell's descendants. Thus, at various stages after injection, the embryos are fixed with 4 per cent paraformaldehyde and embedded in plastic or frozen, for sectioning. The descendants of the original blastomere are identified by their fluorescence; both the variety of cell types labelled and their spatial distribution are noted.

In our lineage studies, individual blastomeres were injected with LRD or LFD at the 16-cell stage (Fig. 3.1.). When assayed at stage 39, the four dorsal, animal pole blastomeres (DA and EA of both sides; see Fig. 3.1) were found to give rise to both the bulk of the central nervous system (CNS) and to a large variety of other tissues derived from all three germ layers. For the most part, the distribution of labelled cells that we observed was very similar to that reported using HRP as the lineage tracer (Hirose and Jacobson 1979). Unlike the previous HRP work, the use of fluorescent dyes made it possible to determine how this pattern arose by following individual cases over time and also by double-labelling animals with both LRD and LFD. In the latter cases, LFD was injected into either EA or DA on the left side of the grey crescent, and LRD was injected into the other blastomere. To get a dynamic picture of development, animals were examined at several stages leading up to stage 39. The results show a dramatic coherence initially of the descendants of each injected blastomere, which becomes significantly distorted by cell mixing with time.

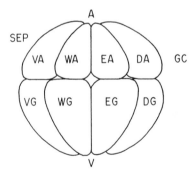

Fig. 3.1. Identification of blastomeres at the 16-cell stage. This is a view of the left side of the embryo with the animal pole (A) at the top, the vegetal pole (V) at the bottom, the sperm entry point (SEP) at the left, and the grey crescent (GC) at the right. After fertilization, the egg is free to rotate within the vitelline membrane, and the heavier, yolky vegetal pole always moves to the bottom. The high yolk content makes the vegetal pole blastomeres (DG, EG, WG and VG) yellow–white in colour, while pigment granules make the animal cells brown or black. The animal blastomeres at the grey crescent (DA and EA) are relatively less pigmented than the ventral blastomeres (VA and WA) due to cortical movements after fertilization. The DA and EA blastomeres give rise to the dorsal structures, including the bulk of the CNS.

Prior to gastrulation (stage 9), both the LRD and LFD descendants form single coherent groups (Fig. 3.2) which include all layers from the surface down to the blastocoele. However, the boundaries between LRD, LFD, and unlabelled cells are not absolute; a small degree of mixing can be seen. At the

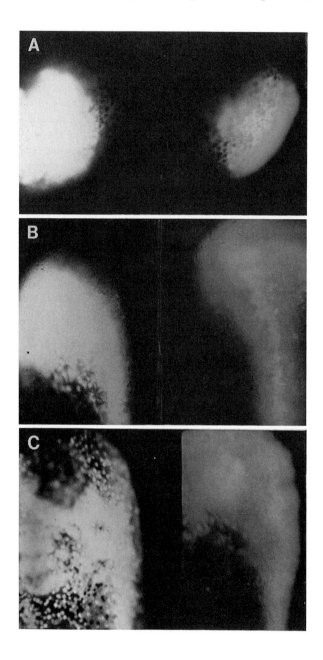

end of gastrulation (approximately stage 16), the labelled cells still form coherent groups, though individual cells can clearly be seen violating the boundary of the group and spreading further into neighbouring areas (Fig. 3.2). Both labelled areas involve the anterior region of the animal and are elongated rostro–caudally along the dorsal midline. In general, the area derived from labelling the dorsal most blastomere (DA) is more anterior and closer to the dorsal midline than the clones formed from more ventral blastomeres (in order: EA, WA, and then VA). Often each clone shows a co-distribution of the labelled cells in all three germ layers. In the ectoderm, the label in the neural plate is continuous with labelled epidermis. Immediately adjacent to the labelled ectoderm is the labelled mesoderm (somite and sometimes notochord). Sometimes the endoderm subjacent to the notochord and somites is also labelled. The amount of endoderm label is highly variable from none to a significant contribution, perhaps reflecting variability in the distance of the third cleavage from the equator (see below). With the conclusion of gastrulation, the basic body plan of the embryo is established; the location and extent of labelled cells at this time have a tremendous impact on which tissues will be labelled in the larva and adult. Since the labelled area can encompass all three germ layers at this stage, it is thus less surprising that these cells contribute to a large variety of different structures.

After neurulation (stage 23), the clones have become very extended along the rostro–caudal axis. A little more cell mixing is observed, but the coherence of the clones is still quite striking, especially in the CNS. Completely labelled areas (LRD or LFD) are often separated from unlabelled (or other labelled) areas by a sharp boundary, although some mixing of the labelled cells is evident. The boundaries between clones appear to separate the CNS into

---

Fig. 3.2. Live double-labelled *Xenopus* embryos at different stages. The left side of each panel shows the LFD, which had been injected into blastomere EA at the 16 cell stage. The animal remained under the objective while the filter sets were changed to show the LRD (right photographs), which had been injected into blastomere DA. Due to the width of these whole animals, not all of the fluorescence is in focus. In (A), stage 9, before gastrulation begins, there is some interdigitation of clones. In sections of other animals at the same stage the beginning of mixing was observed, especially in the deeper layers. In (B), stage 14, a neural plate stage, the view is of the dorsal surface with anterior toward the top of the figure. For each clone, the labelled cells still occupy essentially a single area, with mixing at the edges. In sections of other animals, it can be observed that this coherence extends from the superficial layers down to the deep layers, sometimes involving adjacent portions of all three germ layers. In (C), stage 32, around the time of hatching, the view is of the left side of the animal with anterior toward the top of the figure. In comparison with the photographs in (B) above, the clones occupy the same positions relative to each another. However, because of the mixing which has occurred, the area occupied by each clone is much larger than before, and the two labelled clones overlap more obviously. In these whole-mounts, the overlap is especially apparent in the epidermis.

dorsal and ventral territories, but the positions of the boundaries can vary significantly from animal to animal. Again, this variability is probably due to variations in the locations of the early cleavage planes.

At stage 30, adjacent parts of pharnyx, mesoderm, epidermis, and CNS often contribute to a coherent area of labelled cells. This is most striking in the anterior head region. Further posteriorly, coherent areas within the spinal cord and somites may not be as closely juxtaposed, apparently due to relative movements of the tissues since neurulation. Boundaries are still often seen in the CNS, but are less distinct, suggesting that cell mixing has been progressing. The mixing is suddenly more noticeable at stage 33. Most of the labelled cells in the CNS are seen in clusters (patches). This is probably the result of daughter and grand-daughter cells remaining together for a relatively long time, while more distantly related cells have had time to move away from each other. By stage 39, labelled cells are primarily located anteriorly and along the dorsal midline. However, in these areas, labelled and unlabelled cells are well intermixed within a given structure, and the density of labelled cells decreases smoothly into any unlabelled areas. In the CNS, distinct boundaries between labelled and unlabelled regions are rarely seen, suggesting that the slow, progressive mixing seen at earlier stages has finally become complete.

These results demonstrate that cell mixing is a slow process in *Xenopus*. It begins at gastrulation, continues throughout embryogenesis, and becomes noticeable only after hatching stages. By contrast, the intermixing that occurs in mice (Herrup, Wetts, and Diglio 1984; Rossant 1985) and zebrafish (Kimmel and Warga 1986) is rapid and dramatic (again, beginning at gastrulation). Sometimes clonally related cells differentiate into the same cell type even though they have migrated away from each other. These authors then find it impossible to conceptualize how any extrinsic factors could influence cell fate concurrent with such extensive mixing with unrelated cells. However, all of these investigators agree that ablation or transplantation experiments are required for testing a cell's state of determination.

The importance of testing the mechanisms of lineage restriction is highlighted by considering neural development in invertebrates (such as the leech, nematode, and grasshopper), which is characterized by stereotyped lineages. Uniquely identifiable founder cells undergo a specific sequence of divisions and cell movements, resulting in the formation of specific structures. It is tempting to speculate that the founder cells undergo these stereotyped events because they are determined to do so. To test the determination of the cells, individual nematode cells have been ablated using a laser. The descendants of the ablated cell are absent and the cells of the neighbouring lineages are almost always unchanged, indicating that most progenitors are committed (Sulston and White 1980). Similar inflexibility has been observed in the neuroblasts of the grasshopper nervous system, once the neuroblast population is founded (Doe, Kuwada, and Goodman 1985). However, there is some flexibility in the selection of which epithelial cells become neuroblasts and which become supporting cells. In the leech, a set of four teloblasts (named N, O, P, and Q) on each side of the embryo give rise to a band of blast cells; each bandlet then develops reproducibly into specific parts of the nervous system and other structures (see Weisblat and Shankland 1985). Ablation of any of three teloblast cells (N, O, or Q) leaves the other lineages unaltered. However, ablation of the P teloblast results in the cells of the o bandlet 'transfating' to form derivatives specific to the P lineage. Thus the o blast cells are not completely determined when they are born from the teloblast; it is only after three additional cell divisions that the set of descendants are determined (Shankland and Weisblat 1984). This points to the importance of challenging the stereotyped cell lineages in any system to determine if in fact they reflect a rigidly fixed developmental pathway.

In terms of cell-mixing during development, *Xenopus* resembles the invertebrates. The first six cleavages can be regular and stereotyped, resulting in 64 identifiable blastomeres. Since cell mixing is so slow, each blastomere tends to contribute reproducibly to specific parts of the larva. Thus the somewhat stereotyped lineages in *Xenopus* might lead some investigators to presume, erroneously, that the lineages are restricted. However, the leech studies suggest that ablation or transplantation experiments are required to determine the stage at which *Xenopus* cells are committed to forming specific cell types. The fluorescent dextrans are also useful in this type of experiment. All descendants labelled with LFD can be ablated *in situ* by exposing them to light, whereas other cells labelled with LRD (which is much less phototoxic and is not excited by the blue light used to kill the LFD-filled cells) can be followed during the regeneration. Such experiments can establish when in the lineage the cells are committed to a specific cell phenotype. If it is found that the blastomeres are not committed, they might still be restricted in their cell mingling to a specific domain of the CNS (Jacobson and Klein 1985). Again, because of the regular cleavages and the slow mixing, labelled cells are likely to remain within any arbitrarily drawn boundary, especially if the blastomeres are injected late or if the larvae are examined early, since this allows less time for cell mixing. In our study, many of the embryos did not have absolutely symmetrical cleavages (which has no effect on later development), but they were regular enough to identify the blastomeres; that is, the position of the target cell relative to the other blastomeres was always the same, but the boundaries of the injected cell (determined by the locations of the cleavages) varied relative to the egg as a whole. Later, we observed that the boundaries between labelled and unlabelled areas were not located at the same place in all of the embryos. The regular and reproducible boundaries seen by some investigators are thus likely to be due to their strict selection of embryos displaying perfectly symmetrical cleavages rather than to any fundamental developmental process.

RETINOTECTAL DEVELOPMENT IN *XENOPUS*

A variation of the fluorescent dextran labelling described above can be used for cell marking and fibre tracing within individual embryonic tissues. In these experiments, the embryonic eye was examined by grafting fragments of labelled eye primordia into unlabelled hosts. The fate of the grafted cells can then be followed both *in situ* and in fixed, sectioned material. Because some dextrans are transported down the optic nerve fibres and because the head of the embryo becomes transparent as the yolk stores are utilized, this same vital-dye approach can be used to follow the initial development of the retinotectal projection *in vivo*.

The first series of experiments was designed to characterize the behaviour of large populations of dextran-labelled cells in the developing eye, and it laid the groundwork for investigations into mechanisms of neuronal patterning in the retinotectal projection. Half eye buds from labelled donor embryos were grafted into orthotopic sites in unlabelled hosts. The animals are labelled by injecting them with about 10 nl of either LFD or LRD at the one-cell stage. The embryos treated in this way develop into healthy, but intensely fluorescent, larvae. At stage-32, half eye bud grafts are excised and implanted with watchmakers' forceps and then held in place with small fragments of microscope cover-glass while they heal into the eye over the next two hours. The labelled cells can be clearly followed *in vivo* for about a day, after which the pigmented retinal epithelium obscures the view of the neural retina. Histological sections of the eye are then used to follow the distribution of the labelled cells (Fig. 3.3). Such sections show that the label is visible in all layers of the neural retina and that the grafted cells remain in the positions in which they are grafted. The graft/host border is sharp with only a few scattered labelled graft cells mixed with the unlabelled host cells. In the centre of the retina, the cells withdraw from the mitotic cycle early in development, before the embryo begins to increase in mass; here the dye remains at a relatively high concentration. Around the ciliary margin, at the edge of the eye, cell division continues, and the dye becomes diluted until it is undetectable. This pattern of dilution at the margin of the eye indicates that the normal growth pattern continues in the labelled cells. Because the dye remains visible in the cells for a period of weeks, the positions of defined populations of cells near the centre of the neural retina can be traced throughout larval development.

In previous studies of the eye, pigment mutations were used to mark clones in the pigmented retinal epithelium (Cooke and Gaze, 1983; Conway, Feiock, and Hunt 1980). This marker is present in the cells throughout the life of the animal and is not diluted by cell division; however, it does not mark the cells of the neural retina. Thus, it must be assumed in these studies that the cells of the neural retina have identical behaviour to that of the cells of the outer pigment layers. In more recent years, genetic markers have been developed to map directly the development of the neural retina. Nucleolar markers, such as the

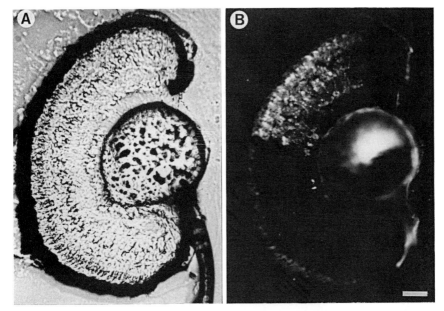

Fig. 3.3. Transverse frozen section through an eye at stage 47 with an LFD-labelled dorsal half. (A) Bright field illumination. (B) Epifluorescent illumination. A labelled half eye bud was grafted into an unlabelled host at stage 32. Label can be seen in all layers of the neural retina in the dorsal half-eye, and the host–graft boundary has remained distinct. In the ciliary margin at the edge of the retina (top), the label has become diluted by cell division. Scale bar: 50 μm.

tetraploid and the anucleolar mutants, provide genetic markers that can be observed in all the cells of the embryo (Conway *et al.* 1980). In addition, the interspecific *borealis–laevis* marker, in which *borealis* cells are clearly distinguishable from *laevis* cells by their distinctive nuclear staining with quinacrine dyes, has also been introduced in *Xenopus* (Thiebaud 1983). One drawback of these genetic markers is that the differences between the strains (or species) in growth parameters or other as yet undefined characteristics may bring unexpected variables into experiments. In some studies, *borealis–laevis* chimaeric eyes have different retinotectal projection patterns than similarly constructed *laevis–laevis* eyes (O'Rourke and Fraser, unpub. results). These differences in projection patterns bring the use of this interspecific marker into question for the study of patterning in the eye, and stress the need for careful controls in the use of genetic markers.

Since some of the dextran dyes fill the axons of developing neurons, the initial appearance of topography in the retinotectal projection can be followed by observing the projection patterns of the optic nerve fibres from labelled half eye bud grafts (O'Rourke and Fraser 1986*a*). The heads of the *Xenopus*

the retinotectal projection maintains the same topographical order during this time, the authors proposed that the optic fibres must continually shift in the tectum to compensate for the differences in growth pattern. Anatomical studies (Gaze, Keating, Ostberg, and Chung 1979; Reh and Constantine-Paton 1984; Easter and Stuermer 1984; Stuermer this volume, Chapter 11) have provided static views of the projection patterns at various time-points during these larval stages. The individual data points can then be reconstructed to provide confirmation of this shift. Electrophysiological assays using light pipe techniques (Fraser 1983; Fraser and Hunt 1986) have been performed several times on one animal, but these techniques do not reveal the underlying anatomical basis of the changes that occur. Taken together, these approaches provide strong evidence for shifting connections in the retinotectal projection, but they can not assay dynamic behaviour directly in the same manner as the LFD fibre tracing technique.

The fibre tracing technique has also been utilized in pattern regulation studies involving perturbation of the normal retinotectal projection pattern. Just as studies of regulation in early amphibian embryos can provide tests of the developmental potential or determination of the embryonic cells, studies of regulation in the eye bud can test hypotheses about positional specification of the retinal cells. In this case, rearrangement or removal of eye bud fragments leads to changes in the pattern of the retinotectal projection. The hope is that analysis of these changes can provide clues to the nature of the positional information which guides the optic fibres to their targets in the tectum. Typically, surgery is performed on the eye buds at embryonic stages, and the resulting projection pattern is assayed once, in the adult, several weeks later (e.g. Hunt and Jacobson 1973; Gaze and Straznicky 1980). This approach provides only limited information on the interactions which take place during development of the regulated pattern. The new fibre tracing technique has the advantage of being able to assay the projection pattern of the heterotopically grafted retinal cells early in development and then to reassay the map at the adult stage. We have used this approach to investigate one particular regulatory interaction in detail (O'Rourke and Fraser 1986b). Labelling of the cell bodies in the retina allowed us to confirm the health of the graft and to verify that the labelled cells remain in their grafted positions. When assayed at early stages, the original grafted cells in the centre of the retina projected according to their original position in the donor eye bud, but later the adult map indicated a regulated projection pattern. Thus the regulated pattern does not involve an immediate change in the positional information of the grafted cells. The regulated pattern was found to appear later in the projections from newly added cells at the periphery of the eye (O'Rourke and Fraser 1986c). Knowledge of the time course of regulation can thus provide insight into the types of interactions involved in the specification of positional information in embryonic tissues.

EXTENSIONS OF PRESENT WORK

The LFD-labelling technique has proven useful in studies of the early development of the eye bud and the retinotectal projection. Observation of the behaviour of fibres from labelled half eye buds has revealed that the initial sorting out of nasotemporal fibres in the tectal neuropil is dynamic. The use of smaller grafted fragments will allow a closer look at the underlying anatomy during this crucial period. Both the projection patterns of small numbers of fibres and the morphology of individual growth cones (Fig. 3.6) can be observed in the tectum of a live tadpole over a period of days. Concurrent use of this anatomical assay with techniques which perturb such factors as neural activity will allow an evaluation of the role of various cellular interactions in fibre rearrangements in the tectal neuropil. Thus these direct anatomical studies should provide clues to the mechanisms of dynamic behaviour in the patterning of neural connections.

In cell lineage studies, analysis of a clone (as a whole) is informative about the potential of the injected cell to intermix and to form different cell types. It is often necessary to focus on a subset of the labelled cells in order to learn

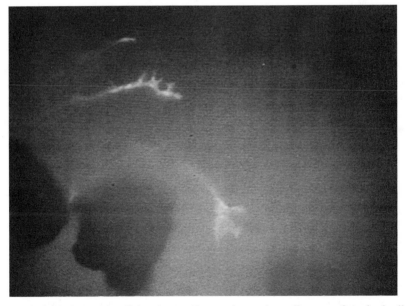

Fig. 3.6. Growth cone in a living, intact *Xenopus* larva. A small group of eye-bud cells were grafted from a LRD-labelled donor into an unlabelled host. The labelled growth cones shown here are typical of those seen and can be classified into: (i) small and elongated (top), (ii) arborized (middle), and (iii) broadened (bottom). To avoid phototoxicity, the photograph was taken from the screen of a SIT image-intensifying video-system. Magnification: × 800.

about later events in the lineage (e.g. in mouse chimaeras—Wetts and Herrup 1982; Schmidt, Wilkinson, and Ponder 1985). However, it can be difficult to draw conclusions about the progenitor of a subset of the clone. This is because any two labelled cells being studied are guaranteed to have only the injected cell as an ancestor. One cannot know with certainty that they share a more recent ancestor. What is required is to inject the dye into cells which arise later in the lineage. Kimmel and Warga (1986) took advantage of the optical clarity of zebrafish embryos to follow the later divisions of individual cells which had been labelled at an earlier stage. In most situations, actually filling a cell at later stages is unavoidable. This implies that the target cell will be smaller and less accessible than most of the cell types filled to date. These technical difficulties can be overcome, as shown by the achievement of Roger Pedersen's group of injecting HRP into the embryonic endoderm of seven-day-old mouse embryos (Lawson, Meneses, and Pedersen 1986). The LFD and LRD are charged molecules, and so these dyes can be iontophoresed into very small cells (Fraser and Bryant, 1985). There is a tremendous number of different cell types in the nervous system; questions about their lineal relationships may soon be addressed for the first time.

SUMMARY

Vital-dye techniques such as those described above offer a new level of refinement in studies of the developing nervous system. New questions can now be raised about the lineages of specific groups of cells, the movements that bring the cells into their final positions in the animal, the details of the morphology of the differentiating cells, and the sequence of events leading to appropriate synaptic connections. While these experiments will be interesting, perhaps more important are the cautions raised by some of the studies that have been performed to date. A major lesson is that events in neurogenesis are dynamic, yet few techniques are available to follow this dynamic behaviour adequately. When observations are made at only one time-point, incomplete or erroneous conclusions can be drawn. For example, after labelling a *Xenopus* blastomere, an analysis of only one developmental age gave the impression of lineage or territorial restrictions in vertebrate neural development. In fact, the examination of a series of stages has now suggested that *Xenopus* cells continually mix during embryogenesis but at a very slow rate. It is only through experiments that follow the lineage of cells and that challenge this lineage in some fashion (i.e. ablation of neighbours) that the question of restrictions can be resolved. In another example, dynamic behaviour appears in the formation of topography along the nasotemporal axis of the retinotectal projection. The use of the fluorescent dextrans as fibre tracers in live tadpoles provides a direct approach to analysing the mechanisms of these fibre rearrangements and other dynamic processes in neural development.

REFERENCES

Conway, K., Feiock, K., and Hunt, R. K. (1980). Polyclones and patterns in developing *Xenopus* larvae. *Curr. Topics Dev. Biol.* **15**, pp. 216–317.

Cooke, J. and Gaze, R. M. (1983). The positional coding system in the early eye rudiment of *Xenopus laevis*, and its modification after grafting operations. *J. Embryol. exp. Morphol.* **77**, pp. 53–71.

Dale, L., Smith, J. C. and Slack, J. M. W. (1985). Mesoderm induction in *Xenopus laevis*: a quantitative study using a cell lineage label and tissue-specific antibodies. *J. Embryol. exp. Morphol.* **89**, pp. 289–312.

Doe, C. Q., Kuwada, J. Y., and Goodman, C. S. (1985). From epithelium to neuroblasts to neurons: the role of cell interactions and cell lineage during insect neurogenesis. *Phil. Trans. R. Soc. Lond. B* **312**, pp. 67–81.

Easter, S. S., Jr. and Stuermer, C. A. O. (1984). An evaluation of the hypothesis of shifting terminals in goldfish optic tectum. *J. Neurosci.* **4**, pp. 1052–63.

Eisen, J. S., Myers, P. Z., and Westerfield, M. (1986). Pathway selection by growth cones of identified motoneurones in live zebra fish embryos. *Nature* **320**, pp. 269–71.

Fraser, S. E. (1983). Fiber optic mapping of the *Xenopus* visual system: shift in the retinotectal projection during development. *Dev. Biol.* **95**, pp. 505–11.

Fraser, S. E. and Bryant, P. J. (1986). Patterns of dye coupling in the imaginal disk of *Drosophilia melanogaster*. *Nature* **317**, pp. 533–6.

Fraser, S. E. and Hunt, R. K. (1986). A physiological measure of shifting connections in the *Rana pipiens* retinotectal system. *J. Embryol. exp. Morphol.* **94**, pp. 149–61.

Gaze, R. M. and Straznicky, C. (1980). Stable programming for map orientation in disarranged embryonic eyes in *Xenopus*. *J. Embryol. exp. Morphol.* **55**, pp. 143–65.

Gaze, R. M., Keating, M. J., Ostberg, A., and Chung, S. H. (1979). The relationship between retinal and tectal growth in larval *Xenopus*: implications for the development of the retinotectal projection. *J. Embryol. exp. Morphol.* **53**, pp. 103–43.

Gimlich, R. L. and Braun, J. (1985). Improved fluorescent compounds for tracing cell lineage. *Dev. Biol.* **109**, pp. 509–14.

Gimlich, R. L. and Cooke, J. (1983). Cell lineage and the induction of second nervous systems in amphibian development. *Nature* **306**, pp. 471–73.

Gimlich, R. L. and Gerhart, J. C. (1984). Early cellular interactions promote embryonic axis formation in *Xenopus laevis*. *Dev. Biol.* **104**, pp. 117–30.

Herrup, K., Wetts, R., and Diglio, T. J. (1984). Cell lineage relationships in the development of the mammalian CNS. II. Bilateral independence of CNS clones. *J. Neurogenet.* **1**, pp. 275–88.

Hirose, G. and Jacobson, M. (1979). Clonal organization of the central nervous system of the frog. I. Clones stemming from individual blastomeres of the 16-cell and earlier stages. *Dev. Biol.* **71**, pp. 191–202.

Holt, C. E. and Harris, W. A. (1983). Order in the initial retinotectal map in *Xenopus*: a new technique for labeling growing nerve fibres. *Nature* **301**, pp. 150–2.

Hunt, R. and Jacobson, M. (1973). Neuronal locus specificity: altered pattern of spatial deployment in fused fragments of embryonic *Xenopus* eyes. *Science* **180**, pp. 509–11.

Jacobson, M. (1982). Origins of the nervous system in amphibians. In *Neuronal development* (ed. N. C. Spitzer), pp. 45–99. Plenum Press, New York.

Jacobson, M. (1984). Cell lineage analysis of neural induction: origins of cells forming the induced nervous system. *Dev. Biol.* **102**, pp. 122–9.

Jacobson, M. and Huang, S. (1985). Neurite outgrowth traced by means of horseradish peroxidase inherited from neuronal ancestral cells in frog embryos. *Dev. Biol.* **110**, pp. 102–13.

Jacobson, M. and Klein, S. L. (1985). Analysis of clonal restriction of cell mingling in *Xenopus. Phil. Trans. R. Soc. Lond. B* **312**, pp. 57–65.

Kimmel, C. B. and Warga, R. M. (1986). Tissue-specific cell lineages originate in the gastrula of the zebrafish. *Science* **231**, pp. 365–8.

Lawson, K. A., Meneses, J. J., and Pedersen, R. A. (1986). Cell fate and cell lineage in the endoderm of the presomite mouse embryo, studied with an intracellular tracer. *Dev. Biol.* **115**, pp. 325–39.

Moody, S. A. and Jacobson, M. (1983). Compartmental relationships between anuran primary spinal motoneurons and somitic muscle fibers that they first innervate. *J. Neurosci.* **3**, pp. 1670–82.

O'Rourke, N. A. and Fraser, S. E. (1986*a*). Dynamic aspects of retinotectal map formation revealed by a vital-dye fiber-tracing technique. *Dev. Biol.* **114**, pp. 265–76.

O'Rourke, N. A. and Fraser, S. E. (1986*b*). Pattern regulation in the eyebud of *Xenopus* studied with a vital-dye fiber-tracing technique. *Dev. Biol.* **114**, pp. 277–88.

O'Rourke, N. A. and Fraser, S. E. (1986*c*). Gradual appearance of a regulated projection pattern in the developing eyebud of *Xenopus laevis. Soc. Neurosci. Abstr.* **12**, p. 543.

Reh, T. A. and Constantine-Paton, M. (1984). Retinal ganglion cell terminals change their projection sites during larval development of *Rana pipiens. J. Neurosci.* **4**, pp. 442–57.

Rossant, J. (1985). Interspecific cell markers and lineage in mammals. *Phil. Trans. R. Soc. Lond. B* **312**, pp. 92–100.

Sakaguchi, D. S. and Murphey, R. K. (1985). Map formation in the developing *Xenopus* retinotectal system: an examination of ganglion cell terminal arborizations. *J. Neurosci.* **5**, pp. 3228–45.

Schmidt, G. H., Wilkinson, M. M., and Ponder, B. A. J. (1985). Detection and characterization of spatial pattern in chimaeric tissue. *J. Embryol. exp. Morphol.* **88**, pp. 219–30.

Shankland, M. and Weisblat, D. A. (1984). Stepwise commitment of blast cell fates during the positional specification of the O and P cell lines in the leech embryo. *Dev. Biol.* **106**, pp. 326–42.

Smith, J. C. and Slack, J. M. W. (1983). Dorsalization and neural induction: properties of the organizer in *Xenopus laevis. J. Embryol. exp. Morphol.* **78**, pp. 299–317.

Stuermer, C. A. O. (1987). Navigation of normal and regenerating axons in the goldfish. In *The making of the nervous system* (eds. J. G. Parnavelas, C. D. Stern, and R. V. Stirling), pp. 204–227. Oxford University Press, Oxford.

Sulston, J. E. and Horvitz, H. R. (1977). Post-embryonic cell lineages of the nematode, *Caenorhabditis elegans. Dev. Biol.* **56**, pp. 110–56.

Sulston, J. E. and White, J. G. (1980). Regulation and cell autonomy during postembryonic development of *Caenorhabditis elegans. Dev. Biol.* **78**, pp. 577–97.

Sulston, J. E., Schierenberg, E., White, J. G., and Thomas, J. N. (1983). The embryonic cell lineage of the nematode *Caenorhabditis elegans. Dev. Biol.* **100**, pp. 64–119.

Thiebaud, C. H. (1983). A reliable new cell marker in *Xenopus. Dev. Biol.* **98**, pp. 245–9.

Weisblat, D. A. and Shankland, M. (1985). Cell lineage and segmentation in the leech. *Phil. Trans. R. Soc. Lond. B.* **312,** pp. 39–56.

Weisblat, D. A., Sawyer, R. T., and Stent, G. S. (1978). Cell lineage analysis by intracellular injection of a tracer enzyme. *Science* **202,** pp. 1295–8.

Wetts, R. and Herrup, K. (1982). Cerebellar Purkinje cells are descended from a small number of progenitors during early development: quantitative analysis of Lurcher chimeric mice. *J. Neurosci.* **2,** pp. 1494–8.

White, J. G. (1985). Neuronal connectivity in *Caenorhabditis elegans. Trends Neurosci.* **8,** 277–83.

PART II

Cell interactions and early pattern formation

Introduction

Regardless of which strategy the embryo uses to generate cell diversity, the final pattern must lead to the development of the correct cell types in their appropriate locations. In 1924, Hans Spemann and his graduate student, Hilde Mangold, published a paper for which Spemann was awarded the Nobel Prize and which was to have enormous impact on developmental biologists. They found that if the dorsal lip of the blastopore of an amphibian embryo was transplanted into certain regions of a host embryo, a new, supernumerary, neural axis formed. This new axis is derived from both the graft and the host tissue. The process was christened 'neural induction'.

Neural induction is a good example of cell interactions that lead to the generation of cell diversity. The ectodermal cells near the inducing mesodermal tissue change their fate under the influence of the inducing tissue, from epidermal to neural. In the absence of induction, the ectoderm gives rise mainly to skin; in response to induction, it develops into brain, neural tube (spinal cord), and to the entire peripheral nervous system. Despite the importance of neural induction as an embryonic event, its molecular and cellular bases are not understood. Efforts to identify substances produced by the inducing tissue and which could change the fate of the responding tissue if added to it exogenously have failed. Instead, it has been known since the 1930s that many common laboratory chemicals are able to mimic some of the effects of the inducing tissue. This implies that, whatever induction is, it is unlikely to involve the action of unique RNAs passing from inducer to responding tissue. This conclusion has shifted the attention of some workers towards normal processes that occur in the cells, such as their physiology. Neural induction could be triggered by subtle changes in the responding cells. In Chapter 4, neural induction is separated into several distinct processes based on the response of the embryo to a variety of experimental manipulations.

Once the neural tube has formed, it proceeds to give rise to the central nervous system and to the entire peripheral nervous system. The latter is derived from two components of the neural tube: the neural crest (from which arise the sensory, sympathetic, and parasympathetic nervous systems, most Schwann cells, some cranial structures, and the melanocytes which give the skin its pigment) and the motor nerves and their glia. The migration of these components away from the neural tube is not haphazard, but delicately patterned. What are the mechanisms that lead to the repeated patterns seen in the peripheral nervous system of both invertebrates and vertebrates? Chapter 5 reviews the processes that generate a segmental pattern in the peripheral nervous system. Like neural induction, segmentation relies upon the influence of some of the surrounding tissues.

4

Analysis of induction in the amphibian nervous system

ANNE WARNER

The generation of the adult, fully differentiated nervous system is the outcome of a complex series of events. In vertebrates, the cells destined to form the nervous system are not programmed from early times, as seems to be the case in many invertebrate embryos, but arise as a result of an inductive interaction between dorsal ectoderm cells and underlying mesoderm cells, brought into the appropriate position by the morphogenetic movements of gastrulation. This inductive interaction sets in hand a chain of events, the outcome of which is the fully developed nervous system.

Neural induction therefore plays an essential part in the subsequent development of the nervous system since it precedes and controls neural morphogenesis, the patterning of structures, and the differentiation of neuronal and glial cells. Despite the central role of this inductive process, the mechanism remains obscure. It is often assumed that a single event underlies its initiation and that the success or failure of neural induction can be assessed adequately by monitoring the progress of events such as the formation of a neural tube. This assumption may be false. In this article I consider the evidence that neural induction may be a more complex process, involving a number of signals. The experimental examples mainly relate to the development of the central nervous system (CNS). The development of the peripheral and enteric nervous systems, which arise from neural crest cells, are largely excluded because in these two cases phenotypic differentiation does not occur until some time after the initial phases of neural induction and because the cells undergo considerable migration through the extracellular matrix. This migratory step, which occurs before differentiation, allows interactions between the migrating cells and the extracellular matrix which may modify any programme initiated during neural induction. Most of the experiments relate to work on the amphibian because of the advantages offered by the free-living embryo. However, many of these early events are likely to be common among the vertebrate species. Since my concern is with principles, rather than with experimental details, the work quoted is not described or illustrated in detail. The majority has already been published in full and interested readers should consult the original articles.

THE CONSEQUENCES OF NEURAL INDUCTION

Neural induction probably begins as soon as invaginating mesoderm cells start to move under the dorsal ectoderm. The end-point of neural induction, when all necessary interaction between mesoderm and ectoderm is complete and further neural development is autonomous, is more difficult to define. However it is reasonable to suppose that closure of the neural tube marks the latest likely time-point, since differentiated neurones, capable of generating action potentials, appear very shortly after the neural tube closes.

The successful induction of the nervous system has three obvious consequences:

(i) The initiation of the morphogenetic movements of neurulation, when the dorsal ectoderm folds in and rolls up to form the neural tube. These movements begin almost as soon as gastrulation is over.
(ii) Cells within the neural plate become programmed to differentiate into the neuronal and glial elements of the nervous system.
(iii) The future anatomical organization of the nervous system is laid out on the neural plate: the structures of the nervous system are patterned.

At present we have no notion of the identity of the putative signal(s) or the way(s) in which they are transmitted from mesoderm to ectoderm. Despite this paucity of knowledge, it is often assumed that the various consequences of neural induction are the outcome of a single inductive event. One way of testing whether this assumption is correct is to see whether the various outcomes of neural induction can be separated experimentally from each other. If it is possible to show that some consequences of neural induction can proceed when others are prevented, this would be strong evidence to suggest that more than one separate process is involved. I have therefore chosen to examine the consequences of treatment of early embryos with agents which interfere with the development of the nervous system in rather different ways, to see whether this approach might help to dissect out the various elements of the process of neural induction.

LITHIUM IONS

It has long been recognized that the lithium ion has potent teratogenic effects on development. Treatment of cleavage-stage amphibian embryos with lithium chloride generates embryos with a variety of superficially obvious defects, of which the most striking is failure of the morphogenetic movements of neurulation, although in very severe cases gastrulation is also affected (see Backstrom 1954; Hall 1942). Such effects have been interpreted as reflecting failure of neural induction (e.g. Hall 1942; Smith, Osborne, and Stanistreet 1976). We have recently been examining the consequences of lithium treatment in more detail, in order to test whether this interpretation is correct and to gain insight into its effects on neural development (Breckenridge, Warren, and Warner 1987).

To generate defective embryos we followed the basic protocol determined by others. *Xenopus laevis* embryos at the 2–4 cell stage were soaked in 100 mM LiCl for four hours, during which time they cleaved to early bastula stage. The embryos were then returned to tap water and left until sibling controls had completed neurulation and had begun to elongate (Nieuwkoop and Faber 1956; stage 22–28). Sibling controls were treated with 100 mM NaCl for four hours or left in tap water. As found by others (Hall 1942; Backstrom 1954), the majority of the embryos gastrulated normally, and the consequences of lithium treatment became apparent during neurulation. Severely affected embryos failed to neurulate completely. Less severely affected embryos lifted the neural folds, but these often failed to close and elongation was inhibited. A similar range of defects generated by a different lithium treatment schedule have been reported very recently by Kao, Masui, and Elinson (1986). As also observed by Kao *et al.* (1986), we found that embryos became less susceptible to treatment with lithium after the 32–64 cell stage. Before considering the developmental consequences of lithium treatment for the nervous system, it is convenient first to discuss the intracellular concentrations of lithium which bring about the teratogenic effect.

At the end of the treatment period a few lithium-treated and control embryos were removed and prepared for total ion analysis. The remaining embryos were reared to stage 22–28 and then scored for abnormalities and death. When comparing control and lithium-treated embryos, account was always taken of the batch viability. Both the net lithium uptake (mmole/l embryo) and the proportion of abnormal embryos were related to the length of exposure of embryos to 100 mM LiCl. The threshold for generation of defects lay at about 0.5 mmoles Li/l embryo and was reached after one hour of exposure to LiCl. Three or four hours of exposure to lithium achieved a maximal number of abnormal and dead embryos (85–100 per cent), by which time lithium uptake had reached 2.5 mmoles/l embryo. Thus the teratogenic effects of lithium are brought about by very low intracellular concentrations. The high levels of extra-embryonic lithium necessary to generate the defects are almost certainly required because the outer cell membranes of the amphibian embryo are relatively impermeable. It should be noted that the threshold for the teratogenic effects of lithium treatment is very close to that used clinically for the treatment of depression.

Superficially the abnormalities generated by lithium treatment seem to fit the original interpretation: that lithium interferes with neural induction. But is this true? Histological examination of lithium-treated embryos reveals profound internal disorder. Blocks of scattered, but unidentifiable, tissue are present throughout the embryo. This suggests that, in addition to inhibiting the morphogenetic movements of neurulation, lithium ions interfere with the patterning which leads to the anatomical organization of the nervous system. However, the lack of organization does not necessarily mean that neuronal differentiation has also been inhibited. The question of whether nerve cells are nevertheless able to differentiate can be addressed in two ways. First, by using cell-type-specific antibodies, such as antibodies to neurofilament protein, which allow the recognition of terminally differentiated neurones even in the face of gross disorganization. Second, one can test whether neurons differentiate from lithium-treated embryos when placed into tissue culture. The two approaches have different advantages. The first provides information on neuronal organization, but is not able to indicate whether there is any quantitative reduction in neuronal differentiation. The second provides quantitative information on the degree to which neurons can differentiate autonomously, but cannot answer questions about the anatomical organization of the nervous system.

When frozen sections of control and lithium-treated embryos of the same age stained with an anti-neurofilament antibody and an anti-muscle antibody are compared it immediately becomes clear that, despite the gross internal disorder of lithium-treated embryos, both neurons and muscle cells can be identified unequivocally. Thus, despite the appearance of lithium-treated embryos, neuronal differentiation is still taking place, suggesting that this particular consequence of neural induction is unaffected. This implies that the signal which sets in train the phenotypic differentiation of neuronal cells may be separate from that which initiates the morphogenetic and patterning elements of neural induction.

Quantitative evidence in support of this conclusion comes from experiments in which neuronal differentiation in tissue culture from lithium-treated embryos is compared with that from controls. For these experiments the method previously described by Messenger and Warner (1979) and Breckenridge and Warner (1982) was used. When control embryos reach stage 20 the neural tube, notochord, and somites are dissected out, dissociated into single cells by brief treatment with ethyleneglycol-*bis*-(β-aminoethyl ether)-N-N'-tetraacetic acid (EGTA) followed by mechanical trituration, and plated out in tissue culture dishes in Ringer solution with 10 per cent fetal calf serum. The dorsal portions of sibling lithium-treated embryos of the same age are similarly dissociated and plated. After 24 hours the cultures form a monolayer of differentiated cells. The proportions of nerve and muscle cells which have differentiated are determined by counting the total number of cells, the number of nerve cells, and the number of muscle cells in each of 20–30 fields chosen at random from three petri dishes. The proportion of neurons which have differentiated is then determined by plotting frequency histograms for cultures prepared from the control and the lithium-treated embryos. It is often very difficult to be certain that severely deformed embryos generated by treatment with lithium are still alive at this stage. This problem was overcome by ignoring experiments in which the total number of differentiated cells was significantly different from the controls. In eight experiments in which there was no drop in the total number of differentiated cells in cultures differentiating from lithium-treated embryos there was clearly no decrease in neuronal differentiation. The mean percentage of neurons differentiating from control cultures was 4·03 per cent per field ($\pm 0\cdot1$ per cent, standard error of mean). Parallel cultures from lithium-treated embryos had a mean of 6·7 per cent neurons/field ($\pm 0\cdot2$ per cent), significantly *greater* than from controls ($p < 0\cdot001$, Student's t-test). By contrast, the proportion of differentiated muscle cells was closely similar (control: 8·8 per cent; lithium-treated: 9·7 per cent; $P > 0\cdot1$). Thus treatment with lithium ions during the early cleavage stages does not reduce neuronal differentiation; rather, lithium treatment enhances differentiation.

These findings call into question the original interpretations of the consequences of lithium treatment and suggest that the view that lithium ventralizes amphibian embryos is unlikely to be correct. A similar conclusion was reached by Kao *et al.* (1986), who also noted considerable distortion of pattern in lithium-treated embryos, but considered that the major consequence was enhancement of dorso–anterior structures, rather than ventralization. Our finding that neuronal differentiation is enhanced rather than suppressed in embryos exposed to lithium chloride is, therefore, complementary to the findings of Kao *et al.* (1986).

The conclusion from these experiments is that lithium ions inhibit morphogenesis and interfere with pattern formation, but do not influence neuronal differentiation.

INHIBITION OF THE SODIUM PUMP DURING NEURULATION

Blackshaw and Warner (1976) showed that when the amphibian embryo enters the mid-neural fold stages the resting potential of cells in the neural plate, but not in the ventral ectoderm, begins to increase. By the late neural fold stage cells in the neural plate have resting potentials almost 20 mV more negative than cells of the ventral ectoderm. Various lines of evidence showed that this increase in membrane potential is the consequence of activation of an electrogenic sodium pump, which produces a substantial fall in intracellular sodium in neural plate cells (Breckenridge and Warner 1982). If the sodium pump is inhibited with the cardiac glycoside, strophanthidin, the increase in resting membrane potential is inhibited (Blackshaw and Warner 1976) intracellular sodium no longer falls (Breckenridge and Warner 1982) and neurons fail to differentiate from the neural plate (Messenger and Warner 1979). Thus the inhibition of the sodium pump during the neural-fold stages, when additional sodium pumps are normally activated in neural plate cells, prevents subsequent neuronal differentiation.

What consequences does inhibiting the sodium pump have for other aspects of neural induction? The morphogenetic movements of neurulation proceed unimpaired, and embryos treated with strophanthidin during the neural plate stages only, and then left to develop to the swimming tadpole stage, look, superficially, fairly normal. When such tadpoles are examined histologically it is clear that the defect induced by inhibiting the sodium pump is restricted to the phenotypic differentiation of CNS neurons (Messenger and Warner 1979; Breckenridge and Warner 1982). Patterning of the nervous system does not seem to be affected. Structures such as the eye and otic vesicle form in the normal position, although within the eye, for example, there are few signs of differentiated neurons, and the orderly array of differentiating neurons is also completely lost within the brain.

The overall conclusion to be drawn from these experiments is that inhibiting the sodium pump prevents the expression of the neuronal phenotype, but has no effect on either the morphogenesis or the patterning of the nervous system. The situation with regard to the glial elements of the nervous system is not yet known.

THE CONSEQUENCES OF INHIBITING COMMUNICATION THROUGH GAP JUNCTIONS

Gap junctions are intercellular membrane structures which allow cells to exchange directly ions and a variety of small molecules without recourse to the extracellular space. Cells within the early embryos of all species tested so far are linked to each other by gap junctions at times when other experiments suggest that important cellular interactions are taking place. Consequently it has frequently been suggested that the pathway mediated by gap junctions may play some role in directing important events during development (e.g. Potter, Furshpan, and Lennox 1966). The possibility that gap junctions are involved in the patterning of structures in the developing embryo is particularly attractive, although until very recently little direct evidence was available to support such a role. When proteins are eluted from isolated gap junctions it seems that a 27 kD protein is the major component, although there is evidence to suggest that a 16 kD protein may also be associated with gap junctions. Several groups have been successful in raising polyclonal antibodies to the 27 kD protein, and at least three of these antibodies not only recognize the 27 kD protein on immunoblots but also inhibit communication through gap junctions (Warner, Guthrie, and Gilula 1984; Hertzberg, Spray, and Bennett 1985). The ability to block communication through gap junctions using specific antibodies will greatly improve our understanding of the functional role of gap junctions, both in adult tissues and during embryogenesis. Experiments using such antibodies to test for a functional role for gap junctions during development have provided some interesting information with regard to the development of the nervous system (Warner *et al.* 1984).

In these experiments gap-junction antibody was injected into the right-hand dorsal blastomere in the animal pole of the 8-cell-stage *Xenopus laevis* embryo. This cell is destined to give rise to head ectoderm and mesoderm derivatives on the right-hand side of the tadpole (see Warner 1985). The antibody-containing cell continued to divide at a rate which was indistinguishable from its uninjected neighbours, and the progeny cells maintained normal resting potentials. When the embryo reached the 32-cell-stage, one of the progeny of the injected cell was tested for the presence of both dye coupling (assayed by injection of Lucifer-yellow dye) and ionic coupling (assayed electrophysiologically). Such tests showed the antibody-containing cells to be completely uncoupled; the antibody had blocked functional communication through gap junctions. Antibody-containing cells continued to divide normally; there was no sign of cytolysis or extrusion, and Lucifer-yellow dye injected at the 32-cell-stage was still visible in the living tadpole three days later. The block of functional communication is maintained beyond gastrulation in about 30 per cent of injected embryos and is still at a depressed level in a further 30 per cent (Warner and Gurdon 1987). Thus a substantial proportion of antibody-containing embryos enter the period of neural induction with cells destined to form right-hand anterior neural structures unable to communicate with their neighbours through gap junctions.

What are the developmental consequences of this block of direct cell–cell communication? All embryos proceeded through the morphogenetic movements of neurulation normally, suggesting that this consequence of neural induction was unaffected by the inability to communicate through gap junctions. However, a substantial proportion of injected embryos (about two-thirds) nevertheless showed pronounced defects in the region derived from the antibody-injected cell. In very severe cases structures such as the trigeminal ganglion, the eye, the otic vesicle, and the anterior somites on the right-hand side were completely missing. But in most cases the affected embryos developed with patterning defects. In these cases structures such as the trigeminal ganglion and eyes were present, but of the wrong size and in the wrong position when compared with the uninjected side of the tadpole. The severity of the defects showed a strict rostro–caudal sequence, so that somite defects were always accompanied by incorrect positioning of more anterior structures, while the trigeminal ganglion could be misplaced, with more posterior structures being more or less normal in size and position. Whenever a particular neural structure was present, it always contained differentiated neurons, even when of the wrong size and positioned incorrectly. Thus it seems that blocking intercellular communication mainly influences the anatomical patterning of the nervous system, with morphogenesis and phenotypic differentiation being relatively normal.

CONCLUSIONS

The mechanism by which each of the three treatments considered above leads to the particular defects in the development of the nervous system is not yet known. In some cases the immediate consequence can be identified, as when considering the effects of agents which block activation of the sodium pump, but exactly how prevention of the fall in intracellular sodium which normally takes place at the mid-neural-fold stage of development results in the failure of the phenotypic differentiation of CNS is not yet clear. Nevertheless, consideration of the rather different consequences brought about by lithium, blocking the sodium pump or inhibiting communication through gap junctions, allows some interesting and potentially important conclusions to be drawn about the process of neural induction.

Table 4.1 sets out the effects of each agent on the three main outcomes of neural induction identified on p. 76. Thus lithium ions affect morphogenesis and patterning, but not neuronal differentiation. Inhibiting the sodium pump prevents neuronal differentiation, but not morphogenesis or patterning. Blocking gap-junctional communication interferes with patterning, but not morphogenesis or phenotypic differentiation. It emerges that 'neural induction' is not a single event but the outcome of several interactions, each of which can be separately and independently manipulated by choosing the appropriate experimental conditions. This conclusion rather strongly suggests that mesoderm cells induce dorsal ectoderm cells to form the nervous system either by generating more than one signal or by initiating completely separate events with a single signal. The possibility that further signals may be involved in generating the neural crest elements of the nervous system remains open. The identity of the inducing signal(s) and the mechanism whereby they initiate morphogenesis, patterning, and phenotypic differentiation in the nervous system remain to be elucidated. However, recognition of the potential complexities of neural induction should allow the design of experiments directed more precisely towards an understanding of the making of the nervous system.

Table 4.1.   *Separation of the various consequences of neural induction.*

Treatment	Morphogenesis	Pattern formation	Neuronal differentiation
Lithium ions	Inhibited	Disturbed	Unaffected
Blocking the sodium pump	Unaffected	Unaffected	Inhibited
Blocking intercellular communication	Unaffected	Disturbed	Unaffected

ACKNOWLEDGEMENTS

I am indebted to my colleagues for allowing me to quote the results of as yet unpublished experiments. The work described in this article was made possible by grants from the Medical Research Council, the Wellcome Trust, and Action Research.

REFERENCES

Backstrom, S. (1954). Morphogenetic effects of lithium on the embryonic development of *Xenopus*. *Arkiv. für Zool.* **6,** pp. 527–36.

Blackshaw, S. E. and Warner, A. E. (1976). Alterations in resting membrane properties during neural plate stages of development of the nervous system. *J. Physiol. (Lond.)* **255,** pp. 231–47.

Breckenridge, L. and Warner, A. E. (1982). Intracellular sodium and the differentiation of amphibian embryonic neurones. *J. Physiol. (Lond.)* **332,** pp. 393–413.

Breckenridge, L. J., Warren, R. L., and Warner, A. E. (1987). Lithium inhibits morphogenesis but not neuronal differentiation in the amphibian nervous system. *Development* **99,** pp. 353–70.

Hall, T. S. (1942). The mode of action of lithium salts in amphibian development. *J. exp. Zool.* **89,** pp. 385–416.

Hertzberg, E. L., Spray, D. C., and Bennett, M. V. L. (1985). Reduction of gap junctional conductance by micro-injection of antibodies against the 27,000 dalton liver gap junction polypeptide. *Proc. Natl. Acad. Sci. USA* **82,** pp. 2412–16.

Kao, K. R., Masui, Y., and Elinson, R. (1986). Lithium induced respecification of pattern in *Xenopus laevis* embryos. *Nature* **332,** pp. 371–3.

Messenger, E. A. and Warner, A. E. (1979). The function of the sodium pump during differentiation of amphibian embryonic neurones. *J. Physiol. (Lond.)* **292,** pp. 85–105.

Nieuwkoop, P. D. and Faber, J. (1956). Normal tables of *Xenopus laevis* (Daudin), North-Holland Amsterdam.

Potter, D. D., Furshpan, E. J., and Lennox, E. S. (1966). Connections between cells of the developing squid as revealed by electrophysiological methods. *Proc. Natl. Acad. Sci. USA* **55,** pp. 328–51.

Smith, J. L., Osborne, J. C., and Stanistreet, M. (1976). Scanning electron microscopy of lithium-induced exogastrulae of *Xenopus laevis*. *J. Embryol. exp. Morph.* **36,** pp. 513–22.

Warner, A. E. (1985). The role of gap junctions during development of the early amphibian embryo. *J. Embryol. exp. Morph.* **89** (Suppl.), pp. 365–80.

Warner, A. E. and Gurdon, J. B. (1987). Functional gap junctions are not required for muscle gene activation by induction in *Xenopus* embryos. *J. Cell Biol.* **104,** pp. 557–64.

Warner, A. E., Guthrie, S. C., and Gilula, N. B. (1984). Antibodies to gap junction protein selectivity disrupt junctional communication in the early amphibian embryo. *Nature* **312,** pp. 127–31.

5

The development of neural segmentation in vertebrate embryos

ROGER J. KEYNES AND CLAUDIO D. STERN

Segmentation of the nervous system used to be a subject of considerable interest to vertebrate embryologists because of its implications for vertebrate evolution. More recently, it must be admitted, this interest has tailed off. The problem remains important, though, from the point of view of neural development, and for an obvious reason—if the nervous system is specified on a segmental basis, we might gain useful clues as to the kinds of cellular and molecular mechanisms involved in its construction.

There are really two aspects to neural segmentation in vertebrates: how the peripheral nervous system becomes segmented, and whether the central nervous system is intrinsically segmented. In this review we will address these questions in turn and consider how important the phenomenon of segmentation might be in guiding growing axons to their targets.

THE CELLULAR BASIS OF PERIPHERAL NEURAL SEGMENTATION

One of the simplest forms of neural organization in vertebrates is the repeating segmental pattern of the peripheral nerves as they emerge from the spinal cord. In the earliest experimental attempt to analyse how this arrangement develops, Lehmann (1927) found that removal of several consecutive somites in urodeles leads to a loss of segmentation of sensory ganglia in the operated region. Detwiler (1934) then extended this approach by showing that grafting an additional somite produces an additional spinal nerve and ganglion. They both concluded that segmentation of the peripheral nerves is secondary to segmentation of the mesoderm; they also extrapolated to the conclusion that the spinal cord has no *intrinsic* segmentation, a theme to which we shall return later.

These pioneering studies were not particularly concerned with exactly where the spinal nerves develop in relation to the somites. Contemporary textbooks describe the nerves as growing either opposite the middle of each somite or between somites. However, in the chick embryo, axons in fact traverse the rostral half of each sclerotome (Keynes and Stern 1984) (Fig. 5.1). To test whether this segmented outgrowth occurs because of intrinsic neural tube segmentation or because of some difference between rostral (anterior) and caudal (posterior) sclerotome halves, rotation experiments were carried out (Fig. 5.2). First, a portion of neural tube opposite 2 or 3 somites was rotated 180° rostro–caudally prior to axon outgrowth, so that neural tube previously opposite rostral half-somite came to lie opposite caudal half. After two days of further development axons had still grown out through the rostral halves of those somites opposite the rotated neural tube [Fig. 5.2(a)]. Second, a portion of segmental plate mesoderm, 2–4 presumptive somites long, was rotated 180° rostro–caudally; this time, after further development, axons had traversed the caudal (original rostral) halves of the grafted somites (Keynes and Stern 1984) [Fig. 5.2(b)].

Axons therefore grow through the rostral half-sclerotome, regardless of its position relative to the neural tube or to the rostro–caudal axis of the whole embryo. These experiments confirm Lehmann's (1927) and Detwiler's (1934) conclusion that segmented axonal outgrowth is controlled by the somites. In addition, they show in the chick that segmentation is due to differences between rostral and caudal sclerotome cells.

Does the rostro–caudal subdivision of each segment determine spinal nerve

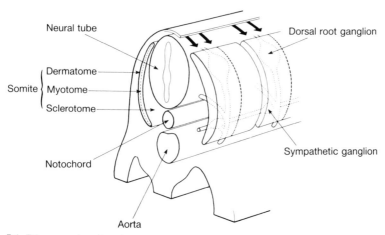

Fig. 5.1. Diagram showing the major pathways of axon growth and trunk neural crest cell migration in the chick embryo. The somite has dispersed into its three components: dermatome (presumptive dermis), myotome (presumptive skeletal muscle), and sclerotome (presumptive vertebral column). Heavy arrows denote the major crest pathway. All the components of the peripheral nervous system are confined to the rostral (left in the diagram) half of each sclerotome. [Reproduced from Keynes and Stern (1985) by kind permission of Elsevier, Amsterdam].

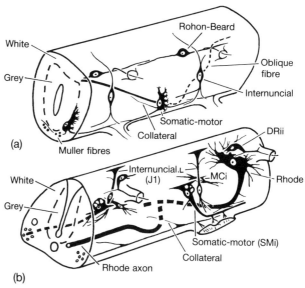

Fig. 5.4. Comparison between the spinal cord neurons of the larval brook-lamprey (a) and those of the adult *Amphioxus* (b). (a) is redrawn from Whiting (1948); (b) is constructed by omitting all cells occurring plurisegmentally, or with no obvious relation to segmentation. In each segment, in both groups, there are single large motor cells, lying in relation to the ventral roots. There are vertical interneurons linking these cells with the dorsal sensory columns, and large dorsal neurons adjacent to the ventral roots, which can probably be regarded as Rohon–Beard cells. Finally there are the Rhode and Muller axons, links between the motor cells and a longitudinal through-conducting mechanism. [Reproduced from Bone (1960) by kind permission of Alan R. Liss, Inc., New York.]

he argues, are probably ancient in the chordate line, being inherited by modern craniates from their ancestors, but becoming obscured as development proceeds. It is worth noting that in the case of *Amphioxus*, motor neurons and certain interneurons are arranged periodically, yet no myelomeres are visible (and the mesoderm is plainly segmented). Perhaps, then, one should not read too much into the presence or otherwise of myelomeres. Moreover, an apparently homogeneous column of neurons extending down the neural tube, such as the motor columns of amniote embryos, could still be determined on a segmental basis: lack of visible boundaries does not necessarily mean lack of segments.

Such segmental specification could provide a basis for the labelling of motor neurons, to allow them both to recognize specific guidance cues in the periphery and to make appropriate connections within the neural tube. While this is obviously speculative, recent observations on the earliest motor neuronal outgrowths in two vertebrate species, the zebrafish and the chick, are of interest. Using Nomarski and fluorescence optics, Eisen *et al* (1986) have found that the primary motor neurons of zebrafish embryos are arranged segmentally, clustered opposite the rostral part of each myotome; furthermore, each primary motor neuron confines its arbor to a specific and characteristic region of each myotome. In the chick embryo, if horseradish peroxidase is applied to the rostral half of a sclerotome to trace the position of the corresponding motor neuron cell bodies, cell bodies are seen to be grouped between the rostral and caudal segment boundaries, despite the asymmetry of their axon projection pattern into the rostral half-sclerotome. Cells placed opposite the caudal half-sclerotome send axons selectively to the rostral half of the same segment, rather than distributing them evenly between this segment and the next-caudal segment (Lim and Keynes 1986). The mechanisms restricting motor axons in these examples have yet to be determined; segmental specification, with perhaps further refinements of specification within each segment, would be an attractive, albeit one, possibility.

There is, as yet, no evidence that the neurons of the peripheral nervous system, other than spinal motor axons, are also positionally specified prior to axon outgrowth. Rostro–caudal selectivity between regenerating preganglionic sympathetic axons and post-ganglionic cells, however, has been demonstrated (Purves, Thompson, and Yip 1981). In addition, in both the sympathetic and parasympathetic systems, the sections of the neural tube that contribute pre-ganglionic and post-ganglionic cells are broadly equivalent along the rostro–caudal axis (Le Douarin, 1982). These phenomena, and the striking segmented pattern of cutaneous innervation (Diamond 1982; Scott 1982), could reflect an underlying segmental matching.

THE GENETIC BASIS OF SEGMENTATION

If there are segmental labels in the vertebrate embryo, how are they specified? In the fruitfly, *Drosophila*, several classes of gene affecting different aspects of segmentation have been identified: for example, homoeotic (e.g. bithorax, *bx*), segment polarity (e.g. engrailed, *en*), and pair-rule genes (e.g. fushitarazu, *ftz*) (Nüsslein-Volhard and Wieschaus 1980). If segmentation-related genes homologous to those of *Drosophila* exist in vertebrates, as the discovery of the vertebrate homoeobox might suggest (McGinnis, Garber, Wirz, Kuroiwa, and Gehring 1984), it is possible to speculate on their functions. Homoeotic-like genes might be concerned with the differences between, say, thoracic and cervical vertebrae, or between different regions of the neural tube along the rostro–caudal axis. Segment polarity genes like engrailed (Joyner, Kornberg, Coleman, Cox, and Martin 1985) could code for the molecular differences between the sclerotome halves and be responsible for the initial pattern of peripheral neural segmentation. Genes expressed repeatedly every two or more segments might help to specify positional addresses using a minimum number of different loci.

Even if this is taking the analogy between *Drosophila* and vertebrates too far, it is interesting that one of the recently identified mouse homoeobox genes, *Hox-3*, has a transcription pattern that is restricted along the length of the neural tube (Awgulewitsch, Utset, Hart, McGinnis, and Ruddle 1986). *Hox-3* messenger RNA is detected in the spinal cord caudal to the level of the third and fourth cervical vertebrae, but not further rostral. Another such gene, *Hox-2.1*, is also preferentially expressed in the neural tube of the mouse embryo, again in the spinal cord (Jackson, Schofield, and Hogan 1985; Jackson, pers. comm.). The role of homoeobox genes in invertebrate, let alone vertebrate, development has yet to be clarified. These observations are at least consistent with the possibility that homoeobox genes are regionally expressed in vertebrates as well as in invertebrates. If so, they are also consistent with the possibility of intrinsic subdivisions of the neural tube.

SEGMENTS AND CELL LINEAGE

In the insects *Drosophila* and *Oncopeltus*, the cells of each segment, and of parts of each segment, are polyclonal in origin. The term 'compartment' refers to *all* the surviving descendants of a small group of founder cells, which do not mix with cells of neighbouring compartments (García-Bellido, Ripoll, and Morata 1973; Lawrence 1975). A segment comprises one or more compartments. Thus, in these organisms, there is a link between cell lineage and segmental arangement.

Could the same be true for vertebrates? At present, there is little decisive information. Experiments using allophenic mice (Gearhart and Mintz 1972) have suggested that somites are polyclonal. We do not know, however, whether they are compartments in the sense defined above. More recently, Kimmel and Warga (1986) have found marked periodicity in the longitudinal arrangements of the central nervous system descendants of single labelled zebrafish blastomeres. However, the period length is variable, ranging from 1·0 to 3·2 segment lengths, and they conclude that 'it is clear that any possible relationship between cell lineage and body segments is more complex than in the leech'. There is some evidence that invariant programmes of cell lineage, such as are found in worms and flies, can exist in vertebrates. A recent example, analysed elegantly by Winklbauer and Hausen (1983, 1985), has been identified in the lateral line system of *Xenopus*.

INTERACTIONS GENERATING THE SEGMENTAL PATTERN

How is the segmentation pattern generated in the first place? If we accept the evidence for intrinsic neural tube segmentation, it is interesting to speculate on the relationship between neural tube and somite segmentation. We have seen how the segmented mesoderm imposes segmentation on the peripheral nervous system. It has also been suggested that, at an earlier stage in development, the nervous system might itself impose segmentation on the mesoderm (Child 1921; Fraser 1960), although the evidence is not compelling (see Bellairs 1963). Interestingly, brief exposure of chick embryos to cytotoxic drugs affecting the cell cycle causes anomalies of both the somites and the neural tube at discrete, identical segmental levels (Primmett, Stern, and Keynes, in prep.). Rather than one element providing the dominating pattern, it is possible that the interactions between the neural tube and the somitic mesoderm that lead to the segmental pattern are reciprocal. Further study of such interactions, using the techniques of cell and molecular biology, should help elucidate the mechanisms of pattern formation in vertebrate embryos.

REFERENCES

Awgulewitsch, A., Utset, M. F., Hart, C. P., McGinnis, W., and Ruddle, F. H. (1986). Spatial restriction in expression of a mouse homoeo box locus within the central nervous system. *Nature* **320**, pp. 328–35.

Bellairs, R. (1963). The development of somites in the chick embryo. *J. Embryol. exp. Morph.* **11**, pp. 697–714.

Bone, Q. (1960). The central nervous system in *Amphioxus. J. Comp. Neurol.* **115**, pp. 27–64.

Bronner-Fraser, M. (1986). Analysis of the early stages of trunk neural crest migration in avian embryos using monoclonal antibody HNK-1. *Dev. Biol.* **115**, pp. 44–55.

Chernoff, E. A. G. and Hilfer, S. R. (1982). Calcium dependence and contraction in somite formation. *Tiss. Cell.* **14**, pp. 435–50.

Chevallier, A., Kieny, M., and Mauger, A. (1977). Limb–somite relationships: origin of the limb musculature. *J. Embryol. exp. Morph.* **41**, pp. 245–58.

Chiarugi, G. (1889). Lo sviluppo dei nervi vago accessorio, ipoglosso e primi cervicali nei sauropsidi e nei mammiferi. *Atti. Soc. Toscana Sc. Nat. in Pisa, Memorie.* **10**, pp. 149–250.

Child, C. M. (1921). *The origin and development of the nervous system.* University of Chicago Press, Chicago, IL.

Cohen, A. M. (1972). Factors directing the expression of sympathetic nerve traits in cells of neural crest origin. *J. exp. Zool.* **179**, pp. 167–82.

Detwiler, S. R. (1934). An experimental study of spinal nerve segmentation in *Amblystoma* with reference to the plurisegmental contribution to the brachial plexus. *J. exp. Zool.* **67**, pp. 395–441.

Diamond, J. (1982). Modelling and competition in the nervous system: clues from the sensory innervation of skin. *Curr. Top. Dev. Biol.* **17**, pp. 147–205.

Eisen, J. S., Myers, P. Z., and Westerfield, M. (1986). Pathway selection by growth cones of identified motoneurones in live zebra fish embryos. *Nature* **320**, pp. 269–71.

Fauquet, M., Smith, J., Ziller, C., and Le Douarin, N. M. (1981). Differentiation of autonomic neuron precursors in vitro; cholinergic and adrenergic traits in cultured neural crest cells. *J. Neurosci.* **1**, pp. 478–92.

Stern, C. D., Sisodiya, S. M., and Keynes, R. J. (1986). Interactions between neurites and somite cells: inhibition and stimulation of nerve growth in the chick embryo. *J. Embryol. exp. Morphol.* **91**, pp. 209–26.

Stirling, R. V. and Summerbell, D. (1985). The behaviour of growing axons invading developing chick wing buds with dorsoventral or anteroposterior axis reversal. *J. Embryol. exp. Morphol.* **85**, pp. 251–69.

Stirling, R. V. and Summerbell, D. (1987). Motor axon guidance in the developing chick limb. In *The Making of the Nervous System* (eds. J. G. Parnavelas, C. D. Stern, and R. V. Stirling), pp. 228–47. Oxford University Press, Oxford.

Streeter, G. L. (1908). The nuclei of origin of the cranial nerves in the 10 mm human embryo. *Anat. Rec.* **2**, pp. 111–15.

Teillet, M. A., Cochard, P., and Le Douarin, N. M. (1978). Relative roles of the mesenchymal tissues and of the complex neural tube–notochord on the expression of adrenergic metabolism in neural crest cells. *Zoon* **6**, pp. 115–22.

Tello, J. F. (1923). Les différenciations neuronales dans l'embryon du poulet pendant le premiers jours de l'incubation. *Trav. Lab. de Rech. Biol.* **21**, pp. 1–93.

Thiery, J. P., Duband, J. L., and Delouvée, A. (1982). Pathways and mechanisms of avian trunk neural crest cell migration and localization. *Dev. Biol.* **93**, pp. 324–43.

Tosney, K. W., Watanabe, M., Landmesser, L. and Rutishauser, U. (1986). The distribution of NCAM in the chick hindlimb during axon outgrowth and synaptogenesis. *Dev. Biol.* **114**, pp. 437–52.

Vaage, S. (1969). The segmentation of the primitive neural tube in chick embryos (*Gallus domesticus*). *Adv. Anat. Embryol. Cell Biol.* **41**, 3, pp. 1–88.

Von Baer, K. E. (1828). *Über die Entwicklungsgeschichte der Thiere.* Königsberg.

Von Ebner, V. (1888). Urwirbel und Neugliederung der Wirbelsäule. *Sitzungsber. Akad. Wiss. Wien (Physiol. Anat. Med.)* **97**, pp. 194–206.

Whiting, H. P. (1948). Nervous structure of the spinal cord of the young larval Brook-lamprey. *Q. J. Microsc. Sci.* **89**, pp. 359–84.

Wigston, D. J. and Sanes, J. R. (1982). Selective reinnervation of adult mammalian muscle by axons from different segmental levels. *Nature* **299**, pp. 464–7.

Winklbauer, R. and Hausen, P. (1983). Development of the lateral line system in *Xenopus laevis.* II. Cell multiplication and organ formation in the supraorbital system. *J. Embryol. exp. Morphol.* **76**, pp. 283–96.

Winklbauer, R. and Hausen, P. (1985). Development of the lateral line system in *Xenopus laevis.* IV. Pattern formation in the supraorbital system. *J. Embryol. exp. Morphol.* **88**, pp. 193–207.

PART III

Molecules and guidance pathways

Introduction

The study of neural induction and of segmentation raise some important questions about specificity. Early neurogenesis in the peripheral nervous system appears to involve relatively non-specific mechanisms, which generate spinal roots and channel them towards roughly the correct regions for subsequent pathfinding. Undoubtedly, there is some specificity in pathfinding and axon–target interactions, although there is little direct evidence for it. The experiments of Lance-Jones and Landmesser (1981) and of Wigston and Sanes (1982) are probably the best examples in the vertebrate peripheral nervous system.

For specificity to exist in axon–target interactions, some 'labelling system' is required to mark the identity or both the axon and of its target. Whether this labelling system resides in the genome or whether it is more stochastic and subtle, perhaps involving a complex co-ordinated timing system of growth pathway selection, remains unknown. Although genetic specification is attractive because of its apparent simplicity, such a system is probably far from simple as far as the embryo itself is concerned (see Stent 1981). To specify every connection uniquely in an organism with 500 neurons, for example, just nine genes are required ($2^9 = 512$); indeed insects do appear to use highly deterministic mechanisms, as has been demonstrated by Bate, Goodman and their collaborators. Even a higher vertebrate, which might have as many as 10 000 000 000 000 connections, could have a unique genetic address for each of these with just 44 genes. However, this solution to the problem of specificity lacks the elegance of the rest of embryonic development and it also lacks flexibility. For example, it would be difficult, if not impossible, to account for a hierarchy of connections.

The question of specificity applies not only to the establishment of connections, but also to the paths that axons take to find their targets. While some pathways are 'public' (i.e. non-specific, or permissive; see Chapters 5, 6, and 12), others may be 'private', in that they can be taken only to be specific axons (Chapter 12). Indeed, axons appear to use a multitude of cues to reach their targets; a multitude of mechanisms act in concert, perhaps indicating that there is some redundancy of information. Chapters 6–8 review the evidence for the involvement of some of the molecules that have been thought to play a role in axonal pathfinding and specificity. Chapters 9–13 review some of the systems in which the general mechanisms of axonal guidance and pathfinding have been investigated, and the problems associated with their study. Chapters 14–16 then assess the roles that glial cells play in axonal guidance in the peripheral and central nervous systems.

6

Guidance of neural crest migration during the early development of the peripheral nervous system

MARIANNE BRONNER-FRASER

The neural crest is a population of cells that exists transiently during development. Neural crest cells originate in the dorsal portion of the neural tube and initiate migration shortly after tube closure. Because the neural tube first closes in the head, and tube closure proceeds progressively tailward, numerous stages of neural crest migration occur simultaneously in a single embryo. Migration is well advanced in rostral regions while just beginning in more caudal regions. After migrating away from the neural tube, neural crest cells migrate extensively and eventually differentiate into a wide variety of cell types (Le Douarin 1982). The pathways followed by neural crest cells are characteristic of their axial level of origin; i.e. cranial neural crest cells follow migratory routes that are distinct in pattern and composition from those in vagal or trunk regions.

At the onset of their migration, neural crest cells appear morphologically similar. After cessation of migration, however, they give rise to a varied array of derivatives. These include several different types of neurons, glial and Schwann cells, pigment cells, adrenomedullary cells, as well as bone and cartilage. The mechanisms that cause this apparently homogeneous population of cells to give rise to divergent derivatives are not completely understood. It is possible that some derivatives exist as 'predetermined' subpopulations in the premigratory neural crest. For example, there are inherent differences in the developmental potential of cranial and trunk neural crest cells, such that the cranial neural crest can give rise to bone and cartilage whereas the truncal neural crest cannot. In other cases, there is evidence that the embryonic environment can affect the decisions made by neural crest cells both during their migration and after overt differentiation (Patterson 1978). Thus neural crest cell differentiation is influenced both by the external environment and by information inherent in the cells themselves.

Because of their numerous derivatives and extensive migratory abilities, the neural crest has been widely studied to investigate the mechanisms involved in both cell movement and differentiation. In the trunk of avian embryos, neural crest cells have been thought to migrate along two primary pathways: dorsally between the somite and ectoderm, the route followed by precursors of melanocytes; and ventrally between the neural tube and somite, the route followed by neuronal, neuroendocrine, and supportive-cell precursors (Fig. 6.1).

This review will examine the pathways and guiding mechanisms that might be involved in neural crest cell migration. A historical overview of several methods for identifying avian neural crest cells will first be discussed. Then, the pathways of neural crest migration and the distribution of extracellular matrix (ECM) molecules along these routes will be reviewed. Last, experiments are presented which examine the importance of interactions between cell surface and ECM molecules in neural crest cell migration.

CELL MARKERS THAT IDENTIFY NEURAL CREST CELLS

Neural crest cells migrate away from the neural tube as a mesenchymal population of cells. In the trunk region, the neural crest cells initially enter a cell-free space containing ECM molecules, but subsequently intermix with other cell types. During most of the migratory phase, neural crest cells cannot be distinguished from the other mesenchymal cells among which they move (Bronner-Fraser 1986a). Therefore it has been necessary to use cell marking techniques to determine the pathways followed by neural crest cells. Neural

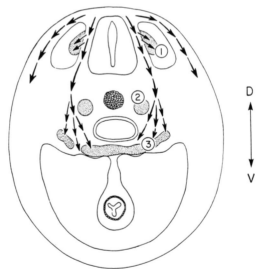

Fig. 6.1. Schematic diagram illustrating the migratory pathways and derivatives of trunk neural crest cells. Cells following the ventral pathway localize in three main areas: (1) the sensory ganglia; (2) the sympathetic ganglia; and (3) the adrenomedullary region. Neural crest cells following the dorsal pathway migrate under the ectoderm and become skin melanocytes. [Reproduced from Bronner and Cohen (1979) by kind permission of the National Academy of Science.]

tube transplantation experiments have been used to implant labelled neural crest cells into unlabelled hosts in order to follow neural crest migratory routes and derivatives. In avian embryos, neural tubes and associated crest cells were marked either with tritiated thymidine (Weston 1963) or by using Japanese quail neural tubes (Le Douarin 1973), and were implanted into unlabelled chickens in place of an appropriate length of host neural tube. In the former case, neural crest cells were followed autoradiographically and, in the latter case, neural crest cells were distinguished from host cells by the condensed heterochromatin which is associated with the quail nucleolus. This heterochromatin marker is stable through cell division and therefore enables long-term identification of implanted cells. These transplantation experiments have established a 'fate map' for the neural crest and have given a general idea of the migratory pathways followed by neural crest cells (see Fig. 6.1). However, details concerning the early stages of migration remained controversial until the advent of non-invasive cell markers.

Recently, monoclonal antibodies that recognize avian neural crest cells have become available. These allow for the paths followed by migrating crest cells to be defined more precisely. The monoclonal antibodies NC-1 and HNK-1 both recognize a carbohydrate epitope on migrating neural crest cells (Tucker, Aoyama, Lipinski, Turz, and Thiery 1984). These antibodies stain trunk crest cells (Vincent and Thiery 1984) and appear to be selective for neural crest cells during the early stages of their migration (Rickmann, Fawcett, and Keynes 1985). At later stages, HNK-1 and NC-1 also recognize mature neurons, glia and Schwann cells, and a subpopulation of leukocytes in addition to neural crest cells (Vincent and Thiery 1984; Tucker *et al.* 1984).

Although avian embryos remain the best studied species for neural crest development, a resurgence of interest has developed in amphibian systems as a result of their accessibility and ease of manipulation. In amphibian embryos, neural tube transplantation experiments have provided ample information concerning the migration of neural crest-derived pigment cells (see Hörstadius 1950). However, information regarding the pathways followed by neural crest precursors to non-pigmented derivatives has been incomplete because of the paucity of useful cell markers. Recently two new cell markers have made it possible to identify neural crest cells during the process of migration: the fluorescent dye, lysinated fluorescein dextran (LFD) (Gimlich and Cooke 1983; O'Rourke and Fraser 1986), and the *Xenopus borealis/laevis* chimeric system (Thiebaud 1983). By grafting neural tubes labelled with one of these markers into unlabelled hosts, it is possible to follow the migration of *Xenopus* neural crest cells emerging from the labelled neural tubes (Krotoski and Bronner-Fraser 1986). *Xenopus borealis* cells can be localized by their characteristic freckled nucleus after quinacrine staining whereas the LFD-labelled cells can be identified by their brightly fluorescent cell bodies. These markers have made it possible to define the pathways of neural crest migration in amphibian embryos (see next section).

PATHWAYS OF NEURAL CREST CELL MIGRATION

In avian embryos, it has been possible to map accurately the early migration of neural crest cells using the monoclonal antibodies NC-1 and HNK-1 (Rickmann *et al.* 1985; Bronner-Fraser 1986*a*; Keynes and Stern this volume, Chapter 5). Unlike neural tube transplantations, the antibody staining techniques require no surgical manipulation of the embryo, thereby allowing observation of neural crest migration through an unperturbed environment. Initially, neural crest cells emerge as a band of cells on the dorsal neural tube, with emigration first occurring in rostral regions; initiation of migration then progresses caudally. In the trunk, neural crest cells can be seen first along the dorsal margin of the neural tube approximately 3–4 somites rostral to the most recently formed somite. As the epithelial somites dissociate to form the dermomyotome and sclerotome, neural crest cells can be seen within the *rostral* half of the sclerotome (Fig. 6.2). This suggests that neural crest cells migrate preferentially through the rostral half of the sclerotome, where they appear to intermix with sclerotomal cells. Neural crest cells have not been observed in the caudal half of the sclerotome or in the region around the notochord, suggesting that they are inhibited or otherwise restricted from these spaces. As the somites mature, the neural crest cells appear to move to progressively ventral positions, surrounding the dorsal aorta. When the neural crest cells have passed through the somites and reached the aorta, differences in the neural crest cell distribution are no longer evident in the rostro–caudal axis. This suggests that the neural crest cells may migrate along the dorsal aorta to fill in the gaps imposed by the caudal sclerotome. In addition to migrating ventrally, some neural crest cells can be seen along the dorso–lateral pathway just underneath the skin and are first seen on that route about eleven somites pairs rostral to the most recently formed somite.

These observations indicate the presence of two major migratory routes in the trunk: a dorso–lateral pathway; and a ventral pathway through the rostral sclerotome. Initiation of neural crest migration begins in the caudal portions of stage-13 embryos and the migratory phase persists in the caudal portions of stage-22 embryos, suggesting that migration occurs for more than 36 hours.

The migration of neural crest cells through the rostral half of the sclerotome parallels that of motoneuron processes emerging from the ventral neural tube (Keynes and Stern 1984). The motor axons emanate from the neural tube as neural crest cells are migrating through that region. Keynes and Stern (1984) determined that the 'guiding' information for the motor axons was within the sclerotome itself and was not inherent to the axons. Neural crest cells do not appear to be necessary for axon outgrowth, since the motor axons continued to migrate through the rostral sclerotome even after ablation of the neural crest (Rickmann *et al.* 1985). This suggests that the guidance cues are intrinsic to the sclerotome rather than caused by migrating neural crest cells or modifications made by these cells to their substrate.

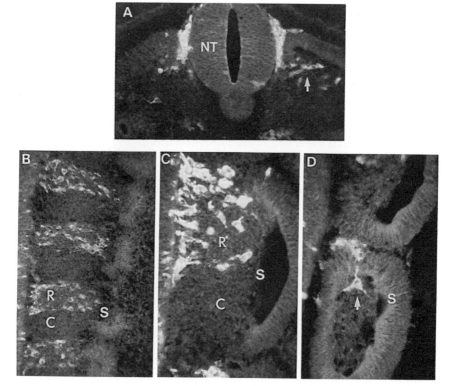

Fig. 6.2. Fluorescence photomicrographs of HNK-1 staining of stage 16–17 chick embryos sectioned in the transverse (A) or longitudinal [(B)–(D)] plane. (A) As seen in cross-section, fluorescently stained neural crest cells leave the dorsal neural tube (NT) and initially are seen between the neural tube and somites. Shortly after the somite breaks up to form the dermomyotome and sclerotome, neural crest cells (indicated by the arrow) can be visualized within the sclerotome (magnification: × 380). (B) In longitudinal section, fluorescently stained neural crest cells are observed within the rostral (R) portion of each somite (S); by contrast, the cells are not detected in the caudal (C) portion of the sclerotome. Some HNK-1 positive cells are also observed within the neural tube (magnification: × 265). (C) High-power photomicrograph of a longitudinal section through the middle of the eighteenth somite of a 30-somite embryo. The remnant of the somitic cavity is still evident in the somite (S), and neural crest cells can be visualized in the rostral half. A sharp border, defined by the neural crest cell staining pattern, is apparent between the rostral (R) and caudal (C) portion of the sclerotome (magnification: × 750). (D) High-power photomicrograph of the twenty-fifth somite of the same 30-somite embryo pictured in (C). A neural crest cell (indicated by the arrow) can be visualized first entering the somite (S) (magnification: × 750). This is the most caudal somite in which neural crest cell staining was detectable in this embryo. [Reproduced from Bronner-Fraser (1986a) by kind permission of Academic Press, New York.]

At cephalic levels, there are no somites through which neural crest cells migrate. Cranial neural crest cells migrate underneath and lateral to the ectoderm and appear to be in close contact, migrating in a sheet-like fashion. At the level of the prosencephalon and rhombencephalon, the neural crest cells encounter physical barriers, such as the optic and otic vesicles which restrict their migration. Vagal neural crest cells arising in the caudal rhombencephalon migrate away from the neural tube and move primarily between the ectoderm and somite (Duband and Thiery 1982). These cells move laterally around the somite and eventually lie ventral to the somitic mesenchyme. Those vagal neural crest cells destined to give rise to parasympathetic ganglia of the gut (Teillet and Le Douarin 1973) then invade the dorsal mesentery and migrate caudally along the gut to give rise to enteric ganglia and other derivatives.

In *Xenopus*, the pathways of trunk neural crest cell migration are quite different from those observed in avian embryos. *Xenopus* neural crest migratory routes were followed by grafting either *borealis* or LFD-labelled neural crest cells (Krotoski and Bronner-Fraser 1986). Labelled trunk neural crest cells were observed on a ventral pathway along the surfaces of the neural tube and notochord, in the narrow space between these structures and the myotome (Fig. 6.3). In addition, neural crest cells were seen above the dorsal mesentery and moving dorsally into the fin. By contrast to birds, few neural crest cells were observed within the somite. We examined the distribution of *Xenopus* neural crest cells in the longitudinal plane to see if any metamerism similar to that observed in avians is evident during amphibian neural crest migration. In longitudinal section, labelled neural crest cells were exclusively observed in the spaces between the neural tube and the *caudal* half of the somite (Fig. 6.3). Thus a metameric pattern of neural crest distribution exists in *Xenopus* but is quite different from the pattern observed in avian embryos.

These studies suggest that neural crest cells in both avian and *Xenopus* embryos migrate along preferential pathways. It seems likely that guiding cues in the somite may be important in determining the patterning of migrating neural crest cells and their derivatives. Whether these cues are permissive or instructive and promote or inhibit migration has yet to be determined.

RELATIONSHIP BETWEEN CELL SURFACE MOLECULES AND THE EXTRACELLULAR MATRIX ALONG NEURAL CREST PATHWAYS

The extracellular matrix

Many aspects of embryonic development are thought to involve interactions between the cell surface and the extracellular matrix (ECM); these include cell growth, cell migration, and cell differentiation (Hay 1982). A variety of ECM

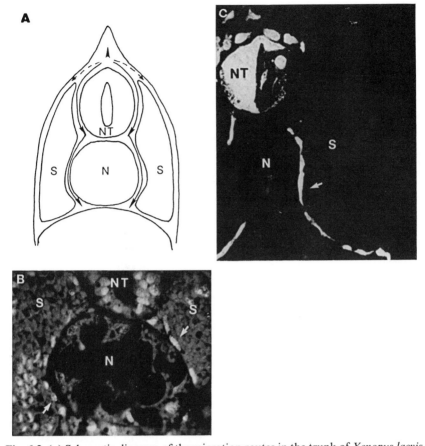

Fig. 6.3. (A) Schematic diagram of the migration routes in the trunk of *Xenopus laevis* embryos. Neural crest cells migrate ventrally between the neural tube (NT) and notochord (N) contributing to the autonomic ganglia, chromaffin cells, and pigment cells. Some cells contribute to the dorsal fin. (B) Section through the trunk of a *X. borealis-laevis* chimaera with neural crest cells (containing freckled grafted nuclei) located around the notochord. (C) Section through the trunk of a *X. laevis* into which a neural tube labelled with lysinated fluorescein dextran (LFD) was grafted. Fluorescent LFD-labelled neural crest cells were seen migrating between the neural tube, notochord, and somite (S). [Reproduced from Krotoski and Bronner-Fraser (1986) by kind permission of Alan R. Liss Inc., New York.]

and cell surface components have been identified in the embryo during neural crest migration. These molecules include fibronectin (FN) (Newgreen and Thiery 1980; Mayer, Hay, and Hynes 1981), hyaluronic acid (HA) (Pintar 1978; Derby 1978), collagen type I (Cohen and Hay 1971), collagen type III, and laminin (LM) (Rogers, Letourneau, Palm, McCarthy, and Furcht 1986; Krotoski, Domingo, and Bronner-Fraser 1986). FN has received particular attention as a candidate for guiding neural crest migration (Duband and Thiery 1982; Newgreen and Thiery 1980; Rogers, Edson, Letourneau, and McLoon 1986; Krotoski and Bronner-Fraser 1986; Krotoski *et al.* 1986). In the cranial regions, there appears to be quite a good correlation between the FN distribution and the routes followed by neural crest cells. However, in the trunk, FN immunoreactivity appears to be more prevalent around tissues where there is little or no neural crest migration than along the routes followed by crest cells (Rickmann *et al.* 1985; Krotoski *et al.* 1986). Recently, LM has also been detected along some of the neural crest pathways and elsewhere in chick embryos. LM has a similar pattern of distribution to that of FN (Rickmann *et al.* 1985; Krotoski *et al.* 1986). In addition to FN and LM, the pathways followed by neural crest cells also contain glycosaminoglycans. For example, high concentrations of HA appear to be present in the trunk region of avian embryos at the time of migration (Pintar 1978; Derby 1978). It is thought that hyaluronate, which is extremely hydrophilic, may promote migration by opening up spaces which facilitate movement of cells through tissues.

To characterize their migratory behaviour on selected extracellular matrix components, neural crest cells can be grown in tissue culture on defined substrates. *In vitro*, avian neural crest cells migrate avidly on FN (Rovasio 1983) and LM (Newgreen 1984), with no apparent preference for either ECM molecule (Goodman and Newgreen 1985). Other molecules may inhibit neural crest migration. For example, some forms of chondroitin sulphate reduce neural crest motility in culture (Newgreen, Gibbins, Sauter, Wallenfels, and Watz 1982). These experiments indicate that FN, LM, HA, and other molecules can serve as permissive substrates for neural crest migration, whereas other less adhesive substrates may inhibit migration. In addition to FN, LM, and glycosaminoglycans, several types of collagen have been detected along some neural crest pathways, though their role in cell migration remains unclear.

Cell surface molecules

Because it is likely that interactions between the cell surface and the ECM are important for neural crest cell migration, it is of value to consider molecules on the surface of neural crest cells at various times in their developmental history. One molecule whose distribution changes during neural crest development is the neural cell adhesion molecule (NCAM). NCAM immuno-reactivity has been detected on the surface of both premigratory and post-migratory neural crest cells in avian embryos, but has not been observed on the surface of migrating neural crest cells (Thiery, Duband, Rutishauser and Edelman 1982). These data have been interpreted to suggest that NCAM, whose binding is Ca^{++}-independent, may be important in normal neural crest cell dispersion. Newgreen and Gibbins (1982) also report a loss of intercellular adhesiveness in neural crest cells *in vitro* when the cells initially migrate away from the neural tube. However, initiation of migration has been shown to involve some Ca^{++}-dependent processes as well (Newgreen and Gooday 1985).

Unlike NCAM, which interacts in a homophilic manner, other surface molecules may be cell surface ligands for ECM molecules. Until recently, little has been known about these receptor molecules. However, the isolation of monoclonal antibodies and peptides which inhibit the binding of cells to tissue culture substrates has resulted in the identification of putative cellular receptors for FN (Neff, Lowrey, Decker, Tovar, Damsky, Buck, and Horwitz 1982; Greve and Gottlieb 1982; Brown and Juliano 1985; Pytela *et al*. 1985) and LM (Malinoff and Wicha 1983; Terranova, Rao, Kalebic, Margulies, and Liotta 1983; Lesot, Kuhl, and von der Mark 1983; Horwitz, Duggans, Creggs, Decker, and Buck 1985; Liotta, Horantland, Rao, Bryant, Barsky, and Schlom 1985).

Two monoclonal antibodies, CSAT (Neff *et al*. 1982) and JG22 (Greve and Gottlieb 1982), both recognize a cell surface receptor complex which is a 'FN receptor' (also called CSAT antigen or CSAT receptor) in avian embryos. The complex, in the molecular weight range of 140 kD (Knudsen, Horwitz, and Buck 1985), co-distributes on cultured fibroblasts with FN and actin in areas of cell–cell contact and along stress fibres (Chen, Hasegawa, Hasegawa, Winstock, and Yamada 1985). On migratory cells such as neural crest cells and somite cells, the distribution of the receptor complex appears to be diffuse and uniform (Duband, Rocher, Chen, Yamada, and Thiery 1986). The CSAT receptor is an integral membrane protein which binds to talin on the cytoplasmic side of the membrane (Horwitz *et al*. 1986) and also binds to LM on the cell surface (Horwitz *et al*. 1985). These observations suggest a possible cellular role for the multifunctional CSAT receptor as part of a cell surface between FN or LM and the cytoskeleton.

Correlations between cell surface and ECM molecules

Both the cell surface receptor and its ligands in the ECM are essential elements for the formation of adhesions between the cell and the substratum. Therefore the spatial and temporal distribution of cell surface and ECM molecules within the embryo may be important during morphogenesis.

To clarify the relationship between one cell surface receptor and its ligands during development, we have analysed the embryonic localization of a FN receptor (recognized by the antibodies CSAT and JG22), together with the ECM molecules FN and LM (Krotoski *et al*. 1986). At the magnification level of the light microscope the distribution of the FN receptor overlapped extensively with the ECM molecules to which it binds. The CSAT antigen was observed on numerous tissues during gastrulation, neurulation, and neural crest migration; for example, the surface of neural crest cells and the basal surface of epithelial tissues such as the ectoderm, neural tube, notochord, and dermomyotome. In turn, FN and LM immunoreactivity were seen in the basement membranes of many of these epithelial tissues, as well as around the otic and optic vesicles.

The pathways followed by cranial neural crest cells are lined with FN and LM, whereas the neural crest cells themselves have the 'FN receptor' on their surfaces. In the mesencephalon, for example, the CSAT antigen has been observed on the surface of premigratory cranial neural crest cells in the dorsal portion of the neural tube and these cells are surrounded by FN and LM (Krotoski *et al.* 1986) (Fig. 6.4). As in mesencephalic neural crest cells, the FN receptor has been seen on migrating trunk neural crest cells. However, FN and LM have only been observed surrounding a subpopulation of trunk neural crest cells (Fig. 6.5).

The parallel distributions between the FN receptor, FN and LM are not, however, absolute. In the trunk, for example, FN and LM immunoreactivity appear to be uniform in both rostral and caudal halves of the sclerotome (Fig. 6.6). In contrast, the CSAT antigen was observed predominantly on the surface of neural crest cells. Because neural crest cells migrate preferentially through the rostral half of the sclerotome (Rickmann *et al.* 1985; Bronner-Fraser 1986*a*), a molecule that 'guides' or 'inhibits' neural crest cell migration would be expected to be in either the rostral or caudal half of the somite, respectively. Since FN and LM are uniformly distributed within the sclerotome, neither FN nor LM appear to have the selective distribution necessary to serve as a guiding molecule for trunk neural crest cells. It remains possible that these molecules serve as substrates for neural crest cell migration, much like asphalt serves as a driving surface for automobiles. Other factors, however, may determine the actual pathways to which the cells are restricted.

The levels of immunoreactivity for FN, LM, and the FN receptor appear to be dynamic at different developmental stages. In our analysis (Krotoski *et al.* 1986), the intensity of FN and LM immunofluorescence in the sclerotome appear to *decrease* somewhat during neural crest migration and return to higher levels after ganglion formation. These observations indicate that either neural crest cells migrate at a time when FN and LM may be reduced on their migratory pathways in comparison to other developmental stages, or some sites of FN and LM are masked at the time of neural crest migration. Levels of CSAT immunoreactivity also change as a function of developmental age and appear to increase on both epithelial and neural crest-derived tissues with increasing age.

These findings suggest that the 'FN receptor' is present on neural crest cells during their migration and that the density of receptor molecules may increase after the cells have ceased migrating. FN and LM are seen on most neural crest pathways, though the levels of immunoreactivity are sometimes lower than those observed on neighbouring tissues. The levels of FN and LM immuno-reactivity also appear to increase after neural crest migration. The balance of

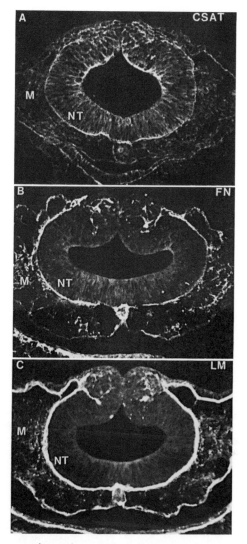

Fig. 6.4. Fluorescence photomicrographs of transverse sections showing CSAT, fibronectin (FN), and laminin (LM) immunoreactivity in the mesencephalon just prior to cranial neural crest migration in stage-10 embryos. (A) CSAT was observed surrounding most cells in the embryo. Immunoreactivity was particularly noticeable around cells of the neural tube (NT), including the premigratory neural crest cells (NC) which were in the dorsal portion of the neural tube. (B) FN was observed on the basal surface of the neural tube, ectoderm, notochord and endoderm, as well as within the cranial mesenchyme (M). FN immunoreactivity was also seen in the area surrounding the premigratory neural crest cells. (C) LM immunoreactivity was observed on the basal surface of the neural tube, ectoderm, endoderm, and notochord. LM was also seen within the cranial mesenchyme and surrounding the premigratory neural crest cells. [Reproduced from Krotoski *et al* (1986) by kind permission of the Rockefeller University Press, New York.]

adhesions between the cell surface and the substrate may be important for cell migration, such that relatively low levels of surface and substrate molecules promote cell movement whereas higher levels of these molecules result in cessation of migration. Though FN and LM line many neural crest pathways, neither molecule has a selective distribution in the trunk region that would suggest a guiding role in neural crest migration.

PERTURBATION EXPERIMENTS: THE ROLE OF CELL SURFACE AND ECM MOLECULES IN NEURAL CREST MIGRATION

One approach for examining the importance of cell surface–ECM interactions is to disrupt one or more of the adhesive interactions and to examine the subsequent effects during development. Antibodies or other reagents that

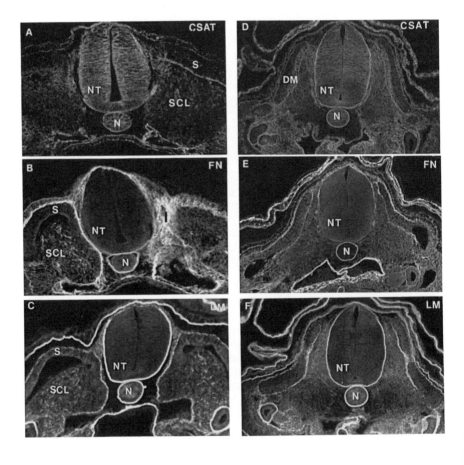

disrupt cell surface–ECM interactions can be used to accomplish such *in vivo* perturbations. This experimental approach has demonstrated the functional importance of NCAM (Thiery, Duband, Rutishauser, and Edelman 1982) in retinal histogenesis, retinotectal map formation (Fraser, Murray, Chuong, and Edelman 1984), and nerve-glia interactions (Silver and Rutishauser 1984). In amphibian embryos, injection of either a decapeptide containing the FN cell-binding sequence or an antibody against FN into the blastocoele caused disruption of normal gastrulation (Boucaut and Darribère 1983; Boucaut, Darribère, Boulekbache, and Thiery 1984a). Similar reagents have been used to disrupt avian neural crest migration *in vitro* (Rovasio, Delouvée, Yamada, Timpl, and Thiery 1983) or *in vivo* in the mesencephalon (Boucaut, Darribère, Poole, Aoyama, Yamada, and Thiery 1984b); the FN decapeptide caused a bilateral inhibition of cranial neural crest migration as well as protrusions of neural crest cells into the lumen of the neural tube (Boucaut *et al.* 1984b). These observations suggest a possible role for FN in gastrulation and cranial neural crest migration.

The role of the extracellular matrix in neural crest migration can also be tested by transplanting matrices from one region of the embryo to another.

Fig. 6.5. Fluorescence photomicrographs of transverse sections through the trunk region showing CSAT, fibronectin (FN), and laminin (LM) immunoreactivity in the trunk region at the onset of neural crest migration [(A)–(C): stage-15 embryos] and during active neural crest migration [(D)–(F): stage-17 embryos]. (A) As neural crest migration was beginning, CSAT was seen surrounding all neural tube (NT) cells, including the premigratory neural crest cells. CSAT was most prominent under the dermomyotome portion of the somite (S) and around the dorsal aorta. Low levels of immunoreactivity were observed under the ectoderm and within the sclerotome (SCL); few neural crest cells have entered the sclerotome at this stage (magnification: × 270). (B) FN was observed around the somite (S), the dorsal portion of the neural tube (NT), and the notochord (N). FN immunoreactivity was particularly strong in the intersomitic space (I), as shown on the right side of this oblique section. Some fibrillar FN staining was noted within the sclerotome (magnification: × 240). (C) LM immunoreactivity was observed around the basal surface of the neural tube, notochord, ectoderm, and somite. Punctate LM staining was also observed within the sclerotome (magnification: × 225). (D) During active neural crest migration, the CSAT staining was more intense than in younger embryos. CSAT was observed around the basal surface of the neural tube, notochord, dermomyotome (DM), ectoderm, and mesonephric tubes. Within the sclerotome, CSAT immunofluorescence was distinct around individual neural crest cells (indicated by arrow) (magnification: × 145). (E) FN immunoreactivity was observed on the dorsal surface of the neural tube, around the dermomyotome, notochord, and dorsal aorta. Low levels of FN immunoreactivity were seen within the sclerotome through which neural crest cells migrate (magnification: × 145). (F) LM immunoreactivity was observed around the neural tube, notochord, ectoderm, dermomyotome, and mesonephric tubules. Low levels of FN immunoreactivity were observed within the sclerotome (magnification: × 145). [Reproduced from Krotoski *et al.* (1986) by kind permission of the Rockefeller University Press, New York.]

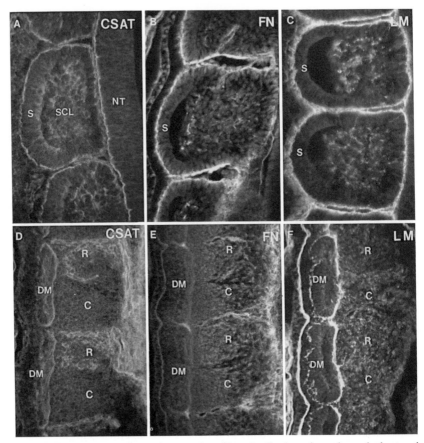

Fig. 6.6. Fluorescence photomicrographs of longitudinal sections through the trunk region showing CSAT, fibronectin (FN), and laminin (LM) immunoreactivity at the onset of neural crest migration [(A)–(C): stage-15 embryos] and during active neural crest migration [(D)–(F): stage-17 embryos]. (A) CSAT outlined the somite (S) and neural tube (NT). Uniform staining was also observed within the sclerotome (SCL) (magnification: × 335). (B) FN immunoreactivity was present around the somite. In addition, some fibrillar FN staining was seen within the sclerotome (magnification: × 360). (C) LM was observed around the somites, as well as in fibrillar form within the somites (magnification: × 375). (D) During active neural crest migration, CSAT was observed around the dermomyotome (DM) and surrounding neural crest cells within the rostral (R) half of the sclerotome. In contrast, only low levels of CSAT reactivity were observed on sclerotomal cells themselves. Consequently, the caudal (C) half of the sclerotome had little CSAT immunoreactivity (magnification: × 250). (E) FN immunoreactivity was observed around the dermomyotome. In addition, low uniform levels of FN were seen within both rostral and caudal halves of the sclerotome (magnification: × 250). (F) LM immunoreactivity was observed around the dermomyotome. Within the sclerotome, uniform LM immunofluorescence was seen in both rostral and caudal halves (magnification: × 250). [Reproduced from Krotoski *et al.* 1986) by kind permission of the Rockefeller University Press, New York.]

Løfberg, Nynas-McCoy, Olsson, Jonsson, and Perris (1985) have elegantly illustrated the importance of the ECM in promoting neural crest migration in axolotl embryos by 'transplanting' conditioned microcarrier filters. The microcarriers contain ECM from donor embryos which is then transplanted to host embryos. These experiments have demonstrated that ECM taken from embryos in which neural crest cells are actively migrating can stimulate premature migration of neural crest cells in younger embryos. Thus the matrix itself appears to promote neural crest emigration from the neural tube of axolotl embryos.

Interactions between the cell surface and the ECM can be perturbed by micro-injecting antibodies into embryos. We have examined the role a 'FN receptor' (JG22/CSAT antigen) plays in neural crest cell migration by implanting function-perturbing antibodies onto neural crest pathways. Using a micro-injection technique, antibodies together with antibody-producing hybridoma cells have been injected lateral to the neural tube in the mesencephalon. The hybridoma cells are labelled with a fluorescent cell marker which is non-deleterious and remains visible after fixation and tissue sectioning. The labelled hybridoma cells, therefore, serve to identify the site of injection. After injection, antibody molecules do not cross the midline, but appear to diffuse throughout the injected half of the mesencephalon, where they remain detectable by immunocytochemistry for about 22 hours (Fig. 6.7).

Antibody-injected embryos were examined either during neural crest migration (up to 24 hours after injection) or after formation of neural crest-derived structures (36–48 hours after injection). In those embryos fixed within the first 24 hours, the major defects were: a reduction in the neural crest cell number on the injected side, a build up of neural crest cells within the lumen of the neural tube, and ectopically localized neural crest cells (Fig. 6.8). In embryos allowed to survive for 36 to 48 hours after injection, the neural crest derivatives appeared normal on both the injected and control side, suggesting that the embryos compensated for the reduction in neural crest cell number on the injected side. However, the embryos often had severely deformed neural tubes and ectopic aggregates of neural crest cells (Fig. 6.9). As the concentration of injected antibody decreased, a downward trend in the percentage of abnormal embryos was observed, suggesting a dose-dependence in the effects of the antibody.

The results show that antibodies to the FN receptor cause severe abnormalities in cranial neural crest cell migration. Synthetic peptides containing the FN cell-binding sequence have also been found to alter cranial neural crest migration (Boucaut *et al.* 1984*a*) in much the same way as the antibodies to the FN receptor. In contrast, several control monoclonal antibodies, which bind to bands of the 140 kD CSAT complex, have little or no influence on cranial neural crest or neural tube development. These findings support the notion that antibody-induced perturbations in cranial

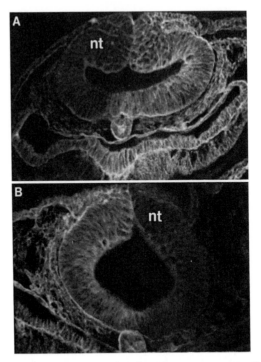

Fig. 6.7. Fluorescence photomicrographs of transverse cryostat sections showing the distribution of the CSAT antibody after injection into the mesencephalon. Embryos pictured in both (A) and (B) were processed six hours after injection. The CSAT antibody was observed around the neural tube (nt), ectoderm, cranial mesenchyme, and surrounding premigratory neural crest cells. Antibodies did not, however, appear to cross the midline (magnification: × 315). [Reproduced from Bronner-Fraser (1986*b*) by kind permission of Academic Press, New York.].

Fig. 6.8. Fluorescence photomicrographs of embryos fixed 11 hours after injection of JG22 antibodies and hybridoma cells into the mesencephalon. The sections were stained with HNK-1 antibodies in order to recognize neural crest cells. Neural crest cells in the mesencephalon normally emigrate away from the neural tube (nt) and into the mesenchyme just beneath the ectoderm. (A) Section through the main injection site, containing the highest concentration of hybridoma cells (magnification: × 330). The brightly fluorescent hybridoma cells that were labelled with CFSE prior to injection are easily visualized on the right-hand side (indicated by the arrow). In the presence of JG22 antibodies, the number of neural crest cells on the injected side was markedly reduced. Quantitative reconstruction of serial sections throughout the mesencephalon of this particular embryo demonstrated a 51 per cent reduction in neural crest cell volume on the injected side relative to the control side. (B) Another section through the posterior mesencephalon of the same embryo illustrated in (A) (magnification: × 330). The reduction in neural crest cell number is more severe and the cells have not migrated as far ventrally on the injected side. In addition, a lobule has formed within the neural

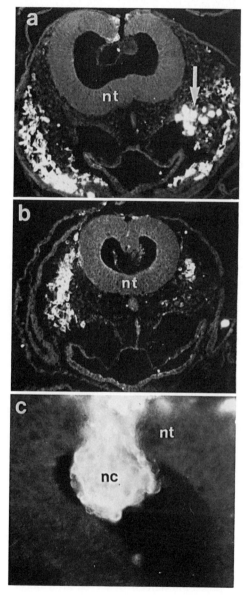

tube (nt) which contains neural crest cells (identified by HNK-1 staining). (c) Another embryo at higher magnification with a profound build up of neural crest cells (nc) in the lumen of the mesencephalic neural tube (magnification: × 1200). [Reproduced from Bonner-Fraser 1985) by kind permission of the Rockefeller University Press, New York.]

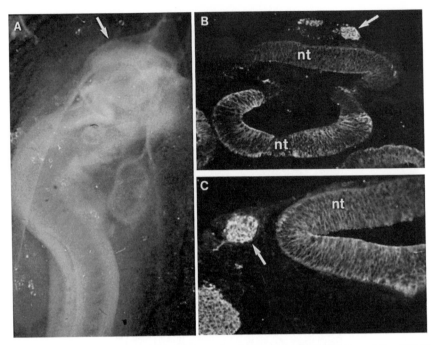

Fig. 6.9. Photomicrographs of an embryo fixed two days after injection of the CSAT antibody into the mesencephalon. (A) Bright field image of the embryo demonstrating that neural tube anomalies such as the open tube (indicated by arrow) can be recognized externally (magnification: × 26). (B) Section at the level of the otic vesicles, stained with HNK-1 to identify neural crest cells; the neural tube (nt) of the embryo is discontinuous in the dorso–ventral plane and aggregates of neural crest cells (indicated by arrow) can be observed dorsal to the neural tube (magnification: × 25). (C) HNK-1 stained section through the mesencephalon of the same embryo; the neural tube (nt) appears normal but an ectopic aggregate of neural cells with a ganglion-like morphology (indicated by arrow) can be observed lateral to the neural tube on the injected side (magnification: × 150). [Reproduced from Bronner-Fraser (1986*b*) by kind permission of Academic Press, New York.]

morphogenesis result from functional blockage of the CSAT receptor and suggest that the receptor complex is important in the normal development of the neural crest and neural tube.

In contrast to the profound defects observed after injection of antibodies into the cranial region, neither antibodies to the FN receptor (Bronner-Fraser 1985) nor FN synthetic peptides (Bronner-Fraser, unpublished obsservations) resulted in comparable alterations in trunk neural crest migration. These results indicate that different molecules are involved in neural crest migration in the trunk and in the head. It is possible that cranial and trunk neural crest cells are inherently different in terms of their migratory mechanisms.

Alternatively, the ECM may be quite different along the pathways followed by cranial and trunk crest cells.

In tissue culture, antibodies to the FN receptor disrupt neural crest cell adhesion and migration (Bronner-Fraser 1985). Furthermore, the purified CSAT receptor binds both FN and LM (Horwitz *et al.* 1985). These *in vitro* observations support the notion that injection of the antibody to the FN receptor *in situ* disrupts neural crest migration on FN and LM. Initiation of cranial neural crest cell migration occurs in a region rich in both LM and FN (Krotoski *et al.* 1986). Injection of the FN receptor antibody into the mesencephalon, therefore, may alter initial emigration of neural crest cells from the neural tube. This may account for the presence of neural crest cells within the neural tube and may be partially responsible for the reduction in neural crest cell numbers. These experiments cannot distinguish, however, between the functional importance of LM and/or FN in cranial neural crest migration since the CSAT antibody interferes with neural crest cell binding both to FN and to LM.

Perturbation experiments of the sort described above form an important correlate to *in vitro* experiments and can be used to test the functional importance of individual molecules *in situ*. However, it is likely that during complicated morphogenetic events several cell surface and/or ECM molecules may work in concert. Perturbation of any one component may result in a functional block of that event. Therefore it is necessary to be aware of possible synergistic effects in designing experiments to test adhesive interactions.

CONCLUDING REMARKS

This chapter has given an overview of methods used to identify migrating neural crest cells and to examine the role of cell interactions in their migration. Neural crest cells migrate along characteristic 'pathways' that contain a variety of ECM molecules including FN, hyaluronate, and LM. The migration of neural crest cells in the trunk region is patterned, i.e. the cells move preferentially through the rostral half of each somite. The interactions leading to this selective distribution of neural crest cells remain unknown.

By micro-injecting antibodies onto cranial neural crest pathways, we found that an antibody to a FN receptor caused severe perturbations in cranial neural crest migration. These results suggest that adhesive interactions between the neural crest cell surface and the ECM may play a role in normal neural crest cell migration. However, many questions remain. Little is known about what causes initiation or cessation of neural crest migration. In addition, the guiding mechanisms involved in the patterning of trunk neural crest cells remain elusive. It seems likely that a variety of molecules will be important as cell- and substratum-adhesion-promoting molecules involved in neural crest morphogenesis; many of these are yet to be identified. Our current understanding of neural crest cell migration is largely descriptive, and future research must delve into the physical and molecular mechanisms underlying the interesting patterns of cell migration.

ACKNOWLEDGEMENTS

I thank Dr J. Coulombe and T. Lallier for helpful comments on the manuscript. This work was supported by USPHS HD-15527 and by a Basic Research Grant from the March of Dimes Birth Defects Foundation.

REFERENCES

Boucaut, J. C. and Darribere, T. (1983). Fibronectin in early amphibian embryos. Migrating mesodermal cells contact fibronectin established prior to gastrulation. *Cell Tiss. Res.* **234,** pp. 135–45.

Boucaut, J. C., Darribere, T., Boulekbache, H., and Thiery, J. P. (1984*a*). Prevention of gastrulation but not neurulation by antibodies to fibronectin in amphibian embryos. *Nature* **307,** pp. 364–7.

Boucaut, J. C., Darribere, T., Poole, T. J., Aoyama, H., Yamada, K. M., and Thiery, J. P. (1984*b*). Biologically active synthetic synthetic peptides as probes of embryonic development: a competitive peptide inhibitor of fibronectin function inhibits gastrulation in amphibian embryos and neural crest migration in avian embryos. *J. Cell. Biol.* **99,** pp. 1822–30.

Bronner, M. and Cohen, A. M. (1979). Migratory patterns of cloned neural crest melanocytes injected into host chicken embryos. *Proc. Natl. Acad. Sci. USA* **76,** pp. 1843–7.

Bronner-Fraser, M. (1985). Alterations in neural crest migration by a monoclonal antibody that affects cell adhesion. *J. Cell Biol.* **101,** pp. 610–17.

Bronner-Fraser, M. (1986*a*). Analysis of the early stages of trunk neural crest migration using monoclonal antibody HNK-1. *Dev. Biol.* **115,** pp. 44–55.

Bronner-Fraser, M. (1986*b*). An antibody to a receptor for fibronectin and laminin perturbs cranial neural crest development in vivo. *Dev. Biol.* **117,** pp. 528–36.

Brown, P. J. and Juliano, R. L. (1985). Selective inhibition of fibronectin-mediated cell adhesion by monoclonal to a cell-surface glycoprotein. *Science* **228,** pp. 1448–51.

Chen, W. T., Hasegawa, E., Hasegawa, T., Winstock, C., and Yamada, K. (1985). Development of cell surface linkage complexes in culture fibroblasts. *J. Cell Biol.* **100,** pp. 1103–14.

Cohen, A. M. and Hay, E. D. (1971). Secretion of collagen by embryonic neuroepithelium at the time of spinal cord–somite interaction. *Dev. Biol.* **26,** pp. 578–605.

Derby, M. A. (1978). Analysis of glycosaminoglycans within the extracellular environments encountered by migrating neural crest cells. *Dev. Biol.* **66,** pp. 321–36.

Duband, J. L. and Thiery, J. P. (1982). Distribution of fibronectin in the early phase of avian cephalic neural crest cell migration. *Dev. Biol.* **93,** pp. 308–23.

Duband, J. L., Rocher, S., Chen, W.-T., Yamada, K. M., and Thiery, J. P. (1986). Cell adhesion and migration in the early vertebrate embryo: location and possible role of the putative fibronectin receptor complex. *J. Cell Biol.* **102**, pp. 160–78.

Fraser, S., Murray, B. A., Chuong, C.-M., and Edelman, G. M. (1984). Alteration of the retinotectal map in *Xenopus* by antibodies to neural cell adhesion molecules. *Proc. Natl. Acad. Sci. USA* **81**, pp. 4222–6.

Gimlich, R. L. and Cooke, J. (1983). Cell lineage and the induction of second nervous systems in amphibian development. *Nature* **306**, pp. 471–3.

Goodman, S. and Newgreen, D. F. (1985). Do cells show an inverse locomotory response to fibronectin and laminin substrates? *EMBO J.* **4**, pp. 2769–71.

Greve, J. M. and Gottlieb, D. I. (1982). Monoclonal antibodies which alter the morphology of cultured chick myogenic cells. *J. Cell Biochem.* **18**, pp. 221–9.

Hay, E. D. (1982). *Cell biology of extracellular matrix*. Plenum Press, New York.

Hörstadius, S. (1950). *The neural crest: its properties and derivatives in the light of experimental research*. Oxford University Press, Oxford.

Horwitz, R., Duggan, K., Buck, C., Beckerle, M., and Burridge, K. (1986). The CSAT antigen is a dual receptor for talin and fibronectin. *Nature* **320**, pp. 531–3.

Horwitz, A. F., Duggan, K., Greggs, R., Decker, C., and Buck, C. (1985). The CSAT antigen has properties of a receptor for laminin and fibronectin. *J. Cell Biol.* **101**, pp. 2134–44.

Hynes, R. O. and Yamada, K. M. (1982). Fibronectins: multifunctional modular glycoproteins. *J. Cell Biol.* **95**, pp. 369–77.

Keynes, R. J. and Stern, C. D. (1984). Segmentation in the vertebrate nervous system. *Nature* **310**, pp. 786–9.

Keynes, R. J. and Stern, C. D. (1987). The development of neural segmentation in vertebrate embryos. In *The making of the nervous system* (eds, J. G. Parnavelas, C. D. Stern, and R. V. Stirling), pp. 84–100. Oxford University Press, Oxford.

Knudsen, K., Horwitz, A., and Buck, C. (1985). A monoclonal antibody identifies glycoprotein complex involved in cell-substratum adhesion. *Exp. Cell Res.* **157**, pp. 218–26.

Krotoski, D. and Bronner-Fraser, M. (1986). Mapping of neural crest pathways in the trunk of *Xenopus laevis*. In *New discoveries and technologies in developmental biology* (ed. H. Slavkin), pp. 229–33. Alan R. Liss Inc., New York.

Krotoski, D., Domingo, C., and Bronner-Fraser, M. (1986). Distribution of a putative cell surface receptor for fibronectin and laminin in avian embryos. *J. Cell Biol.* **103**, pp. 1061–71.

Le Douarin, N. M. (1973). A biological cell labelling technique and its use in experimental embryology. *Dev. Biol.* **30**, pp. 217–22.

Le Douarin, N. M. (1982). *The neural crest*. Cambridge University Press, New York.

Lesot, H., Kuhl, U., and von der Mark, K. (1983). Isolation of a laminin-binding protein from muscle cell membranes. *EMBO J.* **2**, pp. 861–5.

Liotta, L. A., Horan Hand, P., Rao, C. N., Bryant, G., Barsky, S. H. and Schlom, J. (1985). Monoclonal antibodies to the human laminin receptor recognize structurally distinct sites. *Exp. Cell Res.* **156**, pp. 117–26.

Løfberg, J., Nynas-McCoy, A., Olsson, C., Jonsson, L., and Perris, R. (1985). Stimulation of initial neural crest cell migration in the axolotl embryo by tissue grafts and extracellular matrix transplanted on microcarriers. *Dev. Biol.* **107**, pp. 442–59.

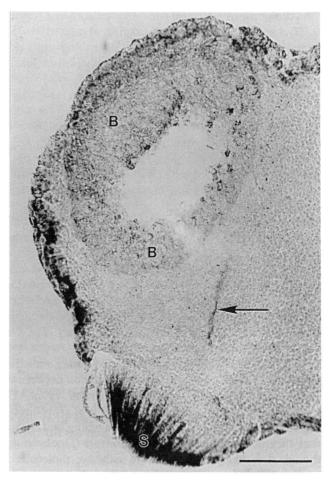

Fig. 7.3. Parasaggital section through the head of a stage-26 *Xenopus* embryo. The section has been stained using polyclonal anti-NCAM and the biotin–avidin–HRP method. Immunoreactivity is seen in the brain (**B**) and the trigeminal nerve (arrow). The dark pigment in the epidermis and sucker (**S**) is melanin. (Scale bar: 100 μm).

formation of specific neuromuscular connections in *Xenopus* has not been published. However, the sequence of events in development of the hind limb seems to be as follows (Muntz 1975; Lamb 1976; Sheard 1985). Myoblasts (premyogenic cells) detach from the somites and migrate into the hind limb bud at about stage 49 (Nieuwkoop and Faber 1967). At about the same time the axons of lateral motoneurons start growing out of the spinal cord, initially guided by the axons of primary motoneurons that have innervated the axial muscles at earlier stages. Our observation that a trail of myoblasts, which express NCAM, extends from the somite to the base of the limb bud suggests

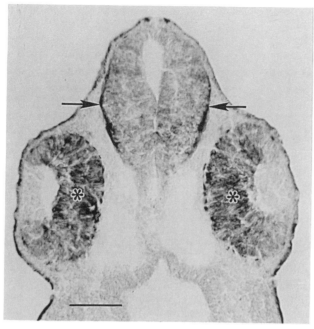

Fig. 7.5. Coronal section through the head of a stage-32 *Xenopus* embryo at the level of the diencephalon and eyes. The section has been stained using polyclonal anti-NCAM primary antibody and the biotin–avidin–HRP method. In the retina the most intense immunoreactivity is over the central region (star) consisting of newly formed neurons. The germinal zone at the retinal periphery is weakly immunoreactive. Axons of the optic tracts (arrows) are intensely immunoreactive. (Scale bar: 100 μm.)

external appearance. However, the level of NCAM in the central retina of ectopic eyes remained much higher than in the normal eyes of the same embryo [Fig. 7.6(C)]. These results show that the formation of central connections is required for the down-regulation of NCAM expression that normally occurs in retinal ganglion cells after they form connections in the tectum. We do not yet know whether the down-regulation occurs in eyes that have projected axons into the spinal cord or whether the effect requires formation of specific retinotectal connections.

In the tectum NCAM is expressed in a pattern that closely parallels that in the retina. The entire tectum stains moderately strongly for NCAM at stages 38–40 during the initial arrival of retinal axons. From stage 40 to stage 50 the level of NCAM diminishes greatly in the tectum except at its caudal region (Fig. 7.7). In other words, NCAM is down-regulated in the region of the tectum that has formed connections with the retina but it is strongly expressed in the most recently formed tectal region that has not yet received retinal axons or that is in the process of being innervated by retinal axons (Jacobson

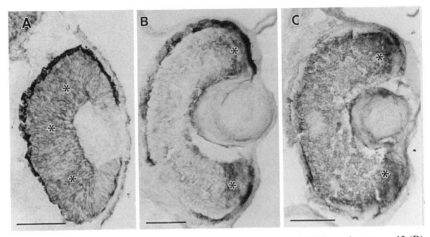

Fig. 7.6. Coronal sections of *Xenopus* embryo eyes at stage 35 (A), and at stage 43 (B), and of an eye at stage 43 (C) that had been transplanted to the abdomen at stage 24. The sections have been stained using polyclonal anti-NCAM primary antibody and the biotin–avidin–HRP method. Intense immunoreactivity is seen over the newly formed neurons (stars). In (A) the peripheral retinal region, containing proliferating germinal cells, is lightly immunoreactive. In (B) the central retinal region, containing the oldest neurons, is least immunoreactive, but the level of immunoreactivity has remained high in the central retinal region of the transplanted eye (C). (All scale bars: 100 μm.)

1977). This pattern persists at later stages: the region of tectum that has formed retinal connections is NCAM-negative, while the tectal region that is in the process of receiving new retinal axons expresses NCAM strongly (Fig. 7.7). These findings indicate that new retinal axons entering the tectum avoid the NCAM-poor regions that have already connected with retinal axons, and target specifically on the NCAM-rich region of tectum. In this way the newly formed axons from the retinal peripheral zone, which express NCAM strongly, target on a broad band of NCAM-positive cells in the caudal margin of the tectum. Possible explanations of the inability to detect NCAM in the older region of tectum are that NCAM epitopes or tectal neurons may be modified or lost or that NCAM epitopes may be hidden by synaptic connections between retinal axons and tectal neurons.

These observations are consistent with others that show that the tectum plays an essential role in the formation of an orderly, continuous, and properly aligned retinotectal map. This evidence suggests that the tectum aligns the map, establishes its polarity, and also provides positional markers that serve as targets for retinal axons (see the review, in Jacobson 1978, pp. 392–403). NCAM appears to play a role in alignment and polarity of the map in the rostro–caudal axis of the tectum which corresponds with the naso–

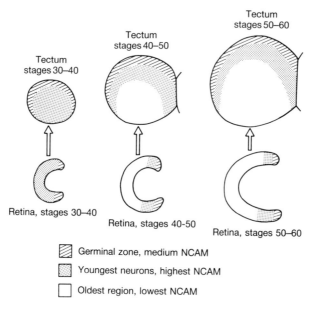

Tectum
stages 50–60

Tectum
stages 40–50

Tectum
stages 30–40

Retina, stages 30–40

Retina, stages 40-50

Retina, stages 50–60

Germinal zone, medium NCAM

Youngest neurons, highest NCAM

Oldest region, lowest NCAM

Fig. 7.7. Patterns of expression of NCAM immunoreactivity in the retina (coronal section) and tectum (surface view) at different stages of embryonic development in *Xenopus*.

temporal retinal axis. Additional positional information may be provided by modulation of the sialic acid content of NCAM, and thus its adhesivity, in the medio–lateral axis of the tectum, and a corresponding pattern of modulation of NCAM sialic acid content in the dorso-ventral axis of the retina. These findings are consistent with earlier reports implicating NCAM in the mechanisms of retinotectal map formation (Thanos, Bonhoeffer, and Rutishauser 1984; Fraser *et al.* 1984).

SUMMARY AND CONCLUSIONS

1. NCAM can first be detected in *Xenopus* embryos in the neural plate after the end of gastrulation. Its absence at the appropriate time and place indicates that it does not play a role in primary neural induction. But primary neural induction is required, indirectly, for the subsequent expression of NCAM on neural cells.

2. Expression of NCAM at moderately high levels occurs on all neuroepithelial cells. The highest level of NCAM expression is seen on young neurons in the process of axon outgrowth, on the elongating axons and their growth cones, and in newly formed zones in the CNS and at neuromuscular junctions. The level of NCAM diminishes rapidly in neurons and axons after they have

formed synaptic connections. We propose that down-regulation of NCAM expression results from trans-synaptic signalling between pre-synaptic neuron and post-synaptic cell.

3. Increase of the sialic acid content of NCAM in *Xenopus* at later stages of development seems to be correlated with the transition from early embryos in which neuroepithelial cell proliferation predominates (in which most of the NCAM is lightly sialylated) to the later embryonic stages and adults in which axogenesis and synaptogenesis are predominant (in which the major form of NCAM is heavily polysialylated). We propose a hypothesis that relates the form of NCAM to its functions at different stages of development of the vertebrate nervous system (Table 7.1). The persistence of the so called 'embryonic' form of NCAM in adult *Xenopus* may be a basis for their ability to regenerate axons in the CNS.

4. Absence of NCAM in the presumptive peripheral nerve pathways but high levels of NCAM on the shafts and growth cones of elongating axons indicates that NCAM is involved in axon fasciculation but not in guidance of axons along specific pathways. High levels of NCAM on axonal targets in the central and peripheral nervous systems and persistence of NCAM at synapses, implicates NCAM in the mechanism of selection of targets and formation of synaptic connections.

5. An example of the level at which NCAM may work is seen during innervation of the limb bud. High levels of NCAM are expressed on the outgrowing motor axons and on their targets, the myoblasts of the limb bud, so that the gross initial connections with the premuscle mass may be mediated by NCAM. NCAM diminishes rapidly to undetectable levels in the muscle cells after they are innervated. This may be the result of trans-synaptic trophic regulation of muscle NCAM by the motor neurons or may result from muscle contraction.

6. In the retinotectal system the patterns of NCAM expression in retina and tectum are correlated with the spatio–temporal patterns of histogenesis and axonal outgrowth. NCAM is sparse in regions of retina and tectum containing the oldest neurons that have previously formed connections. Moderate levels are found in the peripheral retinal and tectal zones containing proliferating neuroepithelial cells which have not initiated axogenesis. The highest levels of NCAM are found in the intermediate zone containing young neurons in the process of axon outgrowth in the retina and in the tectal zone containing their target neurons. A hypothesis is proposed in which the gross formation of the retinotectal map is based on the spatio-temporal pattern of expression of NCAM in retinal ganglion cell axons and their tectal targets, followed by down-regulation of NCAM expression in the retinal and tectal neurons that have formed connections. NCAM expression remains high in the retina in eye rudiments transplanted to the abdomen, showing that down-regulation of NCAM expression depends on retinal axons connecting in the CNS. This is the first evidence of retrograde trans-synaptic regulation of NCAM expression in the CNS.

ACKNOWLEDGEMENTS

This research is supported by grants from the National Science Foundation (BNS 851964) and National Institutes of Health (NS 20569-04). I thank Ken Balak for his collaboration with parts of this work, Urs Rutishauser for encouragement and advice and for a gift of antibodies used in these experiments, and Alan Smith and Philip Sheard for their comments on the manuscript.

REFERENCES

Balak, K., Jacobson, M., Sunshine, J., and Rutishauser, U. (1987). Neural cell adhesion molecule (NCAM) immunoreactivity during embryonic development in *Xenopus. Dev. Biol.* **119**, pp. 540–50.

Beach, D. H. and Jacobson, M. (1978a). Patterns of cell proliferation in the developing retina of the clawed frog in relation to blood supply and position of choroidal fissure. *J. Comp. Neurol.* **183**, pp. 603–13.

Beach, D. H. and Jacobson, M. (1978b). Patterns of cell proliferation in the retina of the clawed frog during development. *J. Comp. Neurol.* **183**, pp. 625–32.

Bertolotti, R., Rutishauser, U., and Edelman, G. M. (1980). A cell surface molecule involved in aggregation of embryonic liver cells. *Proc. Natl. Acad. Sci. USA* **77**, pp. 4831–5.

Buskirk, D. R., Thiery, J.-P., Rutishuaser, U., and Edelman, G. M. (1980). Antibodies to a neural cell adhesion molecule disrupt histogenesis in cultured chick retinae. *Nature* **285**, pp. 488–9.

Chuong, C. M. and Edelman, G. M. (1984). Alterations in neural cell adhesion molecules during development of different regions of nervous system. *J. Neurosci.* **4**, pp. 2354–68.

Chuong, C. M. and Edelman, G. M. (1985a). Expression of cell-adhesion molecules in embryonic induction. I. Morphogenesis of nestling feathers. *J. Cell. Biol.* **101**, pp. 1009–26.

Chuong, C. M. and Edelman, G. M. (1985b). Expression of cell-adhesion molecules in embryonic induction. II. Morphogenesis of adult feathers. *J. Cell. Biol.* **101**, pp. 1027–43.

Covault, J. and Sanes, J. R. (1985). Neural cell adhesion molecule (N-CAM) accumulates in denervated and paralyzed skeletal muscle. *Proc. Natl. Acad. Sci. USA* **82**, pp. 4544–8.

Crossin, K. L., Chuong, C.-M., and Edelman, G. M. (1985). Expression sequences of cell adhesion molecules. *Proc. Natl. Acad. Sci. USA* **82**, pp. 6942–6.

Cunningham, B. A. S., Hoffman, S., Rutishauser, U., Hemperly, J. J., and Edelman, G. M. (1983). Molecular topography of NCAM: surface orientation and the location of sialic acid-rich and binding regions. *Proc. Natl. Acad. Sci. USA* **80**, pp. 3116–20.

Deuchar, E. M. (1975). *Xenopus: the South African clawed frog.* Wiley, Chichester.

Edelman, G. M. (1983). Cell adhesion molecules. *Science* **219**, pp. 450–7.

Edelman, G. M. (1984*a*). Modulation of cell adhesion during induction, histogenesis and perinatal development of the nervous system. *Ann. Rev. Neurosci.* **7**, pp. 339–77.

Edelman, G. M. (1984*b*). Cell adhesion and morphogenesis: the regulator hypothesis. *Proc. Natl. Acad. Sci. USA* **81**, pp. 1460–4.

Edelman, G. M. (1985). Cell adhesion and the molecular processes of morphogenesis. *Ann. Rev. Biochem.* **54**, pp. 135–69.

Edelman, G. M. and Chuong, C. M. (1982). Embryonic to adult conversion of neural cell adhesion molecules in normal and staggerer mice. *Proc. Natl. Acad. Sci. USA* **79**, pp. 7036–40.

Edelman, G. M., Gallin, W. J., Delouvée, A., Cunningham, B. A., and Thiery, J. -P. (1983). Early epochal maps of two different cell adhesion molecules. *Proc. Natl. Acad. Sci USA* **80**, pp. 4384–8.

Fawcett, J. W. (1987). Retinotopic maps, cell death, and electrical activity in the retinotectal and retinocollicular projections. In *The making of the nervous system* (eds. J. G. Parnavelas, C. D. Stern, and R. V. Stirling), pp. 395–416. Oxford University Press, Oxford.

Finne, J., Finne, U., Deagostini-Bazin, H., and Goridis, C. (1983). Occurrence of alpha-2-8 linked polysialosyl units in a neural cell adhesion molecule. *Biochem. Biophys. Res. Comm.* **112**, pp. 482–7.

Fraser, S. E., Murray, B. A., Chuong, C. M., and Edelman, G. M. (1984). Alteration of the retinotectal map in *Xenopus* by antibodies to neural cell adhesion molecules. *Proc. Natl. Acad. Sci. USA* **81**, pp. 4222–6.

Gaze, R. M., Chung, S. H., and Keating, M. J. (1972). Development of the retinotectal projection in *Xenopus*. *Nature* **236**, pp. 133–5.

Gaze, R. M., Keating, M. J., and Chung, S. H. (1974). The evolution of the retinotectal map during development in *Xenopus*. *Proc. Roy. Soc. Lond. B* **185**, pp. 305–30.

Gerisch, G. (1977). Univalent antibody fragments as tools for the analysis of cell interactions in *Dictyostelium*. *Curr. Top. Dev. Biol.* **14**, pp. 243–70.

Goridis, C., Deagostino-Bazin, H., Hirn, M., Rougon, G., Sadoul, R., Langley, O. K., Gombos, B., and Finne, J. (1983). Neural surface antigens during nervous system development. *Cold Spring Harbor Symp. Quant. Biol.* **48**, pp. 527–37.

Grant, P., Rubin, E., and Cima, C. (1980). Ontogeny of the retina and optic nerve in *Xenopus lavis*. I. Stages in the early development of the retina. *J. Comp. Neurol.* **189**, pp. 593–613.

Grumet, M., Rutishuaser, U., and Edelman, G. M. (1982). NCAM mediates adhesion between embryonic nerve and muscle *in vitro*. *Nature* **295**, pp. 693–5.

Hall, A. K. and Rutishauser, U. (1985). Phylogeny of a neural cell adhesion molecule. *Dev. Biol.* **110**, pp. 39–46.

Hoffman, S. and Edelman, G. M. (1983). Kinetics of homophilic binding by embryonic and adult forms of the neural cell adhesion molecule. *Proc. Natl. Acad. Sci. USA* **80**, pp. 5762–6.

Hoffman, S., Chuong, C. M., and Edelman, G. M. (1984). Evolutionary conservation of key structures and binding functions of neural cell adhesion molecules. *Proc. Natl. Acad. Sci. USA* **81**, pp. 6881–5.

Hoffman, S., Sorkin, B. C., White, P. C., Brackenbury, R., Mailhammer, R., Rutishauser, U., Cunningham, B. A., and Edelman, G. M. (1982). Chemical characterization of a neural cell adhesion molecule purified from embryonic brain membranes. *J. Biol. Chem.* **257**, pp. 7720–9.

Hollyday, M. (1983). Development of motor innervation of chick limbs. *Prog. Clin. Med. Res.* **110a**, 183–93.

Holt, C. E. and Harris, W. A. (1983). Order in the initial retinotectal map in *Xenopus*: a new technique for labelling growing nerve fibers. *Nature* **301**, pp. 150–2.

Holtfreter, J. (1939). Gewebeaffinität, ein Mittel der embryonalen Formbildung. *Arch. Exp. Zellforsch.* **23**, pp. 169–209.

Huang, S. and Jacobson, M. (1986). Neurites show pathway specificity but lack directional specificity or predetermined lengths in *Xenopus* embryos. *J. Neurobiol.* **17**, pp. 593–604.

Hyafil, F., Morello, D., Babinet, C., and Jacob, F. (1980). A cell surface glycoprotein involved in the compaction of embryonal carcinoma cells and cleavage stage embryos. *Cell* **21**, pp. 927–34.

Jacobson, M. (1968). Cessation of DNA synthesis in retinal ganglion cells correlated with the time of specification of their central connections. *Dev. Biol.* **17**, pp. 219–32.

Jacobson, M. (1976). Histogenesis of retina in the clawed frog with implications for the pattern of development of retinotectal connections. *Brain Res.* **103**, pp. 541–5.

Jacobson, M. (1977). Mapping the developing retino-tectal projection in frog tadpoles by a double label autoradiographic technique. *Brain Res.* **127**, pp. 55–67.

Jacobson, M. (1978). *Developmental neurobiology* (2nd edition). Plenum Press, New York.

Jacobson, M. and Huang, S. (1985). Neurite outgrowth traced by means of horseradish peroxidase inherited from neuronal ancestral cells in frog embryos. *Dev. Biol.* **110**, pp. 102–13.

Jacobson, M. and Rutishauser, U. (1986). Induction of neural cell adhesion molecule (NCAM) in *Xenopus* embryos. *Dev. Biol.* **116**, pp. 524–31.

Jorgensen, O. S. (1981). Neuronal membrane D-2 protein during rat brain ontogeny. *J. Neurochem.* **37**, pp. 939–46.

Lamb, A. H. (1976). The projection patterns of the ventral horn to the hind limb during development. *Dev. Biol.* **54**, pp. 82–99.

Lamb, A. H. (1977). Neuronal death in the development of somatotopic projections of the ventral horn in *Xenopus*. *Brain Res.* **134**, pp. 145–50.

Lamb, A. H. (1981). Selective bilateral motor innervation in *Xenopus* tadpoles with one hind limb. *J. Embryol. exp. Morphol.* **65**, pp. 149–63.

Landmesser, L. (1980). The generation of neuromuscular specificity. *Ann. Rev. Neurosci.* **3**, pp. 279–301.

Lumsden, A. G. S. (1987). Diffusible factors and chemotropism in the development of the peripheral nervous system. In *The making of the nervous system* (eds. J. G. Parnavelas, C. D. Stern, and R. V. Stirling). pp. 166–87. Oxford University Press, Oxford.

Moscona, A. A. (1974). Surface specification of embryonic cells: lectin receptors, cell recognition, and specific ligands. In *The cell surface in development* (ed. A. A. Moscona), pp. 67–99. Wiley, New York.

Muntz, L. (1975). Myogenesis in the trunk and leg during development of the tadpole of *Xenopus laevis* (Daudin, 1802). *J. Embryol. exp. Morphol.* **33**, pp. 757–74.

Nieuwkoop, P. D. and Faber, J. (1967). *Normal tables of Xenopus laevis (Daudin)* (2nd edition). North-Holland, Amsterdam.

Noble, M., Albrechtsen, M., Moller, C., Goridis, C., Lyles, J., Bock, E., Watanabe, M., and Rutishauser, U. (1985). Purified astrocytes express NCAM/D2-CAM-like molecules *in vitro*. *Nature* **316**, pp. 725–8.

Prestige, M. C. (1967). The control of cell number in the lumbar ventral horns during the development of *Xenopus laevis* tadpoles. *J. Embryol. exp. Morphol.* **18,** pp. 359–87.

Rathjen, F. G. and Schachner, M. (1984). Immunocytological and biochemical characterization of a new neuronal cell surface component (L1 antigen) which is involved in cell adhesion. *EMBO J.* **3,** pp. 1–10.

Rothbard, J. B., Brackenbury, B. A., Cunningham, B. A., and Edelman, G. M. (1982). Differences in the carbohydrate structures of neural cell adhesion molecules from adult and embryonic brains. *J. Biol. Chem.* **257,** pp. 11064–9.

Rutishauser, U. (1984). Developmental biology of a neural cell adhesion molecule. *Nature* **310,** pp. 549–54.

Rutishauser, U., Gall, W. E., and Edelman, G. M. (1978*a*). Adhesion among neural cells of the chick embryos. IV. Role of the cell surface molecule N-CAM in the formation of neurite bundles in cultures of spinal ganglia. *J. Cell. Biol.* **79,** pp. 386–93.

Rutishauser, U., Grumet, M., and Edelman, G. M. (1983). Neural cell adhesion molecule mediates initial interactions between spinal cord neurons and muscle cells in culture. *J. Cell. Biol.* **97,** pp. 145–52.

Rutishauser, U., Thiery, J. -P., Brackenbury, R., and Edelman, G. M. (1978*b*). Adhesion among neural cells of the chick embryos. III. Relationship of the surface molecule CAM to cell adhesion and the development of histotypic patterns. *J. Cell. Biol.* **79,** pp. 371–81.

Rutishauser, U., Watanabe, M., Silver, J., Troy, F. A., and Vimr, E. R. (1985). Specification of NCAM-mediated cell adhesion by an endoneurominidase. *J. Cell Biol.* **101,** pp. 1842–9.

Sakaguchi, D. S. and Murphy, R. K. (1985). Map formation in the developing *Xenopus* retinotectal system: an examination of ganglion cell terminal arborizations. *J. Neurosci.* **5,** pp. 3228–45.

Schlosshauer, B., Schwartz, U., and Rutishauser, U. (1984). Topological distribution of different forms of N-CAM in the developing chick visual system. *Nature* **310,** pp. 141–3.

Sheard, P. W. (1985). The regulation of cell numbers and properties in the developing motor system of *Xenopus laevis*. PhD thesis, University of Western Australia, Perth, Australia.

Silver, J. and Rutishauser, U. (1984). Guidance of optic axons *in vivo* by a preformed adhesive pathway on neuroepithelial endfeet. *Dev. Biol.* **106,** pp. 485–99.

Steinberg, M. S. (1970). Does differential adhesion govern self-assembly processes in histogenesis? Equilibrium configurations and the emergence of a hierarchy among populations of embryonic cells. *J. Exp. Zool.* **173,** pp. 395–433.

Stirling, R. V. and Summerbell, D. (1987). Motor axon guidance in the developing chick limb. In *The making of the nervous system* (eds. J. G. Parnavelas, C. D. Stern, and R. V. Stirling). pp. 228–47. Oxford University Press, Oxford.

Thanos, S., Bonhoeffer, F., and Rutishauser, U. (1984). Fiber–fiber interactions and tectal clues influence the development of the chick retinotectal projection. *Proc. Natl. Acad. Sci. USA* **81,** pp. 1906–10.

Thiery, J. -P., Brackenbury, R., Rutishauser, U., and Edelman, G. (1977). Adhesion among neural cells of the chick embryo. II. Purification and characterization of a cell adhesion molecule from neural retina. *J. Biol. Chem.* **252,** pp. 6841–5.

Thiery, J. -P., Duband, J. L., Rutishauser, U., and Edelman, G. M. (1982). Cell adhesion molecules in early chick embryogenesis. *Proc. Natl. Acad. Sci. USA* **79,** pp. 6737–41.

Tosney, K. W., Watanabe, M., Landmesser, L., and Rutishauser, U. (1986). The distribution of NCAM in the chick hindlimb during axon outgrowth and synaptogenesis. *Dev. Biol.* **114,** pp. 437–52.

Townes, P. L. and Holtfreter, J. (1955). Directed movements and selective adhesions of embryonic amphibian cells. *J. Exp. Zool.* **128,** pp. 53–120.

The role of neurotrophic growth factors in development, maintenance, and regeneration of sensory neurons

RONALD M. LINDSAY

ROLE OF EPIGENETIC FACTORS IN THE DEVELOPMENT OF THE PERIPHERAL NERVOUS SYSTEM

The development of the vertebrate peripheral nervous system (PNS) and the formation of orderly connections between neurons and their appropriate targets, as found in the adult animal, is increasingly thought to be dependent on epigenetic factors—cues from the environment which dictate, possibly by direct action upon gene expression, the differentiation pathway to be taken by progenitor or immature blast cells. Within the PNS such factors may be involved in the initiation and cessation of neuroblast migration from the neural crest and neural placodes, in the promotion of fibre outgrowth and the guidance of neurites to appropriate targets, and in sustaining the survival and differentiated state of neurons which have already established appropriate connections. At present, studies on putative epigenetic factors are centred on two types of macromolecular signals:

(a) Non-diffusible molecules, which may be either extracellular matrix molecules, such as those of the basal lamina (collagens, proteoglycans, laminin, etc.) involved in cell–substratum adhesion, or plasma membrane molecules, such as the cell–cell adhesion molecules (e.g. NCAM and NgCAM, etc.) (for reviews, see Edelman 1984, and Thiery, Duband, and Tucker 1985). It is postulated that such non-diffusible molecules may function as specific cell–cell recognition signals and as axon guidance cues.

(b) Diffusible molecules, which may act either locally as neurotrophic factors (neurite-promoting factors, survival and maintenance factors, etc.) or over relatively longer distances as chemotropic agents which guide neurites to their targets (see Lumsden this volume, Chapter 9).

It is likely that a combination of epigenetic signals, including those mentioned above, are required at precise time-windows in development in order to establish the appropriate sensory and autonomic innervation pattern of individual peripheral tissues and organs. At present, however, detailed information at the molecular level is still far too fragmentary to permit the establishment of a unifying hypothesis based on present concepts of how a spectrum of immobilized and diffusible factors might act synchronously to orchestrate PNS development. Although the case for extrinsic cues being involved in neurite guidance has been expounded for many years, theoretical views in this field have not yet been fully matched by experimental results. It is only recently that supportive evidence at the molecular level has begun to emerge, through identification of possible candidate molecules such as laminin, etc.

NERVE GROWTH FACTOR—ARCHETYPE NEUROTROPHIC FACTOR

In contrast to the lack of an archetype molecule on which to formulate a detailed theory of guidance mechanisms, the crucial role played by neurotrophic molecules in PNS development has been well established due to the discovery and purification of nerve growth factor (NGF)—for reviews of NGF, see Levi-Montalcini 1966; Levi-Montalcini and Angeletti 1968; and Thoenen and Barde 1980. Although retrospectively it is clear that an element of serendipity aided in the discovery of NGF, the isolation and biochemical characterization of NGF and the initial identification of its neurotrophic properties were greatly facilitated by two key factors: (a) the detection of a rich source of NGF—the adult male mouse submandibular salivary gland, and (b) the development of a simple and sensitive *in vitro* bioassay—the sensory neuron fibre outgrowth assay using explants of chick embryo dorsal root ganglia (DRG). The availability of large (mg) quantities of NGF has permitted not only its widespread use in tissue culture studies but also its use in whole-animal studies—experiments involving injections of NGF or NGF antibodies which have proved to be pivotal in establishing a role for NGF *in vivo*. Such studies have clearly demonstrated that NGF is essential as a survival and maintenance factor for developing and adult sympathetic neurons (Levi-Montalcini and Angeletti 1966; Gorin and Johnson 1980). While it is also well established that NGF is essential as a survival factor for certain populations of neurons within spinal sensory ganglia (DRG), it is now evident that NGF is not a universal neurotrophic factor for all sensory neurons (see below), and a detailed picture of the precise neurotrophic requirements of sub-populations of sensory neurons has still to emerge. With regard to the specificity of NGF towards sub-populations of sensory neurons, questions which have not been addressed until recently, or which have not been answered adequately, include:

(a) Are all DRG neurons responsive to the survival and neurite-promoting effects of NGF, or are there sub-populations of DRG neurons—possibly grouped by their distinct sensory functions such as nociception or proprioception—which differ in their neurotrophic requirements?

(b) Are there other neurotrophic factors which act upon DRG neurons, separately or synergistically with NGF?

(c) Are sensory neurons of the various specialized cranial sensory ganglia equally or at all responsive to NGF, and, if not, do they have requirements for neurotrophic molecules distinct from NGF?

(d) Is NGF required continuously as a survival factor for adult sensory neurons, and, if not, does it possibly have any other role such as influencing terminal sprouting, regeneration, or maintenance of specific functions of adult sensory neurons?

(e) Are neurotrophic molecules other than NGF essential for sustaining the survival of adult sensory neurons? This chapter reviews studies which have attempted to answer some of these questions.

DEVELOPING PERIPHERAL NERVOUS SYSTEM

Differences in the requirements of neural-crest- and neural placode-derived sensory neurons for NGF

Origins of spinal and cranial nerve sensory neurons

Sensory neurons of vertebrate peripheral nerve ganglia are derived from either of two distinct embryological structures: the neural crest or neural placodes. The precise contribution of neuroblasts made by these two sources towards the formation of sensory nerve ganglia has been most extensively studied in birds, most recently utilizing the elegant quail–chick chimaera paradigm (Le Douarin 1973; for a review, see Le Douarin 1982; for earlier experimental appoaches, see the references in Lindsay and Rohrer 1985). It is now established, at least for birds, that the neural crest gives rise to all neurons of spinal nerve ganglia (DRG), to the medio–dorsal neurons of the fifth cranial nerve ganglia (the trigeminal ganglion), to neurons of the fused root ganglia (jugular) of the ninth and tenth cranial nerves, and to the satellite and Schwann cells of *all* sensory ganglia. Neural placodes, on the other hand, give rise to ventro–lateral neurons within the trigeminal ganglion and to the neurons of all other cranial nerve sensory ganglia, i.e. the distal ganglia of the seventh, ninth, and tenth cranial nerves (the geniculate, petrosal, and nodose ganglia, respectively) and the vestibulo-acoustic ganglionic complex of the eighth cranial nerve (D'Amico Martel and Noden 1983).

The NGF requirement of spinal sensory neurons

The relative ease in obtaining large numbers of spinal sensory ganglia from the developing nervous system of either chick embryos or perinatal rodents has led to an extensive literature on the NGF responsiveness of DRG sensory neurons maintained in culture. While explant cultures (Fenton 1970) have proved very useful in qualitative assessment of the responsiveness of ganglia to NGF or other neurotrophic factors (Ebendal and Hedlund 1974, 1975; Lindsay and Tarbit 1979; Lindsay and Peters 1984; Davies and Lindsay 1984, 1985; Davies, Thoenen, and Barde 1986*b*), it is extremely difficult using *in vitro* methods alone to obtain unequivocal quantitative data on the number of responsive neurons at any specific developmental stage. Dissociated mono-layer cultures of ganglionic neurons (Greene 1977; Barde, Lindsay, Monard, and Thoenen 1978; Barde, Edgar, and Thoenen 1982; Lindsay and Peters 1984; Lindsay and Rohrer 1985; Lindsay, Thoenen, and Barde 1985*b*), freed of non-neuronal cells (McCarthy and Partlow 1976), do allow one to obtain comparative quantitative data on the survival and neurite-promoting effect of neurotrophic factors, but it must be borne in mind that most culture studies have utilized chick embryo ganglia at embryonic day 8 (E8) and older, which results in two complicating factors. First, in the developing chick embryo many fibres of DRG neurons have already reached their appropriate targets by E8, and thus, strictly speaking, *in vitro* studies using material of this or older ages test the effects of NGF or other neurotrophic factors for their ability to promote survival and regeneration *in vitro* rather than, as is often assumed, determining the potential of such factors to promote neurite outgrowth *ab initio*. Second, neurogenesis within sensory ganglia, be they neural crest- or neural placode-derived, is not highly synchronized but is a protracted event occurring over 2–3 days; E2 to E5 in placodal ganglia and E4·5–E7·5 in crest-derived ganglia (Carr and Simpson 1978; D'Amico-Martel 1982). Thus, at any early embryonic stage (e.g. E6–E12), the neuronal population within spinal or cranial nerve sensory ganglia is quite heteroge-nous with respect to the post-mitotic developmental stage of individual neurons. The reason that this fact complicates interpretation of the NGF requirements of the entire population is because there is evidence that sensory neurons may only require or be responsive to NGF as a survival factor for a limited period after becoming post-mitotic (Winick and Greenberg 1965; Herrup and Shooter 1975; Greene 1977; Barde, Edgar, and Thoenen 1980). Therefore, when comparing the effects of NGF upon cultured DRG neurons from E6 and E12 chick embryos, for example, the nett responsiveness to NGF at both ages may be similar (Lindsay, Barde, Davies, and Rohrer 1985*a*), but the responsive population may be quite different; i.e. at E6 there may be a population of neuroblasts which are not yet responsive to NGF, while at stage E12 the earliest born neurons may have passed through their phase of NGF requirement and only those cells which appeared late in neurogenesis are now dependent on NGF as a survival factor. This inherent difficulty which is imposed upon the interpretation of quantitative results obtained from *in vitro* studies has been further complicated by progressive changes which have occurred in the culture conditions used in the past few years. Using polyornithine as a substrate on which to culture dissociated chick embryo DRG neurons, Barde *et al.* (1980) observed that saturating levels of NGF promoted survival of about 27 per cent of the neurons at E8 and about 45 per cent at E11, the latter age being the peak age of responsiveness to NGF. Similar results were obtained when collagen was used as a substrate (Lindsay *et al.* 1985*b*). However, in the most recent study (Lindsay *et al.* 1985*a*), using the basement membrane glycoprotein laminin as a cell attachment factor, although the effect of NGF on the survival of E11 chick DRG neurons was unchanged compared to using a collagen or a polyornithine substrate, at E6 as many as 70 per cent of DRG neurons cultured on a laminin-coated substrate were found to be supported by NGF. Laminin by itself does not promote neuron survival, but here, and as previously seen with sympathetic neurons (Edgar, Timpl, and Thoenen 1984), a laminin-coated substrate potentiated the effects of NGF. Bearing in mind the above caveats, it would appear from *in vitro* studies that 70 per cent or more of developing DRG neurons are responsive to NGF. Although specific receptors for NGF have been detected on more than 95 per cent of chick embryo DRG neurons between E8 and E12 (Rohrer and Barde 1982; Lindsay and Rohrer 1985), this in itself cannot be construed as an indication of a requirement for NGF as a survival factor. This caution stems from a recent observation (Davies, Lumsden, and Rohrer 1986*a*) that, although the vast majority of primary sensory neurons in the exclusively neural crest-derived trigeminal mesencephalic nucleus bear NGF-receptors, these neurons are almost entirely refractory, at least *in vitro*, to the survival and neurite-promoting effects of NGF.

Early studies by Levi-Montalcini (1962) and Hamburger (1962) on the requirement of spinal sensory neurons for NGF *in vivo* came to the conclusions that late-forming, small, medio–dorsal neurons of DRG were NGF-dependent while the much larger, early forming ventro–lateral neurons were unresponsive to NGF. However, reinvestigation of this question by Hamburger, Bruno-Bechtold, and Yip (1981) has shown that NGF injections *in ovo* dramatically reduce naturally occurring cell death in both the ventro–lateral and medio–dorsal populations of brachial and thoracic DRG, suggesting that the great majority of chick embryo DRG neurons go through a phase of NGF-dependence. Exposure of neo-natal or adult rodents to anti-NGF antibodies, either by injection of heterologous anti-sera or by creation of auto-immunity (Levi-Montalcini and Angeletti 1966; Schwartz, Pearson, and Johnson 1982; Rich, Yip, Osborne, Schmidt, and Johnson 1984), has little effect on the neuronal number in sensory ganglia (but see Yip, Rich, Lampe, and Johnson 1984). Similar exposure of embryonic sensory neurons to anti-NGF results in: (a) destruction of up to 85 per cent of DRG neurons in developing rats or guinea pigs (Johnson, Gorin, Brandeis, and Pearson 1980), (b) destruction of up to 70 per cent of DRG neurons in developing rabbits (Johnson, Gorin, Osborne, Rydel, and Pearson 1982), and (c) a 90 per cent decrease in unmyelinated fibres and a 35 per cent decrease in myelinated fibres of rat dorsal roots (Goedert, Otten, Hunt, Bond, Chapman, Schlumpf, and Lichtensteiger 1984). Conclusions (a) and (b) are drawn from studies in which trans-placental transfer of maternal antibodies was the source of NGF antibodies. In these cases the fact that not all developing DRG neurons are destroyed by deprivation of NGF, as brought about by exposure to NGF antibodies, may be interpreted as an indication that there is a small population of NGF-independent neurons in DRG. It is possible, however, that such neurons have already undergone a brief phase of NGF-dependence before maternal antibodies can freely pass across the placenta. In the other study cited (Goedert *et al* 1984), NGF antibodies were injected *in utero* into rat foetuses at E16.5., and the observed incomplete loss of myelinated and umyelinated fibres in spinal nerve trunks may again reflect a small NGF-independent DRG population, or a population of DRG neurons which have already passed through their stage of NGF-dependency prior to the experimental onset of NGF deprivation.

In summary, therefore, it would appear from culture studies, largely with chick embryo DRG neurons, and from experimental studies *in vivo*, carried out for the most part with rodents, that the vast majority (at least 80 per cent) of DRG sensory neurons require NGF as a survival factor during a limited period of development. Surprisingly, however, very little detailed information is available on the absolute temporal aspect of this window of NGF-dependence for either avian or rodent DRG neurons.

The response of cranial sensory neurons to NGF

In marked contrast to the extensive literature on the NGF requirements of spinal nerve sensory neurons (DRG), there have, until recently, been very few detailed studies of the neurotrophic requirements of cranial sensory neurons of either neural crest or neural placode origin. The limited study of cranial nerve ganglia *in vitro*, compared to the wide use of DRG, most certainly reflects the very time-consuming dissection required to obtain sufficient cranial ganglia for either explant or dissociated cell culture. It may also reflect the fact that it is only relatively recently that the definitive origin of cranial ganglia has been clarified (Narayanan and Narayanan 1980; Le Douarin 1982; D'Amico-Martel and Noden 1983). Reports by Levi-Montalcini (1962, 1966) and her unpublished observations (pers. comm.) on the chick trigeminal and nodose ganglia in culture and *in vivo* were the first to suggest that placode-derived neurons might be refractory to the survival and neurite-promoting effects of NGF. This view was supported by further studies using explant cultures of both chick and mouse trigeminal ganglia, where it was found that NGF promotes fibre outgrowth from medio–dorsal explants, but does not promote fibre outgrowth from the placode-derived neurons of the ventro–lateral portion of this ganglion (Ebendal and Hedlund 1974, 1975; Davies and Lumsden 1983; Davies and Lindsay 1984). However, any generalized conclusion that placode-derived neurons are refractory to NGF must be tempered with conflicting evidence from culture experiments and *in vivo* studies as to the response or requirement of nodose ganglion neurons for NGF. While NGF has been shown in one case to elicit modest fibre outgrowth from E8 chick embryo nodose ganglion explants (Hedlund and Ebendal 1980), and in another case to slightly increase an already significant level of spontaneous fibre outgrowth from E4 and E5 nodose ganglia (Lindsay and Rohrer 1985), dissociated neuron-enriched cultures of chick embryo nodose ganglia have repeatedly been found to be refractory to the survival and neurite outgrowth-promoting activity of NGF (Lindsay 1979; Lindsay and Wilson 1980; Lindsay and Rohrer 1985; Lindsay *et al.* 1985*a*, 1985*b*). As yet there has been only a single report to suggest that NGF is required as a survival factor for mammalian nodose ganglion neurons (Baccaglini and Cooper 1982), but this is not supported by other tissue culture studies (Lindsay 1979; Lindsay, Barber, Sherwood, Zimmer, and Raisman 1982; Mathieu, Moisand, and Weber 1984; Sato 1985) or by studies *in vivo* (Johnson *et al.* 1980; Pearson, Johnson, and Brandeis 1983) on the effects of exposure to anti-NGF antibodies. These conflicting observations prompted us to undertake a detailed developmental study of the NGF responsiveness of explant and dissociated neuron-enriched cultures of the chick embryo nodose ganglion (Lindsay and Rohrer 1985). We found no evidence of NGF supporting the survival or eliciting neurite outgrowth from nodose ganglion neurons from E6 or older chick embryos. Similarly, and perhaps most convincingly, we have demonstrated by incubating cultures with radioactively labelled (^{125}I) NGF that nodose ganglion neurons are devoid of NGF receptors during this developmental period, when, in marked contrast, more than 95 per cent of DRG neurons possess such receptors (Rohrer and Barde 1982; Lindsay and Rohrer 1985). Although unresponsive to NGF, nodose and other placode-derived sensory neurons do require neurotrophic factors for survival and neurite outgrowth *in vitro*, and we have identified (see below) neurotrophic activity for such cells in target tissue extracts, glial cell co-cultures, and a purified brain-derived neurotrophic factor (BDNF) (Lindsay 1979; Lindsay and Wilson 1980; Lindsay and Peters 1984; Lindsay and Rohrer 1985; Davies and Lindsay 1985; Lindsay *et al.* 1985*a*, 1986*b*). The only hesitation in making a categorical statement that nodose ganglion neurons are unresponsive to NGF is the observation that NGF does stimulate or enhance modest neurite outgrowth from E4 to E8 nodose (and petrosal) ganglion neurons (Hedlund and Ebendal 1980; Lindsay and Rohrer 1985; Davies and Lindsay 1985). However, as we have argued in detail (Lindsay and Rohrer 1985), we believe that this modest response to NGF does not arise from the placode-derived neurons themselves, but is indicative of neurite outgrowth from neural crest-derived cells within the developing nodose ganglion. Although in normal development the neural crest only contributes Schwann cells to placode-derived ganglia, it has been demonstrated by back transplantation experiments, using the quail–chick chimaera system (Ayer-le Lièvre and Le Douarin 1982), that at early stages in ontogeny the nodose ganglion contains neural-crest-derived precursors which have neuronal potentialities. It is not yet clear whether such cells represent a single lineage of bi-potential precursors which migrate as such into the nodose ganglion rudiment and in that location are only permitted, by an unknown mechanism, to differentiate along a Schwann cell lineage, or alternatively whether separate neuronal and glial precursors arrive from the neural crest and only the glial precursors are allowed to survive, proliferate, and co-exist with placode-derived neurons. Regardles of which of these possibilities is the correct one, we suggest that NGF-induced fibre outgrowth from explants of placode-derived ganglia is not representative of normal development, but is an epiphenomenon occurring only *in vitro* where a precursor cell is induced to express neuronal potentialities, potentialities that are normally repressed *in vivo* under the influence of localized epigenetic regulatory factors.

To extend specific observations on the nodose ganglion to a general hypothesis that all placode-derived neurons are refractory to NGF as a survival and neurite-promoting factor, a developmental study was carried out to examine and compare the effects of NGF on explant and dissociated cell cultures of all cranial sensory ganglia of the chick embryo (Davies and Lindsay 1985). From this study it was concluded that all neural-crest-derived cranial nerve sensory ganglia (the dorso–medial trigeminal ganglion and jugular ganglion) contain NGF-responsive neurons, while essentially all placode-derived sensory ganglia are unresponsive to NGF. As with the nodose ganglion, NGF did elicit modest fibre outgrowth from geniculate and petrosal ganglia explanted at early developmental stages, but as discussed above this sparse neurite outgrowth may emanate not from placodal neurons but from neural-crest-derived cells within these ganglia. Neurons of the placode-derived vestibular ganglion and neurons of the ventro–lateral portion of the trigeminal ganglion were entirely refractory to NGF at all developmental stages. With the exception of a recent observation that the entire population of neural-crest-derived trigeminal mesencephalic neurons are refractory to NGF (Davies *et al.* 1986*a*), I would conclude that in marked contrast to most crest-derived sensory neurons, the neurons of placode-derived sensory ganglia, at least in the chick embryo, are unresponsive to NGF but are dependent on other neurotrophic factors. There is presently no evidence from *in vivo* studies on the developing chick embryo to support or refute this contention. However, auto-immune studies with the guinea pig have shown that trans-placental exposure to anti-NGF antibodies has no depleting effect upon the final complement of neurons in nodose or spiral ganglia examined either at birth or at maturity (Johnson *et al.* 1980; Pearson *et al.* 1983), while in the same animals this method of NGF deprivation resulted in a 80 per cent loss of neurons in both spinal and trigeminal ganglia.

Response of neural crest- and placode-derived sensory neurons to non-NGF neurotrophic factors

Response of DRG neurons to a central-nervous-system—derived neurotrophic factor—BDNF

Implicit in the study of neurotrophic factors is the underlying hypothesis that target tissues synthesize and release limited amounts of specific growth factors such as NGF, the level of factor(s) being only sufficient to sustain that complement of neurons required for appropriate innervation of each tissue. Thus matching of sensory neurons with their targets during development is thought to be achieved, not by an excess of growth factor attracting a limited or precise number of sensory fibres, but rather through production of an excess of sensory neurons which are subsequently pruned to the requisite number through competition for a limiting supply of an essential neurotrophic survival factor. This hypothesis is well supported by the observation that extensive cell death occurs throughout the PNS during development (see Berg 1982) and by the experimental findings that the steady-state level of NGF is extremely low in sensory and sympathetic target tissues (Korsching and Thoenen 1983, 1985). While many details still need to be established as to its precise specificity and mode of action, NGF is clearly a key *peripheral* target-derived survival factor for neural crest-derived sensory neurons. Given that each sensory neuron projects not only to a peripheral target but also into the central nervous system (CNS), there is now considerable interest in the possibility that specification of sensory neurons during development may also be influenced not only by epigenetic cues in the periphery but also by trophic factors derived from their central 'target'. This suggestion arises from observations from studies *in vitro* and *in vivo*. Tissue culture studies using explant and dissociated neuronal cultures have indicated that tissue extracts and medium that has been conditioned by a variety of cell types contain neurotrophic activities which are distinct from NGF and which act upon both peripheral and central neurons (for reviews, see Varon and Adler, 1981; Barde, Edgar, and Thoenen 1983; Berg 1982, 1984). The first indication that the survival of DRG neurons might be partially dependent on a CNS-derived neurotrophic factor came from a study which showed that conditioned medium from a rat C-6 glioma cell line contained neurotrophic activity which supported the survival and outgrowth of neurites from dissociated neuron-enriched cultures of chick embryo DRG (Barde *et al.* 1978). Further studies demonstrated that similar activity was present in cultures of adult rat brain astroglial cells (Lindsay 1979; Lindsay *et al.* 1982) and in extracts of chick and rat brain (Lindsay and Tarbit 1979; Barde *et al.* 1980). In all the above cases the inability of anti-NGF antibodies to block or to neutralize the CNS-derived neurotrophic activity has been taken as an indication that this factor is distinct from NGF. While this argument is probably valid for neurotrophic activity detected in rat tissue extracts and in cultures derived from rat tissues, as *in vivo* studies with rats have clearly shown that antibodies to mouse NGF cross-react and neutralize rat NGF (Levi-Montalcini and Angeletti 1966), with chick tissue this may be a questionable conclusion as it would appear from all studies to date that there is no endogenous chick NGF which exhibits immunological cross-reactivity with antibodies to mouse NGF.

The purification of BDNF from pig brain (Barde *et al.* 1982) has provided the most compelling evidence to date that DRG sensory neurons may require both a peripheral (NGF) and a central (BDNF) target-derived neurotrophic factor. While it was initially thought that NGF and BDNF might act upon DRG neurons at different stages in development (Barde *et al.* 1980), it has recently been shown that chick embryo DRG neurons are equally responsive to NGF and BDNF as early as E6 in development when grown in culture on a laminin-coated substrate (Lindsay *et al.*, 1985a). Between ages E6 and E12, saturating levels of either NGF or BDNF alone sustain survival and fibre outgrowth from approximately 50 per cent of DRG neurons, while in combination both factors can promote almost 100 per cent survival of chick DRG neurons in culture. The observed additive effect of NGF and BDNF makes it tempting to draw the conclusion that there are two populations of DRG neurons, one dependent on NGF and the other dependent on BDNF. However, other interpretations of these results are possible, especially in view of the heterogeneous developmental stages of individual neurons within the E6 to E12 chick DRG, as discussed above. The present lack of antibodies to BDNF or a cDNA probe to the BDNF message currently limits our knowledge about the distribution of this neurotrophic factor and its site of synthesis. To act, however, as a CNS 'target-derived' factor for DRG neurons, one would expect BDNF to be present in the spinal cord. Although when assayed in tissue culture on a variety of peripheral neurons, developing spinal cord appears to be one of the poorest tissue sources of neurotrophic activity (Lindsay and Tarbit 1979; Riopelle and Cameron 1981; Ebendal, Norrgren, and Hedlund 1983), we have observed that there is BDNF-like activity in extracts prepared from four week old chick and adult rat and adult human spinal cord (Lindsay and Peters 1984).

Until recently there was little evidence from *in vivo* studies to indicate that sensory neurons derived any trophic support from their central targets. Indeed, such a notion seemed unlikely in view of the consistent finding that dorsal rhizotomy in adults caused little degeneration and virtually no loss of neuronal cell bodies within spinal ganglia (see Yip and Johnson 1984; Johnson, Rich, and Yip 1986; and references in both). However, in a novel series of lesioning experiments in both neo-natal and adult rodents (experiments involving dorsal rhizotomy, combined central and peripheral lesions, and combined lesions coupled with NGF deprivation or NGF supplement), Johnson and colleagues have now established a good case for a central target growth factor being essential for the survival of early post-natal sensory neurons and for sustaining the recovery of axotomised mature sensory neurons (Yip and Johnson 1984; Johnson and Yip 1985; Johnson *et al.* 1986). On the basis that NGF injected intraspinally has been shown to be retrogradely transported by the central processes of DRG neurons (Richardson and Riopelle 1984; Yip and Johnson 1984), it has been postulated that NGF itself, in addition to its role in the periphery, may act as a central target-derived neurotrophic growth factor for sensory neurons. Although there is indirect support for this view in the recent detection of β NGF messenger RNA in spinal cord tissue (Shelton and Reichardt 1986), there is apparently no detectable NGF protein in either dorsal root nerve segments or in spinal cord tissue (Korsching and Thoenen 1985).

Response of placode-derived sensory neurons to target tissue extracts and BDNF

Although refractory to the survival and neurite-promoting activity of NGF, dissociated cultures of placode-derived sensory neurons are responsive to neurotrophic activity present in tissue extracts and co-cultured astroglial cells (Lindsay 1979; Lindsay and Wilson 1980; Lindsay *et al.* 1982; Lindsay and Peters 1984). To date the most detailed study has been carried out with the chick embryo nodose ganglion (Lindsay and Rohrer 1985). Although present to some degree in extracts of most tissues, neurotrophic activity for nodose ganglion neurons was found to be greatest in extracts of vagal nerve target tissues such as liver and heart and also in brain tissue. Saturating levels of chick liver extract were found to elicit neurite outgrowth from chick nodose neurons as early as embryonic day 5 (25 per cent), with a maximum response of 50–60 per cent of these placodal neurons at E10–E12 (Lindsay and Rohrer 1985). As with neurotrophic activity for nodose ganglion neurons detected in co-cultured astroglial cells (Lindsay 1979), the neurite-promoting activity of tissue extracts such as liver was not blocked by antibodies to mouse NGF. Neurons of the placode-derived petrosal ganglion were also found to be responsive to liver-derived neurotrophic activity (Davies and Lindsay 1985). Although a detailed understanding of the trophic support that placodal neurons derive from their peripheral targets will require purification of the factors involved and demonstration of a role(s) *in vivo*, it would appear that neural crest- and neural placode-derived sensory neurons do not compete with each other for a limited supply of a single neurotrophic growth factor such as NGF. It seems likely that many peripheral tissues will be found to contain two or more neurotrophic factors, factors which may have broad specificity for either crest or placodal neurons (but not both), or perhaps even narrower specificity for sub-populations of either of these two categories. A very obvious reason to predict differences in the neurotrophic growth factor requirements of placodal and crest-derived sensory neurons are the findings that the birth dates of these two populations are fairly well separated in early chick development (Carr and Simpson 1978; D'Amico-Martel 1982). This fact alone makes it difficult to envisage how, within a single target tissue, selection through competition for a limiting supply of a single neurotrophic factor can operate as a mechanism to achieve the appropriate innervation from two distinct populations of sensory fibres which reach this target at developmental stages which are as much as 2–3 days apart. A more reasonable hypothesis would be that placodal sensory neurons compete among themselves for a limited supply of one or more neurotrophic factors, while the later born neural crest-derived sensory neurons compete among themselves for a different neurotrophic factor(s), which is probably NGF.

While putative peripheral target-derived neurotrophic factors for NGF-insensitive placodal neurons await purification, we have recently established that placodal and neural crest-derived sensory neurons are equally responsive to purified BDNF (Lindsay *et al.* 1985*b*). Comparing the response of dissociated cultures of chick embryo DRG and nodose neurons to BDNF, we observed that BDNF supported survival and neurite outgrowth from both types of neurons as early as E6 in embryonic development. Betwen E6 and E12, about half of each population was responsive to BDNF, especially when laminin was used as a substrate. While NGF had an additive effect with BDNF towards DRG neurons, with nodose ganglion neurons the combination of NGF and BDNF was no greater than saturating levels of BDNF alone. These observation have suggested that placodal and crest-derived sensory neurons, while clearly differing in their requirements for peripheral target-derived neurotrophic factors, may share a requirement for the same neurotrophic factor in their central target, the CNS. In support of this, recent results with explant cultures have indicated that there are at least some BDNF-responsive cells in all placodal and crest-derived sensory ganglia (Davies *et al.* 1986*b*). However, with limited quantitative data from tissue culture studies at present, and the absence of any evidence for a role *in vivo*, the physiological significance of BDNF has still to be established.

ADULT PERIPHERAL NERVOUS SYSTEM

Do mature sensory neurons require NGF for survival or maintenance?

Adult sensory neurons in vitro

Although it is almost a decade since Scott (1977) described a procedure for the preparation of cultures of adult mouse dorsal root ganglion neurons, there have been very few *in vitro* studies using cultures of adult mammalian PNS. From the few published studies available (Scott 1977; Kim, Warren, and Kalkia 1979; Fukada and Kameyama 1980; Goldenberg and De Boni 1983; Unsicker, Skaper, Davis, Manthorpe, and Varon 1985) it is not possible to draw any conclusions as to the trophic requirements of adult sensory neurons. Although in several of these studies adult sensory neurons clearly survived for long periods in the absence of exogenous NGF, the presence of chick embryo extract or abundant non-neuronal cells—either being a probable source of NGF and other neurotrophic molecules—may have contributed to this survival. In the only study where neuron enrichment was carried out before plating adult (rabbit) DRG cultures, NGF was always included in the culture medium but no assessment was made as to whether or not NGF was essential for survival or neurite outgrowth (Goldenberg and De Boni 1983). By implementing minor improvements to a dissociation procedure (Scott 1977) and by modifying an established pre-plating procedure (McCarthy and Partlow 1976), I have recently been able to obtain viable adult rat DRG neurons in high yield (80 per cent) and high purity (80–90 per cent) such that the response of these cells to NGF and BDNF etc. can be studied in culture in the absence of possible endogenous neurotrophic support from non-neuronal cells. Initial results (Lindsay 1987) indicate that the vast majority of adult DRG sensory neurons do not require NGF or BDNF for survival even during long periods (30 days) in culture. However, while NGF or BDNF have no apparent effect on survival of adult sensory neurons cultured in the presence or absence of non-neuronal cells, both neurotrophic factors were found to markedly enhance the initial regeneration of neurites in adult cultures. A detailed morphometric study is in progress to determine whether these growth factors enhance sprouting in all or only a sub-population of adult sensory neurons and whether they continue to enhance neurite elongation over several days or longer.

In vivo *studies of the trophic requirements of adult sensory neurons*

Chronic NGF deprivation in neonatal or adult rodents has consistently been found to produce little or no cell death in DRG (Levi-Montalcini and Angeletti 1966, 1968; Schwartz *et al.* 1982; Rich *et al.* 1984; Johnson *et al.* 1986), although a loss of 20 per cent of neurons in lumbar (L_5) DRG has been reported in neo-natal rats treated with NGF antibodies daily for one week (Yip *et al.* 1984). In contrast to this, administration of exogenous NGF or NGF antibodies to post-natal rodents has been shown to have dramatic effects (marked depletion and marked elevation, respectively) on the level of the putative neurotransmitter substance P found in DRG (Kessler and Black 1980; Otten, Goedert, Mayer, and Lembeck 1980). Thus it is now generally thought that although NGF is not required as a survival factor for adult sensory neurons, it may play a continuous role in the maintenance of adult peptidergic sensory neurons in particular. Johnson and Yip (1985) have recently shown, however, that although NGF antibodies do not initiate any destruction of adult DRG neurons nor enhance the loss of DRG neurons caused by peripheral nerve crush, dorsal rhizotomy in NGF-deprived (auto-immune) adult guinea pigs leads to far greater (25 per cent) loss of cells than occurs in control animals receiving such a lesion (3 per cent loss). This observation, and those from similar types of experiments carried out with neo-natal rodents (Yip and Johnson 1984), suggest that the survival of post-natal

DRG neurons and the recovery of injured adult neurons may be dependent on trophic support derived from both the peripheral and central targets of these cells. It is possible that during development the level of neurotrophic factor(s) may be subsaturating in both the peripheral and the central target fields such that the survival of individual sensory neurons is dependent on the combined level of neurotrophic support available to it from both targets. Thus, as has been shown, deprivation from either source will lead to loss of cells. In the adult, however, the level of neurotrophic factor required for survival of individual cells may be less than during development, such that adequate levels (supersaturating) can be derived from either the periphery or the central target field. This could explain why NGF deprivation alone is not sufficient to cause destruction of mature sensory neurons, but why the combined effects of NGF antibodies and dorsal rhizotomy on the survival of adult sensory neurons is much greater (two fold) than dorsal rhizotomy alone (Johnson and Yip 1985; Johnson *et al.* 1986).

CONCLUSIONS

The wide access to purified NGF and NGF-antibodies, and more recently the availability of cDNA probes to NGF messenger RNA, have allowed detailed verification of the long-standing hypothesis that development of the vertebrate PNS is greatly tailored by epigenetic factors. Although NGF has proven an excellent archetype molecule to test the principle of neurotrophism, it is clear that our understanding of many aspects of NGF are incomplete, such as its mode of action, its site and regulation of synthesis, its precise specificity, etc. While it is likely that these gaps will be filled in the near future, the identification and purification of other neurotrophic molecules, especially growth factors which may be important in CNS development, remains an exciting challenge in neurobiology. While the dramatic effects of NGF antibodies on PNS development have provided some of the key evidence to establish a physiological role for NGF, it is an open question as to whether such experiments will be so dramatically successful with other neurotrophic growth factors.

ACKNOWLEDGEMENTS

I gratefully acknowledge the contribution of my co-authors to publications cited in this chapter. I am especially grateful to Drs Yves Barde and Herman Rohrer for their enthusiastic collaboration over several years.

REFERENCES

Ayer-le Lièvre, C. S. and Le Douarin, N. M. (1982). The early development of cranial sensory ganglia and the potentialities of their component cells studied in quail-chick chimeras. *Dev. Biol.* **94,** pp. 291–310.

Baccaglini, P. I. and Cooper, E. (1982). Electrophysiological studies of newborn rat nodose neurones in cell culture. *J. Physiol (Lond.)* **324**, pp. 429–39.

Barde, Y. -A., Edgar, D., and Thoenen, H. (1980). Sensory neurons in culture: changing requirements for survival factors during embryonic development. *Proc. Natl. Acad. Sci. USA* **77**, pp. 1199–203.

Barde, Y. -A., Edgar, D., and Thoenen, H. (1982). Purification of a new neurotrophic factor from mammalian brain. *EMBO J.* **1**, pp. 549–53.

Barde, Y. -A., Edgar, D., and Thoenen, H. (1983). New neurotrophic factors. *Ann. Rev. Physiol.* **45**, pp. 601–12.

Barde, Y. -A., Lindsay, R. M., Monard, D., and Thoenen, H. (1978). New factor released by cultured glioma cells supporting survival and growth of sensory neurones. *Nature* **274**, p. 818.

Berg, D. K. (1982). Cell death in neuronal development. Regulation by trophic factors. In *Neuronal development* (ed. N. C. Spitzer), pp. 297–331. Plenum Press, New York.

Berg, D. K. (1984). New neuronal growth factors. *Ann. Rev. Neurosci.* **7**, pp. 140–70.

Carr, V. Mc and Simpson, S. B. (1978). Proliferative and degenerative events in the early development of the chick dorsal root ganglia. 1. Normal development. *J. Comp. Neurol.* **182**, pp. 727–40.

D'Amico Martel, A. (1982). Temporal patterns of neurogenesis in avian cranial sensory and autonomic ganglia. *Amer. J. Anat.* **163**, pp. 351–72.

D'Amico Martel, A. and Noden, D. (1983). Contributions of placodal and neural crest cells to avian cranial peripheral ganglia. *Amer. J. Anat.* **166**, pp. 445–68.

Davies, A. M. and Lindsay, R. M. (1984). Neural crest-derived spinal and cranial sensory neurones are equally sensitive to NGF but differ in their response to tissue extracts. *Dev. Brain Res.* **13**, pp. 121–7.

Davies, A. M. and Lindsay, R. M. (1985). The cranial sensory ganglia in culture: differences in the response of placode-derived and neural crest-derived neurons to nerve growth factor. *Dev. Biol.* **111**, pp. 62–72.

Davies, A. and Lumsden, A. (1983). Influence of nerve growth factor on developing dorso–medial and ventrolateral neurons of chick and mouse trigeminal ganglia. *Int. J. Neurosci* **1**, pp. 171–7.

Davies, A. M., Lumsden, A. G. S., and Rohrer, H. (1986a). Neural crest-derived proprioceptive neurons express NGF receptors but are not supported by NGF in culture. *Neurosci.* **20**, pp. 37–46.

Davies, A. M., Thoenen, H., and Barde, Y. -A. (1986b). The response of chick sensory neurons to brain-derived neurotrophic factor. *J. Neurosci.* **6**, pp. 1897–904.

Ebendal, T. and Hedlund, K. -O. (1974). Histology of the chick embryo trigeminal ganglion and initial effects of its cultivation with and without nerve growth factor. *Zoon* **2**, pp. 25–35.

Ebendal, T. and Hedlund, K. -O. (1975). Effects of nerve growth factor on the chick trigeminal ganglion in culture. *Zoon* **3**, pp. 33–47.

Ebendal, T., Norrgren, G., and Hedlund, K. -O. (1983). Nerve growth-promoting activity in the chick embryo: quantitative aspects. *Med. Biol.* **61**, pp. 65–72.

Edelman, G. M. (1984). Modulation of cell adhesion during induction, histogenesis, and perinatal development of the nervous system. *Ann. Rev. Neurosci.* **7**, pp. 3239–77.

Edgar, D., Timpl, R., and Thoenen, H. (1984). The heparin binding domain of laminin is responsible for its effects on neurite outgrowth and neuronal survival. *EMBO J.* **3**, pp. 1463–8.

Fenton, E. L. (1970). Tissue culture assay of nerve growth factor and of the specific antiserum. *Exp. Cell Res.* **59**, pp. 383–92.

Fukuda, J. and Kameyama, M. (1980). A tissue-culture of nerve cells from adult mammalian ganglia and some electrophysiological properties of nerve cells *in vitro*. *Brain Res.* **202**, pp. 249–55.

Goedert, M., Otten, U., Hunt, S. P., Bond, A., Chapman, D., Schlumpf, M., and Lichtensteiger, W. (1984). Biochemical and anatomical effects of antibodies against nerve growth factor on developing rat sensory ganglia. *Proc. Natl. Acad. Sci. USA* **81**, pp. 1580–4.

Goldenberg, S. S. S. and De Boni, U. (1983). Pure populations of viable neurons from rabbit dorsal root ganglia using gradients of percoll. *J. Neurobiol.* **14**, pp. 195–206.

Gorin, P. D. and Johnson, E. M. (1980). Effects of long term nerve growth factor deprivation on the nervous system of the adult rat: an experimental autoimmune approach. *Brain Res.* **198**, pp. 27–42.

Greene, L. A. (1977). Quantitative *in vitro* studies on the nerve growth factor (NGF) requirement of neurons. II. Sensory neurons. *Dev. Biol.* **58**, pp. 106–13.

Hamburger, V. (1962). Specificity in neurogenesis. *J. Cell. Comp. Physiol.* **60**, pp. 581–92.

Hamburger, V., Bruno-Bechtold, J. K., and Yip, J. W. (1981). Neuronal death in the spinal ganglia of the chick embryo and its reduction by nerve growth factor. *J. Neurosci.* **1**, pp. 60–71.

Hedlund, K. -O. and Ebendal, T. (1980). The chick embryo nodose ganglion: effects of nerve growth factor in culture. *J. Neurocytol.* **9**, pp. 665–82.

Herrup, K. and Shooter, E. M. (1975). Properties of β-NGF receptor in development. *J. Cell Biol.*, **67**, pp. 118–25.

Johnson, E. M., Jr and Yip, H. K. (1985). Central nervous system and peripheral nerve growth factor provide trophic support critical to mature sensory neuronal survival. *Nature* **314**, pp. 751–52.

Johnson, E. M., Rich, M., and Yip, H. K. (1986). The role of NGF in sensory neurons *in vivo*. *Trends Neurosci.* **9**, pp. 33–7.

Johnson, E. M., Gorin, P. D., Brandeis, L. D., and Pearson, J. (1980). Dorsal root ganglion neurons are destroyed by exposure *in utero* to maternal antibody to nerve growth factor. *Science* **210**, pp. 916–18.

Johnson, E. M., Gorin, P. D., Osborne, P. A., Rydel, R. E., and Pearson, J. (1982). Effects of autoimmune NGF deprivation in the adult rabbit and offspring. *Brain Res.* **240**, pp. 131–40.

Kessler, J. A. and Black, I. B. (1980) Nerve growth factor stimulates the development of substance P in sensory ganglia. *Proc. Natl. Acad. Sci. USA.* **77**, pp. 649–52.

Kim, S. U., Warren, K. G., and Kalkia, M. (1979). Tissue culture of adult human neurons. *Neurosci. Lett.* **11**, pp. 137–41.

Korsching, S. and Thoenen, H. (1983). Nerve growth factor in sympathetic ganglia and corresponding target organs of the rat: correlation with density of sympathetic innervation. *Proc. Natl. Acad. Sci. USA* **80**, 3513–16.

Korsching, S. and Thoenen, H. (1985). Nerve growth factor supply for sensory neurons. Site of origin and competition with the sympathetic nervous system. *Neurosci. Lett.* **54**, pp. 201–5.

Le Douarin, N. M. (1982). *The neural crest* . Cambridge University Press, Cambridge.

Le Douarin, N. M. (1973). A biological cell labelling technique and its use in experimental embryology. *Dev. Biol.* **20**, pp. 217–22.

Levi-Montalcini, R. (1962). Analysis of a specific nerve growth factor and its antiserum. *Sci. Rept. Ist. Super Sanita* **2,** pp. 345–68.

Levi-Montalcini, R. (1966). The nerve growth factor: its mode of action on sensory and sympathetic nerve cells. *The Harvey Lectures* **60,** pp. 217–59.

Levi-Montalcini, R. and Angeletti, P. U. (1966). Immunosympathectomy. *Pharmacol. Rev.* **18,** pp. 619–28.

Levi-Montalcini, R. and Angeletti, P. U. (1968). Nerve growth factor. *Physiol. Rev.* **48,** pp. 534–69.

Lindsay, R. M. (1979). Adult rat brain astrocytyes support survival of both NGF-dependent and NGF-insensitive neurones. *Nature* **282,** pp. 80–2.

Lindsay, R. M. (1987). Nerve growth factors enhance axonal regeneration but are not required for survival of adult sensory neurons. (submitted).

Lindsay, R. M. and Peters, C. (1984). Spinal cord contains neurotrophic activity for spinal nerve sensory neurons. Late developmental appearance of a survival factor distinct from nerve growth factor. *Neuroscience* **12,** pp. 45–51.

Lindsay, R. M. and Rohrer, H. (1985). Placodal sensory neurons in culture. Nodose ganglion neurons are unresponsive to NGF, lack NGF receptors but are supported by a liver-derived neurotrophic factor *Dev. Biol.* **112,** pp. 30–48.

Lindsay, R. M. and Tarbit, J. (1979). Developmentally regulated induction of neurite outgrowth from immature chick sensory neurons (DRG) by homogenates of avian and mammalian heart, liver and brain. *Neurosci. Lett.* **12,** pp. 195–200.

Lindsay, R. M. and Wilson, J. (1980). Survival in vitro of nodose ganglion neurons in response to target tissue extracts or glial cells. *Neurosci. Lett.* Suppl. **5,** p. 124.

Lindsay, R. M., Barde, Y. -A., Davies, A. M., and Rohrer, H. (1985*a*). Differences and similarities in the neurotrophic requirements of sensory neurons derived from neural crest and neural placode. *J. Cell Sci.* Suppl. **3,** pp. 115–29.

Lindsay, R. M. and Thoenen, H. and Barde, Y. -A. (1985*b*). Placode and neural crest-derived sensory neurons are responsive at early developmental stages to brain-derived neurotrophic factor (BDNF). *Dev. Biol.* **112,** pp. 319–28.

Lindsay, R. M., Barber, P. C., Sherwood, M. R. C., Zimmer, J., and Raisman, G. (1982). Astrocytes from adult rat brain. Derivation, characterization and neurotrophic properties of pure astrological cells from corpus callosum. *Brain Res.* **243,** pp. 329–43.

Lumsden, A. G. S. (1987). Diffusible factors and chemotropism in the development of the peripheral nervous system. In *The Making of the Nervous System* (eds. J. G. Parnavelas, C. D. Stern, and R. V. Stirling), pp. 166–87. Oxford University Press, Oxford.

Mathieu, C., Moisand, A., and Weber, M. J. (1984). Acetylcholine metabolism by cultured neurons from rat nodose ganlia: regulation by a macromolecule from muscle-conditioned medium. *Neuroscience* **13,** pp. 1373–86.

McCarthy, K. D. and Partlow, L. M. (1976). Preparation of pure neuronal and non-neuronal cultures of embryonic chick sympathetic ganglia: a new method based on both differential cell adhesiveness and the formation of homotypic neuronal aggregates. *Brain Res.* **114,** pp. 392–414.

Narayanan, C. H. and Narayanan, Y. (1980). Neural crest and placodal contributions in the development of the glossopharyngeal-vagal complex in the chick. *Anat. Rec.* **196,** pp. 71–82.

Noden, D. M. (1978). The control of avian cephalic neural crest cytodifferentiation. *Dev. Biol.* **67,** pp. 313–29.

Otten, U., Goedert, M., Mayer, N., and Lembeck, F. (1980). Requirement of nerve growth factor for development of substance P-containing sensory neurones. *Nature* **287**, pp. 158–9.

Pearson, J., Johnson, E. M., and Brandeis, L. (1983). Effects of antibodies to nerve growth factor on intrauterine development of derivatives of cranial neural crest and placode in the guinea pig. *Dev. Biol.* **96**, pp. 32–6.

Rich, K. M., Yip, H. K., Osborne, P. A., Schmidt, R. E., and Johnson, E. M., Jr (1984). Role of nerve growth factor in the adult dorsal root ganglion neuron and its response to injury. *J. Comp. Neurol.* **230**, pp. 110–18.

Richardson, P. M. and Riopelle, R. J. (1984). Uptake of nerve growth factor along peripheral and spinal axons of primary sensory neurons. *J. Neurosci.* **4**, pp. 1683–9.

Riopelle, R. J. and Cameron, D. A. (1981). Neurite growth promoting factors of embryonic chick—ontogeny, regional distribution, and characteristics. *J. Neurobiol.* **12**, pp. 175–86.

Rohrer, H. and Barde, Y. -A. (1982). Presence and disappearance of nerve growth factor receptors on sensory neurons in culture. *Dev. Biol.* **89**, pp. 309–15.

Sato, M. (1985). Different effects of nerve growth factor on cultured sympathetic and sensory neurons. *Brain Res.* **345**, pp. 192–5.

Schwartz, J. P., Pearson, J., and Johnson, E. M., Jr (1982). Effect of exposure to anti-NGF on sensory neurons of adult rats and guinea pigs. *Brain Res.* **244**, pp. 378–81.

Scott, B. S. (1977). Adult mouse dorsal root ganglia neurons in cell culture. *J. Neurobiol.* **8**, pp. 417–27.

Shelton, D. L. and Reichardt, L. F. (1986). Studies on the expression of the beta nerve growth factor (NGF) gene in the central nervous system: level and regional distribution of NGF mRNA suggest that NGF functions as a trophic factor for several distinct populations of neurons. *Proc. Natl. Acad. Sci. USA.* **83**, pp. 2714–8.

Thiery, J. P., Duband, J. L., and Tucker, G. C. (1985). Cell migration in the vertebrate embryo: role of cell adhesion and tissue environment in pattern formation. *Ann. Rev. Cell Biol.* **1**, pp. 91–113.

Thoenen, H. and Barde, Y. -A. (1980) Physiology of nerve growth factor. *Physiol. Rev.* **60**, pp. 1284–335.

Unsicker, K., Skaper, S. D., Davis, G. E., Manthorpe, M., and Varon, S. (1985) Comparison of the effects of laminin and polyornithine-binding neurite promoting factor from RN22 Schwannoma cells on neurite regeneration from cultured newborn and adult rat dorsal root ganglion neurons. *Dev. Brain Res.* **17**, pp. 304–8.

Varon, S. and Adler, R. (1981). Trophic and specifying factors directed to neuronal cells. *Adv. Cellular Neurobiol.* **2**, pp. 115–63.

Winick, M. and Greenberg, R. E. (1965). Chemical study of sensory ganglia during a critical period of development. *Nature* **205**, pp. 180–1.

Yip, H. K. and Johnson, E. M. (1984). Developing dorsal root ganglion neurons require trophic support from their central processes: evidence for a role of retrogradely transported nerve growth factor from the central nervous system to the periphery. *Proc. Natl. Acad. Sci. USA* **81**, pp. 6245–9.

Yip, H. K., Rich, K. M., Lampe, P. A., and Johnson, E. M. (1984). The effects of nerve growth factor and its antiserum on the postnatal development and survival after injury of sensory neurons in dorsal root ganglia. *J. Neurosci.* **4**, pp. 2986–92.

from the side of a sensory ganglion explant facing an NGF-producing tumour (Lamont 1968) or a capillary tube containing NGF (Charlwood, Lamont and Banks 1972; Ebendal and Jacobson 1977*a*; Rutishauser and Edelman 1980). Neurites regenerating from sympathetic neurons cultured with NGF did not cross a silicone grease barrier and enter a medium to which no NGF had been added, while neurites readily crossed such a barrier when NGF was present on both sides (Campenot 1977). Letourneau (1978) has demonstrated a slight but consistent preferred orientation of chick dorsal root ganglion (DRG) growth cones up a concentration gradient of NGF in an agar matrix. Gundersen and Barrett (1979) observed that when growth cones of chick DRG neurons are presented, at a distance of less than 25 μm, with a micropipette releasing a high concentration of NGF, they turn and grow towards that source. The rapidity of this re-orientation (about 20 minutes), together with the facts that it did not involve an increased growth rate as compared with that of neurites growing at a distance from the source and that it was not abolished by background levels of NGF, led Gundersen and Barrett (1980) to conclude that the turning response was not due to the trophic effect of NGF.

An important consideration when evaluating the above *in vitro* studies is that although NGF is required for survival and growth of the late, axotomized neurons used for these experiments, NGF is not required by early sensory neurons during their initial growth to the periphery (Davies, Lumsden, Slavkin, and Burnstock 1981; Lumsden and Davies 1983; Lindsay, Thoenen, and Barde 1985).

NGF DOES NOT MEET THE REQUIREMENTS OF A NATURAL CHEMOATTRACTANT

The above observations, taken together, demonstrate that neurons are capable of making a chemotropic response (for discussion, see Dunn 1981 and Bray 1982), but they do not show that NGF has a long-range chemotropic role in development. Indeed, there are cogent reasons for considering that NGF is not a natural chemoattractant. To produce the highly organized and stereotyped patterns of peripheral nerves, such agents must fulfil three requirements; they must be regionally specific, they must be available at the appropriate time in development, and they should be produced at a level sufficient for free diffusion and the establishment of a gradient over the distance that nerve fibres grow to reach their targets. The directional response to NGF, however, is not restricted to one subpopulation of neurons with a single target specificity, but appears to be elicited from many populations of both sympathetic (Menesini-Chen *et al.* 1978) and DRG neurons (Gundersen and Barrett 1980) whose targets *in vivo* are virtually ubiquitous. In the only early developing system so far studied with an assay method of adequate resolution (the mouse embryo trigeminal, using two-site enzyme immuno-assay), NGF is detectable in the maxillary process target field at and after the time of innervation but is not detectable in this target field earlier, during the critical period of primary peripheral outgrowth from the trigeminal ganglion (Davies and Korsching, pers. comm.). Even at its peak level, which is reached shortly after target encounter at embryonic day 13 (E13), the amount of NGF in the maxillary process is approximately eight orders of magnitude less than that used to demonstrate a turning response *in vitro* (about 50 μg/ml; Gundersen and Barrett 1979). Since NGF at such high concentrations increases the adhesion of NGF-receptor-bearing growth cones to the substratum (Schubert and Whitlock 1977), and growth cones move preferentially from less to more adhesive substrata (Letourneau 1975), the possibility exists that the turning response, rather than being evidence of a chemotropic mechanism, was an artefact involving abnormal adhesive interactions. An adhesion gradient has itself been widely considered as a possible guidance mechanism (Letourneau 1982), although the evidence for haptotaxis is scant and difficult to adduce (Trinkaus 1985).

Notwithstanding these objections, experiments with NGF have shown that this molecule can diffuse from a source and establish effective gradients over a considerable distance both *in vitro* (Letourneau 1978) and, presumably, *in vivo* (Menesini-Chen *et al.* 1978), and thereby demonstrate the feasibility of chemotropism as a long-range guidance mechanism in the embryo.

Objections to the putative involvement of NGF in developmental nerve guidance, founded on its lack of neuronal specificity, could be overcome if it were assumed that its role is merely to stimulate the growth of nerve fibres along preferred steric guidance pathways (Purves 1982). This action, however, would not be tropic since it would be the pathway rather than the gradient which gives direction, and the lack of NGF at the appropriate time in development suggests that even this trophic role would be limited to local stimulation once nerve fibres have reached the general vicinity of their target.

That NGF may indeed operate locally to modulate axonal arborizations by a trophic mechanism has been shown by Campenot (1982*a*, 1982*b*); sympathetic ganglion cells cultured with NGF in the central compartment of a three-compartment chamber extended neurites along avenues of collagen through a grease seal into the side compartments. Although the rate of neurite elongation in the side compartments was independent of the local NGF concentration, this did influence neurite density (Campenot 1982*a*). Withdrawal of NGF from a side compartment caused a local regression of neurites without affecting survival of their parent neurons in the central compartment (Campenot 1982*b*).

Final elucidation of the role of NGF during the period of nerve guidance, whether it operates at long-range, short-range, or not at all, will require the observation of developing projections in embryos in which the effect of any endogenous NGF has been eliminated by antibody blockade.

PERIPHERAL TARGET ORGANS HAVE A TROPHIC BUT NOT NECESSARILY A TROPIC EFFECT ON NEURONS

A second line of evidence which has been held to support Cajal's chemotropic theory comes from observations of neurite outgrowth from explanted neural tissue in co-culture with peripheral target organs. For example, an increased outgrowth of neurites was observed from rat sympathetic ganglia on the side of the explant facing vas deferens (Chamley, Goller, and Burnstock 1973; Chamley and Dowel 1975), from frog spinal cord facing limb-bud mesenchyme (Pollack, Muhlach, and Liebig 1981), and from various sensory, sympathetic, and parasympathetic ganglia of the chick embryo facing a number of tissues (Ebendal and Jacobson 1977*b*; Ebendal, Jordell-Kylberg, and Soderstrom 1978; Ebendal 1981). In these studies, however, neurite outgrowth was not confined to the target-facing side of the neural explant, nor was the outgrowth on this side consistently directed towards the target tissue; rather, the presence of the target caused an increase in the vigour or profusion of radially extending neurites. This pattern of growth is suggestive of a scalar response to a trophic (in the sense of growth-stimulating) activity enhancing the growth of neurons which happen to be nearest its source. A tropic response, on the other hand, is characterized by a vector field, which is described by both the magnitude and the direction of the concentration gradient (Dunn 1981).

One reason why trophic responses have been mistaken for tropic responses is that co-culture studies have mostly been conducted between denervated targets and regenerating neurons. It is questionable whether tissues which have already become innervated can be regarded as developmental targets and it may be that neurons which have already encountered their targets would have become dependent on a target-derived trophic factor for their survival and growth. Amongst the few exceptions to this general use of inappropriately aged explants is Coughlin's (1975) study of the effects of mouse embryo submandibular gland epithelium on neurite outgrowth from the parasympathetic submandibular ganglion. Here, neurites grew towards target epithelium co-cultured in juxtaposition with the ganglion, but, because the ganglion cells are dispersed within and were evidently inseparable from capsular mesenchyme, it was not possible to test whether this was a tropic response such as would prevail in the absence of the normal pathway.

Compelling evidence of developmental chemotropism from co-culture studies will thus require the demonstration of the effect between virgin target tissues and their respective neurons growing *ab initio*, and the demonstration that the growth of neurites has been preferentially oriented towards the target by a chemical gradient acting at an appropriate distance across an isotropic matrix.

STUDIES ON A TARGET TROPIC EFFECT IN THE MOUSE EMBRYO TRIGEMINAL SYSTEM

Normal development

The trigeminal system in the mouse embryo presents some clear advantages for the study of early target influences on nerve fibre growth. The trigeminal ganglion contains primary sensory neurons, 60 per cent of which project to the whisker field at the rostral end of the maxillary process (Davies and Lumsden 1984). The target tissue of the majority of whisker afferents in the maxillary nerve is the prospective sensory epithelium; in the adult, fibres terminate as intra-epithelial disc endings in association with mechano-receptive Merkel cells in the external root sheaths of whiskers (Vincent 1913; Patrizi and Munger 1966). The maxillary nerve contains only sensory fibres from the trigeminal ganglion; analysis of its growth is thus not complicated by the presence of a contingent of motor axons (these travel in the mandibular nerve) which differ in their target specificities. The time course for development of the trigeminal whisker field projection has been documented in the mouse (Davies and Lumsden 1984); the ganglion appears at embryonic day 9 (E9 —the vaginal plug appears on day 0), and by E10 both the ganglion and the whisker field can be easily visualized and lie approximately 200 μm apart. Peripheral nerve fibre outgrowth commences at E9·5, and by E10 about 1200 fibres extend a short distance into the maxillary process. Fibres first reach the target epithelium during E11 and invade the differentiating whisker follicles during E12–13. At this time the fibre content of the maxillary nerve is maximal (about 26 000), thereafter declining to a stable complement (about 13 000) by E19. Both the ganglion and its principal target field thus form well-defined structures; the feasibility of explanting both at an appropriately early embryonic stage enables the influence of the virgin target on the growth of primary neurites to be studied *in vitro*. The final advantage in using mouse tissues for such studies is that possible synthesis of NGF by target cells in culture, which would complicate the analysis of a tropic response to some other target-derived agent, can be eliminated by direct blockade using anti-serum raised to mouse submandibular gland NGF.

The virgin maxillary process has a chemotropic influence on trigeminal ganglion neurites which is not due to NGF

Mouse embryo trigeminal ganglia have been co-cultured in collagen gels both with their own target field (the whisker field) and with an alternative inappropriate cutaneous field, the distal tip of the forelimb bud (Lumsden and Davies 1983). In three sets of experiments, tissues were explanted from E10, E11, and E12 embryos representing, respectively, the periods of initial outgrowth, mass outgrowth, and target encounter (Fig. 9.1). When cultured alone by this method, for any of the three stages, trigeminal ganglia never extended neurites. When co-cultured, however, they did extend neurites which, in the large majority of both E10 and E11 co-cultures, grew exclusively from the quadrant of the ganglion which faced the natural target, and, in this quadrant, the neurites were consistently directed towards the target. In none of these co-cultures did neurites grow towards the inappropriate cutaneous tissue. This pattern of exclusively target-directed neurite outgrowth persisted throughout the period of observation (up to 72 hours), with few or no neurites growing from lateral-facing quadrants of the ganglion.

Explants were usually spaced by between 200 and 500 μm, equivalent to the normal distance between the trigeminal ganglion and the maxillary process at E10 and E11. At a greater spacing the exclusively target-directed outgrowth still appeared but the number of neurites progressively reduced with distance up to 1 mm, beyond which the target had no detectable influence.

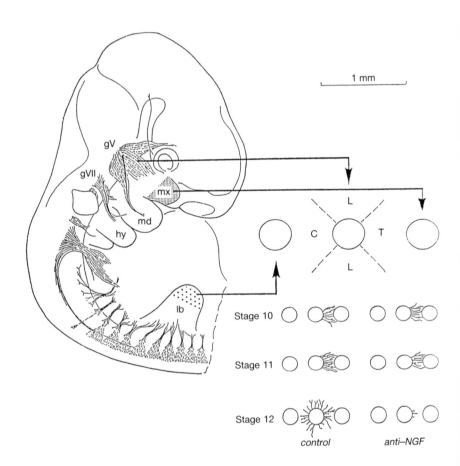

In E12 co-cultures there was a much lower incidence of exclusively target-directed outgrowth, a higher incidence of outgrowth in lateral quadrants, and, for the first time, there was outgrowth towards the inappropriate tissue. In general, the pattern of outgrowth in these later co-cultures was radial.

The addition of anti-NGF at the commencement of the culture period did not significantly influence the pattern or magnitude of neurite outgrowth in E10 co-cultures (Fig. 9.2). In E11 co-cultures anti-NGF resulted in both a small reduction in the overall number of ganglia which extended neurites and a small but significant reduction in the magnitude of outgrowth in the remainder. In E12 co-cultures, however, anti-NGF greatly reduced the number of ganglia which extended neurites and greatly reduced the lengths and number of neurites in the remainder.

The above results demonstrate the existence of an agent, immuno-chemically distinct from NGF, which is produced by the peripheral region of the maxillary process target field, and which both elicits and orients the growth of very early trigeminal neurites.

The pattern of outgrowth in E12 co-cultures (Fig. 9.4(a)) and its virtual suppression by anti-NGF indicates that at this age NGF is released by the target (and possibly also the limb bud), an interpretation which is consistent with the results of direct two-site enzyme immuno-assay of NGF in the maxillary process (Davies and Korsching, pers. comm.). That the E12 effect is not also due to the maturation of neuronal responsiveness is shown by earlier experiments (Davies *et al.* 1981; Davies and Lumsden 1984) in which NGF was shown to produce an increase in the extent of neurite outgrowth from E10

Fig. 9.1. Schema of procedure (to scale) in which the trigeminal ganglion (gV), maxillary process whisker field target tissue (mx), and limb-bud control tissue (lb) were explanted from E10 (shown), E11 and E12 mouse embryos, and co-cultured in three-dimensional hydrated collagen gels. The three explants, each one oriented at random, were aligned with the ganglion flanked by maxillary process and limb-bud explants. These were submerged in collagen gel medium (Lumsden and Davies 1983), with or without the inclusion of anti-NGF antiserum (sheep anti-mouse submandibular gland 2.5S NGF, courtesy of Dr Yves Barde), at a concentration (1 in 100) sufficient to block the activity of 2 BU/ml 2.5S NGF in the standard biological assay. The limb-bud explants provided an inappropriate target and also controlled for possible non-specific contact guidance effects mediated by alignment of fibrils in the collagen gel matrix which can result from mechanical stresses (Ebendal 1976) and cell traction (Stopak and Harris 1982). Cultures were examined after incubating for 24, 48 and 72 hours and the orientation, length, and density of neurite outgrowth in each quadrant of the ganglion measured (T, target quadrant; L, lateral quadrants; C, control quadrant). For quantitation methods see Lumsden and Davies (1983) and Davies and Lumsden (1984). A cartoon summary of the results, depicting patterns of neurite outgrowth typical of each of the six age/medium groups, is also shown. md, mandibular process; gVII, geniculate ganglion; hy, hyoid process. [Reproduced from Lumsden and Davies (1987) by kind permission of Springer-Verlag, Berlin.]

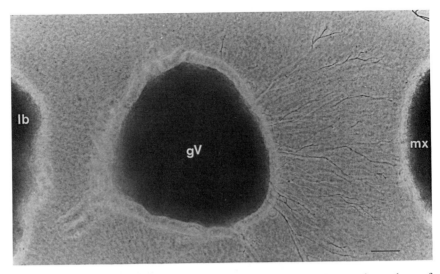

Fig. 9.2. Phase contrast photomicrograph of a representative collagen gel co-culture of E10 trigeminal ganglion (gV), maxillary process (mx), and limb-bud (lb) explants after incubating for 48 hours in medium containing a blocking level of anti-NGF anti-serum. Cytosine arabinoside (AraC, 10^{-5} M) was added at 24 hours to suppress non-neuronal cell proliferation. Neurites have extended directly and exclusively to the maxillary process target but none has emerged in the ganglion quadrants which face laterally or towards the control tissue. Scale bar: 100 μm. [Reproduced from Lumsden and Davies (1987) by kind permission of Springer-Verlag, Berlin.]

trigeminal ganglia cultured on a planar substratum. The unavailability of NGF in the maxillary process during the period of primary outgrowth, together with its production being coincident with target-field innervation (E11·5–E12), adds to the considerable body of evidence that the biological role of NGF is in the mediation of selective survival during the ensuing period of natural neuronal death (Hamburger, Brunso-Bechtold, and Yip 1981; Johnson, Gorin, Brandeis, and Pearson 1980) and further underscores the contention that it has no biological role in directing primary outgrowth.

Target field production of the agent is restricted to the period of normal primary outgrowth

The almost total suppression by anti-NGF of neurite outgrowth from E12 ganglia co-cultured with E12 maxillary processes compared with the only partial suppression of outgrowth in E11 co-cultures indicates that the NGF-independent directed outgrowth begins to decline after E11 and ceases by E12, when nerve fibres have reached the periphery during normal development. Heterochronic co-cultures indicate that the decline in the effect is probably due both to decreasing production of the agent and to decreasing reponsive-ness of trigeminal ganglion neurons (Lumsden, in prep.). It is not known whether all trigeminal ganglion neurons are responsive to the agent during E10–11 or whether its effects are restricted to a sub-population of pioneer neurons. It is interesting to speculate that innervation of the target might be responsible for down-regulating production of the agent. Similarly, NGF synthesis might be initiated by innervation; NGF messenger RNA is first detectable in the maxillary process at precisely the time that the first maxillary nerve fibres reach the periphery (Davies and Heumann, pers. comm.).

The agent is a diffusible molecule

Three-dimensional collagen gel matrices have been shown to be capable of stabilizing gradients of diffusible molecules (Ebendal *et al.* 1978; Harris, Holt, Smith, and Gallenson 1985); in our experiments, it can be presumed that the agent emanating from the E10–11 maxillary process formed a stable gradient in the gel.

The importance of the gel and the presumed gradient within it are illustrated by a further series of experiments (Lumsden, Davies, unpub. obs.) in which explants were co-cultured (with the ganglion flanked by target and control tissues and spaced as before) on a planar collagen substratum rather than in a three-dimensional collagen gel. Under these conditions the E10 and E11 targets had no directional influence on outgrowth from equivalent aged ganglia. E12 targets, however, elicited a radial outgrowth pattern similar to that which formed in the gel. An effective gradient of the agent was evidently not formed either in the medium overlying a planar substratum or adsorbed to the substratum itself.

The diffusible nature of the agent is also implied by the results of recent experiments (Lumsden and Davies 1987) which have shown that maxillary process explants can condition a liquid medium with the neurite-promoting and -orienting activity which is retained following immuno-absorption by solid phase-bound anti-laminin antiserum. By growing maxillary processes alone for 48 hours in collagen gels it is possible to precondition these with the activity, so that ganglia introduced after removal of the target exhibited outgrowth directed to the position in the gel formerly occupied by the latter. There was no outgrowth, however, when such preconditioned gels are washed with saline before introduction of ganglia (Lumsden, in prep.).

The agent has both trophic and tropic effects

The pattern of exclusively target-directed neurite outgrowth in E10 and E11 co-cultures suggests that the agent has both trophic (growth-stimulating) and tropic (neurite-orienting) effects. The trophic effect is demonstrated by the finding that neurites did not grow in the absence of appropriate target tissue.

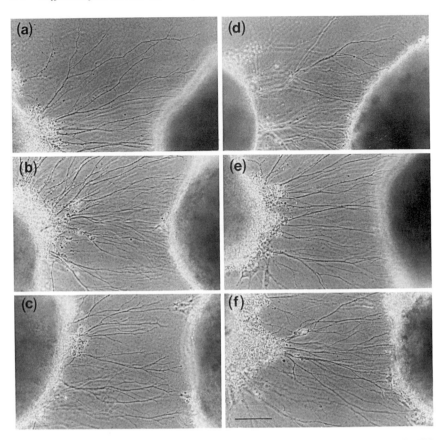

Fig. 9.3. Phase contrast photomicrographs of E10 [(a)–(c)] and E11 [(d)–(f)] co-cultures after incubating for 48 hours in medium containing a blocking level of anti-NGF antiserum and AraC, showing the pattern of target-directed neurites. Scale bar: 100 μm. [Reproduced from Lumsden and Davies (1987) by kind permission of Springer-Verlag, Berlin.]

The tropic component was deduced from several aspects of the pattern of neurite growth. First, growth cones displayed a consistent preferred orientation towards the target (Fig. 9.3). Second, neurites whose initial orientation was tangential to the target, and which would have missed it if they had continued to grow straight, consistently bent towards the target [Fig. 9.3(a) and (d)]. The shape of a neurite in a collagen gel is a faithful record of the progressive changes in direction taken by its growing tip as it threads its way through the fibrillar matrix; thus changes in direction during outgrowth can be deduced from the final pattern of growth. Third, the observation that the exclusively target-directed pattern of outgrowth persisted for a further 24–48 hours after it had become established also favours a chemotropic interpretation since it would be expected that an agent with solely trophic activity would elicit (radial) outgrowth from the lateral and away-facing surface of the ganglion as it diffused away from the source.

That this was not simply because the agent had not diffused beyond the target-facing surface of the ganglion is shown by a series of experiments in which E10 and E11 targets were co-cultured with two trigeminal ganglia in tandem (Lumsden and Davies 1983). In these, the magnitude of neurite outgrowth in the target-facing quadrant of the distal ganglion was significantly greater than that in the away-facing quadrant of the proximal ganglion. This result is not unequivocal since neurites did appear, albeit sparsely and to short extents, on the away-facing side of the proximal ganglion—which they did not when the ganglion faced a limb-bud explant. It is possible that the ganglion itself elicits some sort of trophic response, but the significantly more luxuriant growth from the distal ganglion shows that the mutual effects of the ganglia are minor compared with the target effect. This result thus demonstrates that the agent had effectively diffused beyond the proximal ganglion and that most neurite outgrowth was directed up a concentration gradient to the target. Presumably neurons on the control-facing side of ganglia in E10 and E11 co-cultures send their neurites through the ganglion to emerge on the target-facing side, but this has not been shown.

The agent is regionally specific

To estimate the role of the chemotropic agent in normal development it is necessary to establish whether there is specificity in the regional extent of the agent's production and whether there is a corresponding specificity in the neuronal populations which respond. The above experiments have indicated that the agent has some degree of regional specificity as it is not produced by the limb bud, which, although also a presumptive cutaneous field, derives sensory innervation from DRG.

A more stringent test for regional specificity of the agent would be to compare the effects of trigeminal ganglion territory (the first branchial arch) with that of the adjoining geniculate ganglion territory (the second branchial arch, Fig. 9.1) which becomes innervated during the same period of development, E10–11. Accordingly, both the trigeminal ganglion and the geniculate ganglion were each co-cultured in collagen gels with both their own and adjoining virgin target fields, the maxillary process (or mandibular process—also first arch) and the hyoid process. In all trigeminal ganglion co-cultures in which neurites grew, these were confined to the quadrant facing the first-arch explant. Although geniculate ganglia, unlike trigeminal, extended neurites when cultured alone both at E10 and E11, this outgrowth was neither augmented by, nor oriented to, co-cultured target tissue of either arch. These findings (Lumsden and Davies 1986) show that production of the agent (hereafter referred to as maxillary process chemotropic factor or Max Factor (MF)) is precisely limited to the trigeminal field; it is not detectable in the adjoining target field, and it affects the population of neurons appropriate to its field but not those of the adjoining field. An equivalent chemotropic effect in the second arch was not detected.

The source of MF is within the target epithelium

The identity of the cells in the target field which synthesize MF has been preliminarily investigated by culturing E10 and E11 trigeminal ganglia with the epithelial and mesenchymal components of the maxillary process, separated by enzyme digestion of the intervening basement membrane (Lumsden and Davies 1986). When co-cultured in three-dimensional gels, neurites appeared within 48 hours in the epithelium-facing quadrant and were directed to this tissue (Fig. 9.4(b)). No neurites grew in lateral- and mesenchyme-facing quadrants. In a second set of experiments, co-cultures were set up in which the mesenchymal masses and epithelial sheets were allowed to adhere to the bottom of the plastic dish before being overlain with collagen solution in which ganglia were positioned as before. Under these conditions the target tissues attached and spread and epithelium-directed neurite outgrowth was enhanced, compared with that which grew to the suspended tissue (Fig. 9.4(c)). As before, there was no outgrowth towards the mesenchyme.

Fig. 9.4. (a) Phase contrast photomicrograph of a representative collagen gel co-culture of E12 explants after incubating for 48 hours in control medium (no added anti-NGF). Neurites have extended radially from all quadrants of the ganglion. In co-cultures of the same age incubated with anti-NGF antiserum, there was little or no neurite outgrowth. lb, limb-bud control tissue; gV, trigeminal ganglion; mx, maxillary process, whisker field target tissue. Scale bar: 200 μm.

(b) Phase contrast photomicrograph of a representative collagen gel co-culture of an E10 trigeminal ganglion (gV), maxillary process epithelium (E), and mesenchyme (M). For tissue separation and culture techniques, see Lumsden and Davies (1986). Neurites have extended directly and exclusively to the epithelium. In this co-culture, collagen fibrils have become aligned on the mesenchyme side of the ganglion, presumably through cell traction, and non-neuronal cells have grown out of the ganglion on the target side. There was no correlation, however, between cell outgrowth (which was variously at one location, all around the ganglion, or non-existent) and neurite outgrowth which, when present, was invariably target directed. Scale bar: 100 μm.

(c) Epithelium-directed E10 trigeminal ganglion neurites growing in a collagen gel towards a monolayer of E11 maxillary process epithelium (E); neurites have been stained by the indirect immunoperoxidase method using monoclonal anti-neurofila-ment antibody RT 97 (courtesy of Dr John Wood). Scale bar: 100 μm. [Reproduced from Lumsden and Davies (1987) by kind permission of Springer-Verlag, Berlin.]

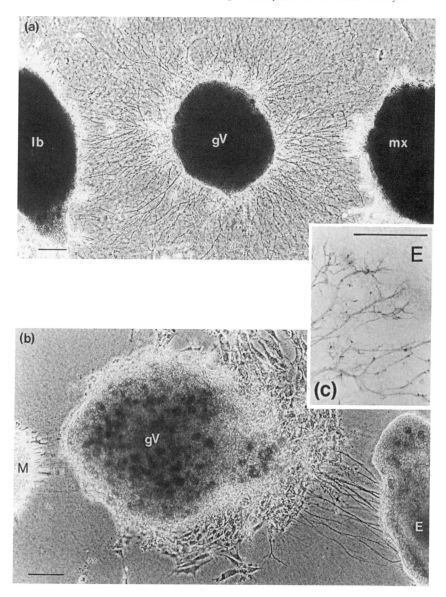

DOES CHEMOTROPISM OPERATE IN NORMAL TRIGEMINAL DEVELOPMENT?

Developing nerve fibres may be guided to their targets by two general mechanisms: either they respond to cues which are laid down along the route to the target (and which may also be distributed more widely), or they respond by chemotropism to a long-range target-derived diffusible signal. In a given system either one or both mechanisms could be involved, in parallel or in series.

Although MF has yet to be shown to have a role in the second of these mechanisms during normal development, this possibility is suggested by its temporal and spatial specificities together with the finding that the site of MF synthesis in the embryo (target epithelium) broadly coincides with the normal location of the majority of whisker afferent nerve endings in the adult (intra-epithelial Merkel discs).

That the target field can exert a long-range growth-stimulating and orienting effect on its appropriate innervating neurons suggests that the whisker field target is specified to attract its correct sensory innervation at a distance. Since, in our culture system, the normal pathway mesenchyme is substituted by a collagen matrix which can be presumed not to contain the specific directional cues such as have been postulated in the normal pathway (Al-Ghaith and Lewis 1982; Ebendal 1977; Rogers *et al.* 1986), it can be reasoned that the pathway need provide no more than a permissive environment for nerve fibre growth.

That MF is synthesized by the most distant part of the target field (epithelium), and can exert its effect over a distance *in vitro* which is comparable to that which normally spaces the early trigeminal ganglion from its epithelial target field, further emphasizes the possibility that MF could exert its effect through a mesenchymal matrix *in vivo*. The maximum distance over which the epithelial target need exert its influence *in vivo* lies well within the theoretical limit (1 mm) over which an effective concentration gradient could be set up in a developing organism within the time available (Crick 1970).

INFLUENCE OF THE PERIPHERY DURING TRIGEMINAL DEVELOPMENT—A POSSIBLE ROLE FOR MF

The trigeminal territory plays a very important part in tactile exploration, especially in the many orders of mammal in which whiskers are prominent; it is by far the most densely innervated region of the integument. In spite of the very large number of trigeminal nerve fibres which grow to the periphery during normal development, the receptive field of the trigeminal ganglion is precisely circumscribed in contrast to the considerable overlap between the receptive fields of DRG in the trunk and limbs.

The characteristic pattern of whisker follicles on the rodent face is anatomically and functionally related to homeomorphic arrays of multineuronal units in the brain stem, thalamus, and cortex (Woolsey and van der Loos 1970). Although the terminations of nerve fibres within the peripheral trigeminal territory ultimately become highly ordered, the maxillary nerve is not initially ordered in relation to the emerging whisker pattern (Davies and Lumsden 1986). The demonstration that isolated maxillary processes can generate this pattern in the absence of innervation (Andres and van der Loos 1982), together with the sequential emergence of the pattern at ascending levels in the CNS during normal development, suggest that the periphery provides spatial information for organizing the central synaptic stations (van der Loos and Dorfl 1978). The release of MF by the epithelium of presumptive whisker follicles could direct profuse peripheral nerve fibre growth into the whisker field and thus establish diffuse projection to this target. Regionally specific chemotropism may thus be one mechanism whereby the periphery exerts an early organizing influence on the centre.

IS THE TRIGEMINAL A SPECIAL CASE?

In addition to the absence of a detectable serial homologue of first-arch chemotropism in the second arch of the mouse embryo (Lumsden and Davies 1986), there is a lack of evidence for regionally specific chemotropism in some systems (e.g. the retinotectal system of *Xenopus*; Harris *et al.* 1985) and counter-evidence from others; in the development of hind-limb innervation in the chick, for example, appropriate sorting of axons into dorsal and ventral positions in the lumbosacral plexus occurs even when the limb bud is ablated prior to axon outgrowth (Tosney and Landmesser 1984). In the complete absence of distal targets these axons are restricted to the plexus region. When target remnants are present, however, axons are enticed to grow out of the plexus into the deficient limb and innervate developing muscles in a segmentally appropriate manner (Tosney and Landmesser 1984). These findings suggest that, whereas pathway selection in the plexus appears to depend on influences of local origin, i.e. restrictive regions of dense precartilaginous mesenchyme and specific local cues confined to the mesenchyme of the limb base, pathway selection distal to the plexus, where axons diverge to their respective premuscles, appears to depend on the target or target-associated mesenchyme.

The nature of the specific target cues is unknown but the possibility exists that axons respond to local portions of a gradient that is produced by a distant source. McCaig (1986) has shown that neurites from dissociated *Xenopus* embryo neural tube motoneurons, in co-culture with virgin skeletal myoblasts and ventral skin, exhibit a preferred orientation towards myoblasts and that the attraction is mediated by a soluble factor. This factor, however, is possibly unrelated to the specific cues implicated in the later stages of motoneuron projection to specific developing muscles (Landmesser 1984) because motoneurons in co-culture showed no ability to discriminate between myoblasts of the appropriate segmental level and those of different levels.

During the development of lumbosacral spinal nerves in the chick, cutaneous sensory fibres from DRG grow directly to their target skin along a defined set of pathways and establish their respective dermatome precisely at its characteristic location (Scott 1982). Whereas sensory nerve growth cones follow the motoneuron pathways for the early part of their course, and may normally be guided by the spatially defined substratum provided by motoneurons (Tosney and Landmesser 1985*b*), this mechanical influence is not required for successful cutaneous projections; sensory nerve fibres can follow the usual paths of the main nerve trunks and form cutaneous branches in an almost normal way when the precursors of motoneurons are destroyed at an early stage (Swanson and Lewis 1986). Nerve fibres from lumbar DRG implanted into aneural chick wing buds also grow, in some cases, along paths resembling the normal highways (Swanson 1985). Thus sensory fibres can act as pioneers and respond correctly to local guidance cues which, proximally, appear to be non-specific. The specificity of segmental cutaneous projections (Honig 1982; Scott 1982), however, suggests that spinal sensory neurons, as motoneurons, are specified with respect to their individual target fields (Scott 1984) and that distal cues, whose nature is presently unknown, may be specific and, possibly, target derived.

Homing behaviour by axons of displaced or misdirected axons (Lance-Jones and Landmesser 1980; Ferguson 1983; Harris 1986) indicates that specific directional cues are not confined to particular pathways but are widely distributed in the embryo. Although discussion of the distributed guidance mechanism has considered the notion of positional information to be a more likely explanation than chemotropism, this is a bias which reflects the lack of direct evidence for the latter in these systems rather than any inherent improbability in the chemotropic mechanism itself (for discussion, see Trinkaus 1985). The evidence for region-specific chemotropism in guiding trigeminal neurites may give substance to the possibility that other nerves may be guided by this mechanism. As Trinkaus (1985) has argued, chemotactic mechanisms are so efficient for giving directionality to moving cells (and presumably also growth cones) that it is 'not improbable that selection would have favoured such a mechanism, wherever it appeared'.

SUMMARY

Developing nerve fibres navigate by following specific cues which are not confined to outgrowth routes. The tropic response of growth cones to a specific attractant diffusing from the target field is one possible distributed guidance mechanism. Some *in vitro* effects of NGF, however, which have been advanced as evidence that NGF has a chemotropic role in development, do not justify this presumption. Compelling evidence for neuronal chemotropism is also lacking from neural-target co-culture studies. When early mouse embryo trigeminal ganglia, however, are co-cultured in collagen gels with their appropriate target (the developing whisker field), neurites grow exclusively to this tissue. The attractant is produced during the normal period of initial outgrowth, declines after normal growth-cone–target-field encounter, is distinct from both NGF and laminin, and is not produced by the adjoining cutaneous field. When co-cultured with components of the whisker field, trigeminal neurites grow directly to the epithelium, but not to the mesenchyme. Epithelia may thus be specified to attract their correct sensory innervation at a distance, and mesenchyme, through which nerves grow to reach epithelial targets and in which preformed pathways have been postulated, may play only a permissive role in trigeminal sensory nerve fibre growth.

ACKNOWLEDGEMENTS

This work is supported by a project grant from the Medical Research Council. I wish to thank Dr W. A. Harris for reading the manuscript and Vanessa Harrison for technical assistance.

REFERENCES

Al-Ghaith, L. K. and Lewis, J. H. (1982). Pioneer growth cones in virgin mesenchyme: an electron microscope study in the developing chick wing. *J. Embryol. exp. Morphol.* **68**, pp. 149–60.

Andres, F. L. and van der Loos, H. (1982). Cultured embryonic non-innervated muzzle skin is capable of generating a whisker pattern. *Int. J. Dev. Neurosci.* **1**, pp. 310–38.

Bonhoeffer, F. and Huf, J. (1982). *In vitro* experiments on axon guidance demonstrating an anterior–posterior gradient on the tectum. *EMBO J.* **1**, pp. 427–31.

Bray, D. (1982). Filopodial contraction and growth cone guidance. In *Cell behaviour* (eds. R. Bellairs, A. Curtis, and G. Dunn), pp. 299–317. Cambridge University Press, Cambridge.

Cajal, S. R. (1910). Algunas observaciones favorables a la hipótesis neurotrópica, *Trab. Lab. Invest. biol. Univ. Madr.* **8**, pp. 63–134.

Cajal, S. R. (1919). Acción neurotrópica de los epitelios, *Trab. Lab. Invest. biol. Univ. Madr.* **17**, pp. 181–228.

Campenot, R. B. (1977). Local control of neurite development by nerve growth factor. *Proc. Natl. Acad. Sci. USA* **74**, pp. 4516–19.

Campenot, R. B. (1982*a*). Development of sympathetic neurons in compartmentalized cultures. I. Local control of neurite growth by nerve growth factor, *Dev. Biol.* **93**, pp. 1–12.

Campenot, R. B. (1982*b*). Development of sympathetic neurons in compartmentalized cultures. II. Local control of neurite survival by nerve growth factor. *Dev. Biol.* **93**, pp. 13–21.

Chamley, J. H. and Dowel, J. J. (1975). Specificity of nerve fibre 'attraction' to autonomic effector organs in tissue culture. *Exp. Cell Res.* **90**, pp. 1–7.

Chamley, J. H., Goller, I., and Burnstock, G. (1973). Selective growth of sympathetic nerve fibers to explants of normally densely innervated autonomic effector organs in tissue culture. *Dev. Biol.* **31**, pp. 362–79.

Charlwood, K. A., Lamont, D. M., and Banks, B. (1972). Apparent orienting effects produced by nerve growth factor. In *Nerve growth factor and its antiserum* (eds. E. Zaimis and J. Knight), pp. 102–7. Athlone Press.

Cohen, J., Burne, J. F., Winter, J., and Bartlett, P. (1986). Retinal ganglion cells lose response to laminin with maturation. *Nature* **332**: pp. 465–7.

Cohen, J., Burne, J. F., Winter, J., and McKinley, C. (1987). The role of laminin and the laminin/fibronectin receptor complex in the outgrowth of retinal ganglion cell axons. *Dev. Biol.* **122**, pp. 407–418.

Coughlin, M. D. (1975). Target organ stimulation of parasympathetic nerve growth in the developing mouse submandibular gland. *Dev. Biol.* **43**, pp. 140–58.

Crick, F. (1970). Diffusion in embryogenesis. *Nature* **225**, pp. 420–2.

Davies, A. M. and Lumsden, A. G. S. (1984). Relation of target encounter and neuronal death to nerve growth factor responsiveness in the developing mouse trigeminal ganglion. *J. Comp. Neurol.* **223**, pp. 124–37.

Davies, A. M. and Lumsden, A. G. S. (1986). Fasciculation in the early mouse trigeminal nerve is not ordered in relation to the emerging pattern of whisker follicles. *J. Comp. Neurol.* **253**, pp. 13–24.

Davies, A. M., Lumsden, A. G. S., Slavkin, H. C., and Burnstock, G. (1981). Influence of nerve growth factor on the embryonic mouse trigeminal ganglion in culture. *Dev. Neurosci.* **4**, pp. 150–6.

Dunn, G. A. (1981). Chemotaxis as a form of directed cell behaviour: some theoretical considerations. In *Biology of the chemotactic response* (eds. J. M. Lackie and P. C. Wilkinson), pp. 1–26. Cambridge University Press, Cambridge.

Ebendal, T. (1976). The relative roles of contact inhibition and contact guidance in orientation of axons extending on aligned collagen fibrils *in vitro*. *Exp. Cell Res.* **98**, pp. 159–69.

Ebendal, T. (1977). Extracellular matrix fibrils and cell contacts in the chick embryo: possible roles in orientation of cell migration and axon extension. *Cell Tissue Res.* **175**, pp. 439–58.

Ebendal, T. (1981). Control of neurite extension by embryonic heart explants. *J. Embryol. exp. Morphol.* **61**, pp. 289–301.

Ebendal, T. and Jacobson, C. O. (1977*a*). Tests of possible role of NGF in neurite outgrowth stimulation exerted by glial cells and heart explants in culture. *Brain Res.* **131**, pp. 373–8.

Ebendal, T. and Jacobson, C. O. (1977*b*). Tissue explants affecting extension and orientation of axons in cultured chick embryo ganglia. *Exp. Cell Res.* **105**, pp. 379–87.

Ebendal, T., Jordell-Kylberg, A., and Soderstrom, S. (1978). Stimulation by tissue explants on nerve fibre outgrowth in culture. *Zoon* **6**, pp. 235–43.

Ferguson, B. A. (1983). Development of motor innervation of the chick following dorso–ventral limb bud rotations. *J. Neurosci.* **3**, pp. 1760–72.

Geraudie, J. and Singer, M. (1982). Axonal guidance in the neuroepithelium of the tail trout *Salmo gairdneri. J. Exp. Zool.* **219**, pp. 355–60.

Gundersen, R. W. and Barrett, J. N. (1979). Neuronal chemotaxis: chick dorsal root axons turn towards high concentrations of nerve growth factor. *Science* **206**, pp. 1079–80.

Gundersen, R. W. and Barrett, J. N. (1980). Characterisation of the turning response of dorsal root neurites towards nerve growth factor. *J. Cell Biol.* **87**, pp. 546–54.

Hamburger, V., Brunso-Bechtold, J. K., and Yip, J. W. (1981). Neuronal death in the spinal ganglia of the chick embryo and its reduction by nerve growth factor. *J. Neurosci.* **1**, pp. 60–71.

Hammarback, J. A., Palm, S. L., Furcht, L. T., and Letourneau, P. C. (1985). Guidance of neurite outgrowth by pathways of substratum-adsorbed laminin. *J. Neurosci. Res.* **13**, pp. 213–20.

Harris, W. A. (1986). Homing behaviour of axons in the embryonic vertebrate brain. *Nature* **320**, pp. 266–9.

Harris, W. A., Holt, C. E., Smith, T. A., and Gallenson, N. J. (1985). Growth cones of developing retinal cells *in vivo*, on culture surfaces, and in collagen matrices. *J. Neurosci. Res.* **13**, pp. 101–22.

Honig, M. G. (1982). The development of sensory projection patterns in embryonic chick hind limb. *J. Physiol. (Lond.)* **330**, pp. 175–202.

Jacobson, M. and Huang, S. (1985). Neurite outgrowth traced by means of horseradish peroxidase inherited from neuronal ancestral cells in frog embryos. *Dev. Biol.* **110**, pp. 102–13.

Johnson, E. M., Gorin, P. D., Brandeis, L. D., and Pearson, J. (1980). Dorsal root ganglion neurons are destroyed by exposure *in utero* to maternal antibody to nerve growth factor. *Science* **210**, pp. 916–8.

Katz, M. and Lasek, R. (1979). Substrate pathways which guide growing axons in *Xenopus* embryos. *J. Comp. Neurol.* **183**, pp. 817–32.

Lamont, D. M. (1968). Some studies of proteins that affect the growth of dorsal root ganglia in culture. PhD thesis, University of London, London, UK.

Lance-Jones, C. and Landmesser, L. (1980). Motoneuron projection patterns in the chick hind limb following early partial spinal cord reversals. *J. Physiol. (Lond).* **302**, pp. 581–602.

Lance-Jones, C. and Landmesser, L. (1981). Pathway selection by chick lumbosacral motoneurons during normal development. *Proc. R. Soc. Lond. B* **214**, pp. 1–18.

Landmesser, L. (1984). The development of specific motor pathways in the chick embryo. *Trends Neurosci.* **7**, pp. 336–9.

Letourneau, P. C. (1975). Cell to substratum adhesion and guidance of axonal elongation. *Dev. Biol.* **44**, pp. 92–101.

Letourneau, P. C. (1978). Chemotactic response of nerve fiber elongation to nerve growth factor. *Dev. Biol.* **66**, pp. 183–96.

Letourneau, P. C. (1982). Nerve fiber growth and its regulation by extrinsic factors. In *Neuronal development* (ed. N. C. Spitzer), pp. 213–54. Plenum Press, New York.

Levi-Montalcini, R. (1982). Developmental neurobiology and the natural history of nerve growth factor. *Ann. Rev. Neurosci.* **5**, pp. 341–62.

Lindsay, R. M., Thoenen, H., and Barde, Y.-A. (1985). Placode and neural crest-derived sensory neurones are responsive at early developmental stages to brain-derived neurotrophic factor. *Dev. Biol.* **112**, pp. 319–28.

Lumsden, A. G. S. and Davies, A. M. (1983). Earliest sensory nerve fibres are guided to peripheral targets by attractants other than nerve growth factor. *Nature* **306**, pp. 786–8.

Lumsden, A. G. S. and Davies, A. M. (1987). Chemotropic influence of specific target epithelium on the growth of embryonic sensory neurites. In *Epithelial–mesenchymal interactions in neural development* (eds. J. R. Wolff and Sievers), pp. 323–340. NATO–ASI series, Springer-Verlag, Berlin.

Lumsden, A. G. S. and Davies, A. M. (1986). Chemotropic effect of specific target epithelium in development of the mammalian nervous system. *Nature* **323**, pp. 538–9.

McCaig, C. D. (1986). Myoblasts and myoblast-conditioned medium attract the earliest spinal neurites from frog embryos. *J. Physiol. (Lond.)* **375**, pp. 39–54.

Menesini-Chen, M. G., Chen, J. S., and Levi-Montalcini, R. (1978). Sympathetic nerve fiber ingrowth in the central nervous system of neonatal rodents upon intracerebral NGF injections. *Arch. Ital.Biol.* **116**, pp. 53–84.

Patrizi, G. and Munger, B. L. (1966). The ultrastructure and innervation of rat vibrissae. *J. Comp. Neurol.* **126**, pp. 423–36.

Pollack, E. D., Muhlach, W. L., and Liebig, V. (1981). Neurotropic influence of mesenchymal limb target tissue on spinal cord neurite growth *in vitro*. *J. Comp. Neurol.* **200**, pp. 393–405.

Purves, D. (1982). Guidance of axons during development and after nerve injury. In *Repair and regeneration of the nervous system* (ed. J. G. Nicholls), pp. 107–25. Springer-Verlag, Berlin.

Rogers, S. L., Edson, K. J., Letourneau, P. C. and McLoon, S. C. (1986). Distribution of laminin in the developing peripheral nervous system of the chick. *Dev. Biol.* **113**, pp. 429–35.

Rutishauser, U. and Edelman, G. M. (1980). Effects of fasciculation on the outgrowth of neurites from spinal ganglia in culture. *J. Cell Biol.* **87**, pp. 370–8.

Schubert, D. and Whitlock, C. (1977). Alteration of cellular adhesion by nerve growth factor. *Proc. Natl. Acad. Sci. USA* **74**, pp. 4055–8.

Scott, S. A. (1982). The development of the segmental pattern of skin sensory innervation in embryonic chick hind limb. *J. Physiol. (Lond.)* **330**, pp. 203–30.

Scott, S. A. (1984). The effects of neural crest deletions on the development of sensory innervation patterns in embryonic chick hind limb. *J. Physiol. (Lond.)* **352**, pp. 285–304.

Silver, J. and Ogawa, M. Y. (1983). Postnatally induced formation of the corpus callosum in acallosal mice on glia-coated cellulose bridges. *Science* **220**, pp. 1067–9.

Silver, J. and Robb, R. M. (1979). Studies on the development of the eye cup and optic nerve in normal mice and in mutants with congenital optic nerve aplasia. *Dev. Biol.* **68**, pp. 175–90.

Silver, J. and Sidman, R. L. (1980). A mechanism for the guidance and topographic patterning of retinal ganglion axons. *J. Comp. Neurol.* **189**, pp. 101–11.

Singer, M., Nordländer, R. H., and Egar, M. (1979). Axonal guidance during embryogenesis and regeneration in the spinal cord of the newt: the blueprint hypothesis of neuronal pathway patterning. *J. Comp. Neurol.* **185**, pp. 1–22.

Stopak, D. and Harris, A. K. (1982). Connective tissue morphogenesis by fibroblast traction. *Dev. Biol.* **90,** pp. 383–98.

Swanson, G. J. (1985). Paths taken by sensory nerve fibres in aneural chick wing buds. *J. Embryol. exp. Morphol.* **86,** pp. 109–24.

Swanson, G. J. and Lewis, J. H. (1986). Sensory nerve routes in chick wing buds deprived of motor innervation. *J. Embryol. exp. Morphol.* **95,** pp. 37–52.

Tosney, K. W. and Landmesser, L. (1984). Pattern and specificity of axonal outgrowth following varying degrees of chick limb bud ablation. *J. Neurosci.* **4,** pp. 2518–27.

Tosney, K. W. and Landmesser, L. (1985a). Specificity of early motoneuron growth cone outgrowth in the chick embryo. *J. Neurosci.* **5,** pp. 2336–44.

Tosney, K. W. and Landmesser, L. (1985b). Growth cone morphology and trajectory in the lumbosacral region of the chick embryo. *J. Neurosci.* **5,** pp. 2345–58.

Trinkaus, J. P. (1985). Further thoughts on directional cell movement during morphogenesis. *J. Neurosci. Res.* **13,** pp. 1–19.

Van der Loos, H. and Dorfl, J. (1978). Does the skin tell the somatosensory cortex how to construct a map of the periphery? *Neurosci. Lett.* **7,** pp. 23–30.

Vincent, S. B. (1913). The tactile hair of the white rat. *J. Comp. Neurol.* **23,** pp. 1–34.

Wolpert, L. (1969). Positional information and the spatial pattern of cellular differentiation. *J. Theor. Biol.* **25,** pp. 1–47.

Woolsey, T. A. and van der Loos, H. (1970). The structural organisation of layer IV in the somatosensory region (SI) of mouse cerebral cortex. *Brain Res.* **17,** pp. 205–42.

10

Growth cone guidance and labelled axons

JONATHAN A. RAPER, SUSANNAH CHANG,
JOSEF P. KAPFHAMMER, AND FRITZ G. RATHJEN

Growth cones navigate accurately through extremely complex environments *in vivo*. A great variety of environmental cues may serve growth cones as navigational aids. Simplest among them are mechanical constraints. Small oriented extracellular channels have been hypothesized to orient fibres growing in the spinal cord (Singer, Nordländer, and Edgar 1979) and retinal fibres growing towards the optic disc (Silver and Sidman 1980). The developing pelvic girdle of the chick leg excludes outgrowing motoneurons and canalizes them into their major peripheral trunks (Tosney and Landmesser 1984). Even anisotropic collagen matrices can affect growth cone orientation (Ebendal 1976). However, mechanical constraints by themselves cannot provide the specificity required for growth cones to find their individual ways.

Several other cues relevant to growth cone guidance have been identified by experiments *in vitro*. Extracellular matrix molecules like fibronectin and laminin are able to promote neurite outgrowth (Akers, Mosher, and Lilien 1981; Baron-Van Evercooren, Kleinman, Ohro, Marangos, Schwartz, and Dubois-Dalq 1982) and, when localized in defined tracks, can orient growth cone extension (Collins and Garrett 1980; Hammarback, Palm, Furcht, and Letourneau 1985). Neurite-promoting molecules on the surfaces of specific non-neuronal cells, and the distributions of the cells themselves, could act in a similar way (Silver, Lorenz, Wahlsten, and Koughlin 1982; Noble, Fok-Seang, and Cohen 1984; Silver and Rutishauser 1984; Fallon 1985). Electric fields (Hinkle, McCaig, and Robinson 1981; Patel and Poo 1984) can orient growth cones over long distances. Inhomogeneous distributions of soluble factors have also been shown to orient growth cones (Coughlin 1975; Letourneau 1978; Gundersen and Barrett 1980; Lumsden and Davies 1983; Gundersen and Park 1984). Most of the factors which have been described attract growth cones, but epidermal cells secrete a factor which repels dorsal root ganglion neurites (Verna 1985). Thus far, it is unclear to what extent many of these insoluble and soluble factors affect specific growth cone subpopulations. One example of a soluble factor that does have a specific effect on growth cone behaviour is the neurotransmitter serotonin. It inhibits the motility of a specific snail growth cone in culture, and its absence influences the development of the same neuron *in vivo* (Haydon, McCobb, and Kater 1984; Goldberg and Kater 1985).

If these environmental cues are present in graded distributions *in vivo*, they could theoretically generate global addressing systems (Wolpert 1969; Nardi and Kafotos 1976; Gierer 1981; Bonhoeffer and Huf 1982; Nardi 1983; Berlot and Goodman 1984; Harris 1986). Alternatively, they could be distributed in defined tracks connecting a source to its target (Katz and Lasek 1979; Silver *et al.* 1982; Silver and Rutishauser 1984). Some of these cues may be particularly important in orienting and guiding the very first axons to extend in an embryo.

Another environmental feature in the developing nervous system that contains considerable information is provided by the axon pathways of early differentiating neurons. If these pathways have labels associated with them, and if growth cones choose to grow in association with particular labels, early axonal pathways could serve as a highway system for later extending growth cones (Goodman, Raper, Ho, and Chang 1982; Raper, Bastiani, and Goodman 1983*a*). Supporting this hypothesis is the observation that particular growth cones prefer to grow upon specific axonal substrates in both invertebrate and vertebrate preparations.

The growth cones of many identified neurons have been found to extend on specific and reproducible sequences of axonal substrates in the peripheral and central nervous systems of the grasshopper (Ho and Goodman 1982; Keshishian and Bentley 1983; Raper *et al.* 1983*a*; Bastiani, Raper, and Goodman 1984). For example, the A and P neurons pioneer a lateral axon fascicle in the neuropil of each segmental ganglion. Normally, the growth cone of the G neuron grows anteriorly through the neuropil within this fascicle [Fig. 10.1.(a)]. If the P cells are killed, and the A axons prevented from growing forward, the behaviour of the G cell's growth cone is affected (Raper *et al.* 1983*b*; Raper, Bastiani, and Goodman 1984). It has difficulty extending anteriorly, and is more likely to extend too far laterally [Fig. 10.1.(b)]. Transmission electron micrographs reveal an unusually high number of G cell processes scattered in abnormal locations throughout the neurophil. Deletion of only the P cells has a similar effect. Similar results have been obtained with other cells in the grasshopper (Bentley and Caudy 1983; du Lac and Goodman 1984; Goodman, Bastiani, Doe, du Lac, Helfard, Kuwada, and Thomas 1984) and in a fish (Kuwada 1986). These findings indicate that growth cones can recognize specific axons and, moreover, require their presence to extend normally.

Vertebrate growth cones are also able to recognize and respond to specific axonal substrates. In an elegant experiment (Bonhoeffer and Huf 1985) the axons from nasal and temporal chick retinal explants are forced to grow down the arms and to the base of a 'Y'. The growth cones from a third fluorescently labelled explant are forced to grow, starting from the base of the 'Y', in the opposite direction. When the explant at the base of the 'Y' is from the

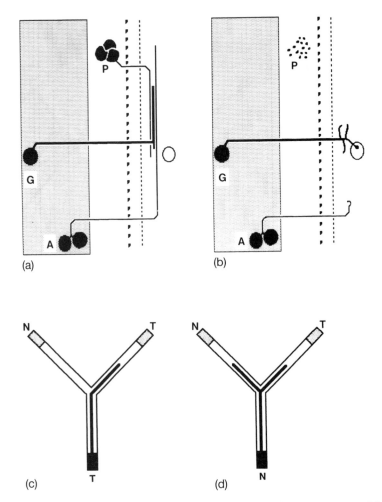

Fig. 10.1. *Selective fasciculation in the grasshopper central nervous system.* (a) The major axon of the G neuron crosses from one side of a ventral ganglion (shaded) to the other side (open). It grows past several axon fascicles (dotted lines), and turns anteriorly on a fascicle formed by the axons of the A and P neurons. (b) If the A and P axons are prevented from extending by cutting the A axons and killing the P neurons, G is unable to grow on its normal route (from Raper *et al.* 1984).

Selective fasciculation of embryonic chick retinal tissues in culture. (c) The growth cones from a fluorescently labelled temporal explant (T—solid) extend on the axons of a second temporal explant (T—shaded) in preference to the axons of a nasal explant (N—shaded). (d) The growth cones from a nasal explant show no preference. [Reproduced from Bonhoeffer and Huf (1985) by kind permission of Macmillan Press, London.]

temporal retina, its growth cones choose to grow on the temporal branch of the 'Y' [Fig 10.1.(c)]. Nasal growth cones have no preference for one branch rather than the other [Fig. 10.1.(d)]. This suggests that temporal growth cones have a specific affinity for temporal axons.

Another example of neurite–neurite recognition between cultured vertebrate tissues has been described by Bray, Wood, and Bunge (1980). Using rat retinal and superior cervical ganglia grown on collagen, they found that retinal neurites mix freely with other retinal neurites, sympathetic neurites mix freely with other sympathetic neurites, but retinal neurites do not mix with sympathetic neurites. We have replicated this experiment with embryonic chick retinal and sympathetic explants grown on laminin-coated glass (Kapfhammer, Grünewald, and Raper 1986). The neurites from two opposed retinal and sympathetic explants are deflected from one another and form two separate territories [Fig. 10.2.(a)]. The territories are sometimes separated by a relatively axon-free zone. Some sympathetic axons invade retinal territory, but they remain unnaturally fasciculated instead of splitting into ever finer fascicles as they do on laminin alone. The neurites from two opposed retinal explants mix without forming separate territories [Fig. 10.2.(b)], as do the neurites from two opposed sympathetic explants [Fig. 10.2.(c)].

We have made a time-lapse study of encounters between individual growth cones and neurites in these cultures (Kapfhammer *et al.* 1986; Kapfhammer and Raper, 1987). Growth cones maintain their normal, flattened, motile morphologies when retinal growth cones contact retinal neurites or when sympathetic growth cones contact sympathetic neurites. They continue to advance at a steady pace before [Fig. 10.3.(a) and (b)], during [Fig. 10.3.(c) and (d)], and after contact [Fig. 10.3.(e) and (f)]. In the conditions in which our cultures grow, retinal growth cones cross retinal neurites and sympathetic growth cones cross sympathetic neurites with little or no delay.

A very different result is obtained when growth cones meet unlike neurites. Retinal growth cones collapse on contact with sympathetic neurites, and sympathetic growth cones collapse on contact with retinal neurites. An encounter between a retinal growth cone and a sympathetic neurite is shown in Fig. 10.4. A flattened, motile retinal growth cone advances rapidly towards a sympathetic neurite [Fig. 10.4.(a) and (b)]. After making contact along the entire leading edge of its lamellipodium [Fig. 10.4.(b)], its filopodia thicken while its lamellipodium shrinks in size [Fig. 10.4.(c)]. The entire motile region of the growth cone is resorbed as the trailing neurite retracts away from the sympathetic neurite [Fig. 10.4.(d)]. A few fine cytoplasmic strands span the gap between the collapsed growth cone and the sympathetic neurite [arrow, Fig. 10.4.(d)]. A new growth cone is organized [arrow, Fig. 10.4.(e)] and begins a new advance [Fig. 10.4.(f)]. These events exactly parallel those which occur in contact-mediated inhibition of locomotion 'type I' between some cultured non-neuronal cells (Abercrombie and Heaysman 1954; Abercrombie 1970; Vésely and Weiss 1973; Heaysman 1978). We find that retinal growth cones

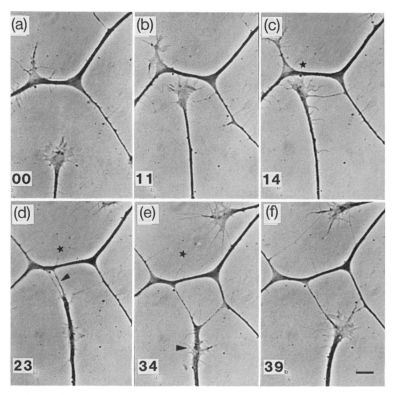

Fig. 10.4. A retinal growth cone retracts on contact with a sympathetic neurite. (a) A retinal growth cone approaches and (b) touches a sympathetic neurite. Its filopodia become shorter and thicker while the lamellipodium shrinks (c) and (d). (d) The trailing neurite retracts when the growth cone is fully collapsed. Fine cytoplasmic strands connect the growth cone and the neurite (arrow). (e) A new growth cone is then formed (arrow) and (f) re-advances. A star marks a fixed location on the substrate. Scale bar: 10 μm; time in minutes. [Reproduced from Kapfhammer and Raper (1987) by kind permission of the Society for Neuroscience, Bethesda, MD.]

surface antigens (Chang, Rathjen, and Raper 1987). Ultimately, we hope to find antibodies which (i) slow down or halt growth cone extension on axons in the assay, (ii) do not effect the extension of the same growth cones on polylysine, collagen, or laminin substrates, and (iii) stain the surfaces of axon subpopulations early in the developing nervous system. Surface antigens present on subpopulations of axons have been described (Cohen and Selvendran 1981; Vulliamy, Rattray, and Mirsky, 1981; Henke-Fahle and Bonhoeffer 1983; Goodman *et al.* 1984; Dodd and Jessell 1985). The functions of most of these antigens are unknown. Polyvalent monoclonal antibodies to one of them has been shown to impair the outgrowth of retinal axons on collagen, laminin, and an intact basement membrane preparation (Henke-Fahle, Rechhaus, and Babiel 1984).

To force growth cones to extend on a purely axonal substrate we have devised the following procedure. We first plate and fix dissociated chick brain cells in an annulus around the perimeter of a small glass coverslip. The central portion of the coverslip is coated with laminin. An embryonic chick sympathetic ganglion is placed in the centre of the coverslip and cultured for five days in the presence of anti-mitotic drugs. Anti-laminin antibodies are then added to the cultures to neutralize the neurite promoting effects of laminin adsorbed onto the glass. The tips of the neurites radiating from the explant are held in place by the annulus of fixed cells [Fig. 10.5.(a)]. A small number of dissociated, fluorescently labelled sympathetic neurons are then sprinkled onto the explant. Some stick to and grow on the axons radiating from it [Fig. 10.5.(b) and (c)]. One group of explants is cultured for 14 hours in the presence of test antibodies, while a matched group is cultured in the absence of antibodies. The preparations are fixed and the neurite lengths of the individual labelled neurons are measured and compared.

Among the antibodies we have tested are polyclonal Fabs against the neural cell adhesion molecule (NCAM) and polyclonal Fabs against the glycoproteins immuno-purified by a monoclonal antibody named G4. NCAM is a well characterized adhesive cell surface glycoprotein that is widely distributed in the nervous system (Edelman 1984; Rutishauser 1984). It is likely to play a role 'in the formation of side-to-side adhesions between individual neurites' (Rutishauser, Einar, and Edelman 1978) and in the extension of motor axons on myotubes (Rutishauser, Grumet and Edelman 1983). The G4 immuno-isolate is related to L1 by N-terminal sequence analysis and consists of a major component of 135 kD and minor components of 190 and 65 kD (Rathjen and Schachner 1984). The Fab polyclonal antibodies raised against the G4 immuno-isolate stain the surfaces of living sympathetic axons in culture.

Polyclonal Fabs against NCAM have little or no effect on the lengths of sympathetic neurites growing on sympathetic axons. The distributions of antibody-treated neurite lengths and control lengths are very similar [Fig. 10.6.(a)]. This is in spite of the fact that abundant NCAM is present on the surfaces of cultured sympathetic axons, and each of the three anti-NCAM antibody preparations we used were effective in preventing retinal cell aggregation. If the same experiment is performed on laminin-coated glass instead of on axonal substrates, the distributions of antibody-treated and control lengths are superimposable [Fig. 10.6.(b)].

Polyclonal Fabs against the G4 immuno-isolate significantly shorten sympathetic neurites growing on sympathetic axons [Fig. 10.6.(c)]. Since the same antibodies have no significant effect on the lengths of sympathetic neurites growing on laminin-coated glass [Fig. 10.6.(d)], their primary effect does not appear to be on cell viability or the ability of growth cones to locomote. Since anti-NCAM antibodies do not affect sympathetic outgrowth

REFERENCES

Abercrombie, M. (1970). Contact inhibition in tissue culture. *In Vitro* **6**, pp. 128–42.

Abercrombie, M. and Heaysman, J. E. M. (1954). Observations on the behavior of cells in tissue culture: II. Monolayering of fibroblasts. *Exp. Cell Res.* **6**, pp. 293–306.

Akers, R. M., Mosher, D. F., and Lilien, J. E. (1981). Promotion of retinal neurite outgrowth by substratum-bound fibronectin. *Dev. Biol.* **86**, pp. 179–88.

Baron-Van Evercooren, A., Kleinman, H. K., Ohno, S., Marangos, P., Schwartz, J. P., Dubois-Dalq, M. (1982). Nerve growth factor, laminin, and fibronectin promote neurite growth in human fetal sensory ganglion cultures. *J. Neurosci. Res.* **8**, pp. 170–93.

Bastiani, M. J., Raper, J. A., and Goodman, C. S. (1984). Pathfinding by neuronal growth cones in grasshopper embryos: III. Selective affinity of the G growth cone for the P cells within the A/P fascicle. *J. Neurosci.* **4**, pp. 2311–28.

Bentley, D. and Caudy, M. (1983). Navigational substrates for peripheral pioneer growth cones: limb axis polarity cues, limb segments boundaries, and guidepost neurons. *Cold Spring harbor Symp. Quant. Biol.* **48**, pp. 573–85.

Berlot, J. and Goodman, C. S. (1984). Guidance of peripheral pioneer neurons in the grasshopper: adhesive hierarchy of epithelial and neuronal surfaces. *Science* **223**, pp. 493–6.

Bonhoeffer, F. and Huf, J. (1982). In vitro experiments on axon guidance demonstrating an anterior–posterior gradient on the tectum. *EMBO J.* **4**, pp. 427–31.

Bonhoeffer, F. and Huf, J. (1985). Position-dependent properties of retinal axons and their growth cones. *Nature* **315**, pp. 409–10.

Bray, D. (1982). Filopodia contraction and growth cone guidance. In *Cell behaviour* (eds. R. Bellairs, A. Curtis, and G. Dunn), pp. 299–317. Cambridge University Press, Cambridge.

Bray, D., Wood, P., and Bunge, R. P. (1980). Selective fasciculation of nerve fibers in culture. *Exp. Cell Res.* **130**, pp. 241–50.

Chang, S., Rathjen, F. G., and Raper, J. A. (1987). Extension of neurites on axons is impaired by antibodies against specific neural cell surface glycoproteins. *J. Cell Biol.* **104**, 355–62.

Cohen, J. and Selvendran, S. Y. (1981) A neuronal cell-surface antigen is found in the CNS but not in peripheral neurones. *Nature* **291**, pp. 421–3.

Collins, F. and Garrett, J. E. (1980). Elongating nerve fibers are guided by a pathway of material released from embryonic nonneuronal cells. *Proc. Natl. Acad. Sci. USA.* **77**, pp. 6226–8.

Coughlin, M. D. (1975). Target organ stimulation of parasympathetic nerve growth in the developing mouse submandibular gland. *Dev. Biol.* **43**, pp. 140–58.

Daniloff, J. K., Chuong, C. -M., Levi, G. and Edelman, G. M. (1986). Differential distribution of cell adhesion molecules during histogenesis of the chick nervous system. *J. Neurosci.* **6**, pp. 739–58.

Dodd, J. and Jessell, T. M. (1985). Lactoseries carbohydrates specify subsets of dorsal root ganglion neurons projecting to the superficial horn of rat spinal cord. *J. Neurosci.* **5**, pp. 3278–94.

Du Lac, S. and Goodman, C. S. (1984). Selective fasciculation in the grasshopper embryo: experimental test of the labelled pathways hypothesis. *Neurosci. Abstr.* **10**, p. 140.

Ebendal, T. (1976). The relative roles of contact inhibition and contact guidance in orientation of axons extending on aligned collagen fibrils in vitro. *Exp. Cell Res.* **98**, pp. 159–69.

Edelman, G. M. (1984). Modulation of cell adhesion during induction, histogenesis, and perinatal development of the nervous system. *Ann. Rev. Neurosci.* **7**, pp. 339–77.

Fallon, J. R. (1985). Preferential outgrowth of central nervous system neurites on astrocytes and Schwann cells as compared with nonglial cells in vitro. *J. Cell. Biol.* **100**, pp. 198–207.

Gierer, A. (1981). Development of projections between areas of the nervous system. *Biol. Cybern.* **42**, pp. 69–78.

Goldberg, I. I. and Kater, S. B. (1985). Experimental reduction of serotonin content during embryogenesis alters morphology and connectivity of specific identified Helisoma neurons. *Soc. Neurosci. Abstr.* **11**, p. 158.

Goodman, C. S., Raper, J. A., Ho, R., and Chang, S. (1982). Pathfinding by neuronal growth cones during grasshopper embryogenesis. *Symp. Soc. Dev. Biol.* **40**, pp. 275–316.

Goodman, C. S., Bastiani, M. J., Doe, C. Q., du Lac, S., Helfand, S. L., Kuwada, J. Y., and Thomas, J. B. (1984). Cell recognition during neuronal development. *Science* **225**, pp. 1271–9.

Gundersen, R. W. and Barrett, J. N. (1980). Characterization of the turning response of dorsal root neurites toward nerve growth factor. *J. Cell. Biol.* **87**, pp. 546–54.

Gundersen, R. W. and Park, K. H. C. (1984). The effects of conditioned media on spinal neurites: substrate-associated changes in neurite direction and adherence. *Dev. Biol.* **104**, pp. 18–27.

Hammarback, J. A., Palm, S. L., Furcht, L. T., and Letourneau, P. C. (1985). Guidance of neurite outgrowth by pathways of substratum-adsorbed laminin. *J. Neurosci. Res.* **13**, pp. 213–20.

Harris, W. A. (1986). Homing behavior of axons in the embryonic vertebrate brain. *Nature* **320**, pp. 266–8.

Haydon, P. G., McCobb, D. B., and Kater, S. B. (1984). Serotonin selectively inhibits growth cone motility and synaptogenesis of specific identified neurons. *Science* **266**, pp. 561–4.

Heaysman, J. E. M. (1978). Contact inhibition of locomotion: a reappraisal. *Int. Rev. Cytol.* **55**, pp. 49–66.

Henke-Fahle, S. and Bonhoeffer, F. (1983). Inhibition of axonal growth by a monoclonal antibody. *Nature* **303**, pp. 65–7.

Henke-Fahle, S., Reckhaus, W., and Babiel, R. (1984) Influence of various glycoprotein antibodies on axonal outgrowth from the chick retina. In *Developmental neuroscience: physiological, pharmacological and clinical aspects* (eds F. Caciagli, E. Giacobini, and R. Paoletti), pp. 393–8. Elsevier, Amsterdam.

Hinkle, L., McCaig, C. D., and Robinson, K. R. (1981). The direction of growth of differentiating neurones and myoblasts from frog embryos in an applied electric field. *J. Physiol. (Lond.)* **314**, pp. 121–35.

Ho, R. K. and Goodman, C. S. (1982). Peripheral pathways are pioneered by an array of central and peripheral neurones in grasshopper embryos. *Nature* **297**, pp. 404–6.

Kapfhammer, J. P. and Raper, J. A. (1987). The collapse of growth cone structure on contact with specific neurites in culture. *J. Neurosci.* **7**, pp. 201–12.

Kapfhammer, J. P., Grünewald, E. B., and Raper, J. A. (1986). The selective inhibition of growth cone extension by specific neurites in culture. *J. Neurosci.* **9**, pp. 2527–34.

Katz, M. J. and Lasek, R. J. (1979). Substrate pathways which guide growing axons in Xenopus embryos. *J. Comp. Neurol.* **183**, pp. 817–32.

Keshishian, H. and Bentley, D. (1983). Embryogenesis of peripheral nerve pathways in grasshopper legs. II. The major nerve routes. *Dev. Biol.* **96**, pp. 740–6.

Kuwada, J. Y. (1986). Cell recognition by neuronal growth cones in a simple vertebrate embryo. *Science* **233**, pp. 740–6.

Lemmon, V. and McLoon, S. C. (1986). The appearance of an L1-like molecule in the chick primary visual pathway. *J. Neurosci.* **6**, pp. 2987–94.

Letourneau, P. C. (1975). Cell-to-substratum adhesion and guidance of axonal elongation. *Dev. Biol.* **44**, pp. 92–101.

Letourneau, P. C. (1978). Chemotactic response of nerve fiber elongation to nerve growth factor. *Dev. Biol.* **66**, pp. 183–96.

Lumsden, A. G. S. and Davies, A. M. (1983). Earliest sensory nerve fibres are guided to peripheral targets by attractants other than nerve growth factor. *Nature* **396**, pp. 786–8.

Nardi, J. B. (1983). Neuronal pathfinding in developing wings of the moth Manduca sexta. *Dev. Biol.* **95**, pp. 163–74.

Nardi, J. B. and Kafotos, F. C. (1976). Polarity and gradients in lepidopteran wing epidermis: II. The differential adhesiveness model: gradient of a non-diffusible cell surface parameter. *J. Embryol. exp. Morphol.* **36**, pp. 489–512.

Noble, M., Fok-Seang, J., and Cohen, J. (1984). Glia are a unique substrate for the in vitro growth of central nervous system neurons. *J. Neurosci.* **4**, pp. 1892–903.

Patel, M. B. and Poo, M. M. (1984). Perturbation of the direction of neurite growth by pulsed and focal electric fields. *J. Neurosci.* **4**, pp. 2939–47.

Poole, T. J. and Steinberg, M. S. (1982). Evidence for the guidance of pronephric duct migration by a craniocaudally traveling adhesion gradient. *Dev. Biol.* **92**, pp. 144–58.

Raper, J. A., Bastiani, M. J., and Goodman, C. S. (1983a). Pathfinding by neuronal growth cones in grasshopper embryos: II. Selective fasciculation onto specific axonal pathways. *J. Neurosci.* **3**, pp. 31–41.

Raper, J. A., Bastiani, M. J., and Goodman, C. S. (1983b). Guidance of neuronal growth cones: selective fasciculation in the grasshopper embryo. *Cold Spring Harbor Symp. Quant. Biol.* **48**, pp. 587–98.

Raper, J. A., Bastiani, M. J., and Goodman, C. S. (1984). Pathfinding by neuronal growth cones in grasshopper embryos: IV. The effects of ablating the A and P axons upon the behavior of the G growth cone. *J. Neurosci.* **4**, pp. 2329–45.

Rathjen, F. G. and Schachner, M. (1984). Immunocytological and biochemical characterization of a new neurona cell surface component (L1 antigen) which is involved in cell adhesion. *EMBO J.* **3**, pp. 1–10.

Rathjen, F. G., Wolff, J. M., Frank, R., Bonhoeffer, F., and Rutishauser, U. (1987). Membrane glycoproteins involved in neurite fasciculation. *J. Cell Biol.* **104**, pp. 343–53.

Rutishauser, U. (1984). Developmental biology of a neural cell adhesion molecule. *Nature* **310**, pp. 549–54.

Rutishauser, U., Gall, W. E., and Edelman, G. M. (1978). Adhesion among neural cells of the chick embryo: IV. Role of the cell surface molecule CAM in the formation of neurite bundles in cultures of spinal ganglia. *J. Cell Biol.* **79**, p. 391.

Rutishauser, U., Grumet, M., and Edelman, G. M. (1983). Neural cell adhesion molecule mediates initial interactions between spinal cord neurons and muscle cells in culture. *J. Cell Biol.* **145**, pp. 145–52.

Silver, J. and Rutishauser, U. (1984). Guidance of optic axons in vivo by a preformed adhesive pathway on neuroepithelial endfeet. *Dev. Biol.* **106**, pp. 485–99.

Silver, J. and Sidman, R. L. (1980). A mechanism for the guidance and topographic patterning of retinal ganglion cell axons. *J. Comp. Neurol.* **189**, pp. 101–11.

Silver, J., Lorenz, S. E., Wahlsten, D., and Coughlin, J. (1982). Axonal guidance during development of the great cerebral commissures: descriptive and experimental studies, in vivo, on the role of preformed glial pathways. *J. Comp. Neurol.* **210**, pp. 10–29.

Singer, M., Nordlander, R. H., and Egar, M. (1979). Axonal guidance during embryogenesis and regeneration in the spinal chord of the newt: the blueprint hypothesis of neuronal pathway patterning. *J. Comp. Neurol.* **185**, pp. 1–22.

Tosney, K. W. and Landmesser, L. T. (1984). Pattern and specificity of axonal outgrowth following varying degrees of chick limb bud ablation. *J. Neurosci.* **4**, pp. 2518–27.

Verna, J. M. (1985). In vitro analysis of interactions between sensory neurons and skin: evidence for selective innervation of dermis and epidermis. *J. Embryol. Exp. Morphol.* **86**, pp. 53–70.

Vesely, P. and Weiss, R. A. (1973). Cell locomotion and contact inhibition of normal and neoplastic rat cells. *Int. J. Cancer* **11**, pp. 64–76.

Vulliamy, T., Rattray, S., and Mirsky, R. (1981). Cell surface antigen distinguishes sensory and autonomic peripheral neurons from central neurons. *Nature* **291**, pp. 418–20.

Wolpert, L. (1969). Positional information and the spatial pattern of cellular differentiation. *J. theor. Biol.* **25**, pp. 1–47.

11

Navigation of normal and regenerating axons in the goldfish

CLAUDIA A. O. STUERMER

THE PATHWAY OF NORMAL RETINAL AXONS AND THE SHIFTING OF TERMINAL ARBORS

The retinotopic map

The retinotectal system of lower vertebrates has been widely used as a model system (reviewed in Gaze 1970) in search of mechanisms which guide growing axons to their targets. The axons from retinal ganglion cells project to their target, the optic tectum, in a geometrically simple manner, so that the axon terminals from neighbouring ganglion cells in the retina reside in the tectum as neighbours forming the retinotopic map (Gaze 1958; Gaze and Jacobson 1963; Jacobson and Gaze 1965).

Unique to the retinal axons in amphibians and fish is their ability, following transection of the optic nerve, to regenerate and grow back to the tectum to restore a retinotopically ordered projection. The first evidence for the existence of the retinotopic map in normal fish and its restoration in regenerates has been provided by behavioural tests (Arora and Sperry 1963; Northmore and Masino 1984) and electrophysiological recordings (Gaze 1959; Maturana, Lettvin, McCulloch, and Pitts 1959; Jacobson and Gaze 1965; Schmidt and Edwards 1983). The frog's appropriate strike for a lure in certain positions of its visual field (Sperry 1944) and the responses of axons in defined places in the tectum after stimulation of ganglion cells in corresponding positions in the retina showed that functional connections at appropriate sites in the tectum were reformed (Gaze 1959, 1960; Gaze and Jacobson 1963; Jacobson and Gaze 1965).

These methods relate elegantly the position of the ganglion cells to their terminal endings in the target region. They do not, however, provide any clues about the axonal pathways: the question of whether the axons take direct routes or navigate by trial and error to their targets can be answered only by visualizing their trajectories with anatomical methods. Such approaches can provide valuable information on how systems might operate to create patterned connections. In fact, the analysis of the fibre path in the goldfish tectum brought a new perspective to the development of the retinotopic order in fish (Raymond and Easter 1983; Easter and Stuermer 1984). This view differs greatly from the concept of Attardi and Sperry (1963).

For a long time, Attardi and Sperry's (1963) sketches were the only existing documentation on the path of retinal axons. Their drawings originated from experiments which involved ablation of parts of the goldfish retina together with optic nerve transection, and investigation of the regenerating axons of the remainder of the retina as to where they would terminate and which routes they would take. Their results implied that regenerating axons follow normal routes, and that these routes in both normal fish and regenerates take the axons directly to their retinotopic sites (Fig. 11.1).

These implications are not compatible with recent experimental data showing, first, a more complicated organization of the normal pathway (Easter, Rusoff, and Kish 1981; Cook, Rankin, and Stevens 1983; Stuermer and Easter 1984a; Rusoff 1984) as a result of the continuous growth of the retinotectal system in fish (Raymond and Easter 1983), and, second, the existence of aberrant routes in regenerates (Horder 1974; Udin 1978; Fawcett and Gaze 1981; Fujisawa, Tani, Watanabe, and Ibata 1982; Cook 1983; Stuermer and Easter 1984a).

The following discussion will first present a revised interpretation of the normal pathway order in fish. We will then proceed to illustrate some novel findings on the abnormal paths and the striking morphologies of retinal fibres during regeneration.

Growth of the goldfish retinotectal system: implication for the maintenance of the retinotopic map

In the goldfish, the eyes and brain grow continuously throughout most of the life of the fish (Raymond and Easter 1983). The retina grows in rings by adding new cells at its peripheral margin (Johns and Easter 1977; Meyer 1978) while the tectum grows by adding new cells at its caudal pole in crescents (Raymond and Easter 1983). Despite the geometrically different growth, the same geometrically simple and undistorted retinotopic projection is maintained in all fish, small and large. In this system, the centre of the eye projects to the centre of the tectum, the periphery of the eye to the periphery of the tectum (Schwassmann and Kruger 1965). The constancy of this projection is surprising since, during tectal growth, the centre comes to lie at successively more caudal sites, while the centre of the eye remains constant.

This implies that the central ganglion cell axons (and with them all others) cannot remain stationary at their old sites, but instead have to move on to new appropriate sites to keep the projection centred on the tectum (Raymond and Easter 1983).

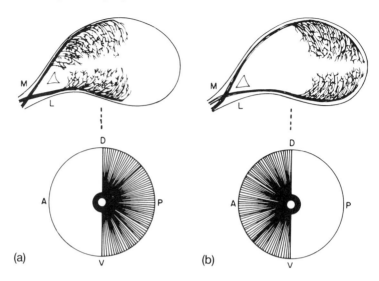

Fig. 11.1. Two pairs of sketches showing the paths and terminations of retinal axons in tectum after partial retina ablation: (a) After removal of temporal (anterior) retina; (b) after removal of nasal (posterior) retina. M, medial; L, lateral; P, posterior; A, anterior; D, dorsal; V, ventral. [Reproduced from Attardi and Sperry (1963) by kind permission of Academic Press, New York.]

A geometrical difference in the growth of the eye and the tectum was found previously in *Xenopus* development by Straznicky and Gaze (1971, 1972). To account for the maintenance of retinotopia, Gaze, Chung, and Keating (1972) and Gaze, Keating, and Chung (1974) proposed the hypothesis of sliding connections: they envisaged that retinal axons in the tectum must abandon their old sites of termination, move, and reconnect at sites which are appropriate with respect to the retinotopic map. More recently, this view was supported by experimental data in the retinotectal system of the frog *Rana pipiens* (Constantine-Paton, Pitts, and Reh 1983).

We believe that our findings on the retinotectal system in goldfish are also consistent with Gaze's hypothesis. Our analysis of the pathway order of the retinal fibres in the goldfish tectum allowed us to reconstruct the route and orientation of the fibres as well as the distances they covered. From these observations we have proposed a general model describing the strategies of retinal axon growth in the tectum (Easter and Stuermer 1984).

The pathway of normal retinal fibres in goldfish

Axon order in tectal fascicles

Before they enter into the tectum, the axons from the dorsal and the ventral portions of the retina grow through separate branches of the optic tract, the ventro–lateral and dorso–medial brachia (Attardi and Sperry 1963; Stuermer and Easter 1984*a*). The fibres arrive at the rostral margin of the tectum and then fan out into numerous fascicles, covering the dorso–medial and ventro–lateral halves of the tectal lobe. These two mirror-symmetrical arrays of fascicles meet at a line, the tectal equator, which is the border between the dorsal and ventral hemitectum. Fascicles within each fan almost never cross one another. They all run parallel to each other, taking curved paths towards the tectal equator. Fascicles have different lengths depending on their location: there are short rostral fascicles which meet the equator in the rostral tectum, and longer, more peripheral fascicles which meet the tectal equator in the caudal tectum. Each fascicle loses fibres along its path so that it becomes thinner as it approaches the tectal equator.

According to Attardi and Sperry's (1963) view, the fibres of these fascicles terminate in the synaptic layer next to their fascicle of entrance, and thus the fascicles are shown as direct routes to the retinotopic termination sites (Fig. 11.1). In their sketches, then, the temporal fibres are shown to travel over rostral fascicles to terminate in rostral tectum, and the fibres of nasal retina over longer periphero–caudal fascicles to terminate in caudal tectum (see Fig. 11.1).

We tested the retinal regional origin of individual fascicles by applying crystals of horseradish peroxidase (HRP) to individual fascicles close to the point of their entrance (Stuermer and Easter 1984*b*). Three of these sites are indicated by A, B, and C in Fig. 11.2. The HRP is taken up by the broken fibres and transported retrogradely to their cells of origin in the retina where they can be visualized in retinal whole mounts.

The HRP-labelled ganglion cells in the retina lay in the appropriate ventral hemiretina, and formed a partial annulus centred on the optic disk (Fig. 11.2). The partial annulus extended from the nasal boundary between dorsal and ventral hemiretina into the temporal retina, and spanned an area of approximately 120°. These partial annuli or arcs were close to the optic disk when a short rostro–central fascicle was labelled (see site A in Fig. 11.2). Labelling of more peripheral fascicles (sites B and C in Fig. 11.2) gave arcs of labelled ganglion cells in more peripheral retina. Thus each of the fascicles, even the very rostral ones, contains fibres from nasal and temporal retina. We did not test the ventral fascicles in this set of experiments. However, other and later experimental data (Stuermer 1984; Rusoff 1984) proved our implication correct; ventral fascicles are also composed of fibres from partial annular regions, but their parent ganglion cells are in the corresponding dorsal hemiretina.

With reference to the fact that the retina grows by adding cells in annuli, it is logical that annuli of cells close to the optic disc are old and that progressively more peripheral rings are younger. Therefore we conclude that each bundle of fascicles from the dorsal and ventral hemitectum contains fibres from cells of

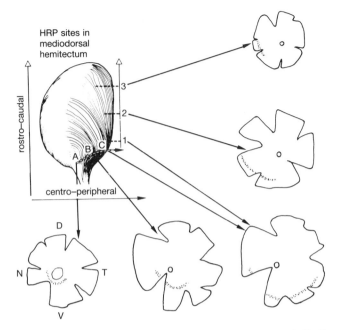

Fig. 11.2. A sketch of a dorso–medial view of fascicles in the tectum. A, B, C, and 1, 2, 3, indicate the sites of HRP applications in different experiments in individual fish. The long arrows point to retinal whole mounts with ganglion cells (black dots) which were labelled as a result of the HRP application to a rostro–central (A), intermediate (B), and a periphero–caudal (C) fascicle and to peripheral fasicles at a rostral (a), middle (2), and caudal (3) site of the fascicle's extent. The open circles mark the position of the optic disc. N, nasal; T, temporal; D, dorsal; V, ventral.

similar ages and that short rostral fascicles are composed of fibres from old retina and more peripheral ones from young retina. Furthermore, this means that each individual fascicle contains fibres with very different tectal addresses, since each is a combination of age-related nasal and temporal fibres, a very different picture than that given by Attardi and Sperry's (1963) sketches. Given this spatial and temporal order, why do fibres take these fasicle routes and how do they get to their retinotopic sites?

Order of fibre exit from tectal fascicles

We first probed the fibre exit from the peripheral fascicles by placing HRP at the rostral, the middle, and further caudal parts of a fascicle's route across the tectum (see sites 1, 2, and 3 in Fig. 11.2) (Stuermer and Easter 1984*b*). The rostral label produced partial annuli of 120° from the nasal boundary, from the middle label roughly 90°, and from the caudal label about 45°. This means that the fibres of different retinal regions leave their peripheral fascicles in sequence. The temporal fibres get off first, the nasal fibres later. Only the fibres from the most temporal portion of the retina (approximately 60° of the retinal circumference) were absent from the fascicle at the points where we labelled them. More recent experiments by Springer and Mednick (1985), Rusoff (1984), and ourselves (Stuermer, unpub. obs.) have revealed that these temporal fibres separate from their age-related partners prior to the point where the fascicles begin their course through the tectum and enter over the rostral tectal pole directly.

Thus, as the bundle of young fibres approaches and courses through the tectum, the fibres for the different tectal addresses depart along the tectal margin in an order that is consistent with the retinotopic map. These routes and modes of departure bring the axons from the peripheral retina close to their retinotopic termination sites in the periphery of the tectum. In fact, fibres in all fascicles, even the old ones in the rostral tectum, follow the same sequence of exit. However, these fibres from central retina do not terminate next to their rostral fascicle of entrance. If they did, the retinotopic order would break down. Instead, retinotopia requires that they terminate close to and around the centre of the tectum. Independent evidence was provided that the terminal arbors of these fascicles are located exactly where we expect them to be (Rusoff 1984; Stuermer 1984; Easter and Stuermer 1984).

Shifting of terminal arbors

The concept for shifting of terminal arbors

Before we turn to the order of terminal arbors, let us recapitulate and evaluate the results mentioned so far. The rules which determine the special path of the fibres are understood in the context of the on-going and geometrically dissimilar growth of the retina and tectum. We propose the following sequence of events. When the eye adds new cells peripherally, the axons from each new generation of ganglion cells travel together in age-related bundles throughout their path from the eye to the tectum. The age-related fibres from dorsal and ventral hemiretina then follow the ventral and dorsal peripheral margins of the tectum. Along their path around the peripheral margin, the fibres leave the fascicle to enter into the synaptic layer in a retinotopic sequence as described above.

We assume that fibres from earlier generations behave similarly. Axons from the periphery of the previously smaller retina followed the margin of the tectum when it was smaller. After retinal and tectal growth, these fascicles remain in place; any given fascicle roughly marks the peripheral boundary the tectum had when the fascicle grew in (Stuermer and Easter 1984b).

At all stages in development, the temporo–nasal sequence of fibre exit from a fascicle guarantees that the peripheral fibres always get close to their retinotopic sites along the rostro–caudal extent of the peripheral tectum. The map created in the periphery is correct and centred on the tectum. The same correct order was laid out by older fibres when they, much earlier, arrived as peripheral fascicles. After tectal growth, the original order can no longer be correct, since the centre of the tectum comes to lie caudally to where it had previously been. To maintain the retinotopic order, the terminal endings of these old fibres must give up their previous connection sites, move, and reconnect at new sites which are consistent with the retinotopic map. The axon terminal arbors must shift.

In Fig. 11.3. we illustrate these events in a scheme for three representative ganglion cells at three successive stages of development. The first panel of Fig. 11.3. shows a small tectum (above) and a small retina (below) with the pathways taken by axons from a temporal, ventral, and nasal ganglion cell (shown as circles in the retina). The axons of these cells travel to the margin of the small tectum, where the temporal axons come to terminate in rostro–peripheral tectum, the ventral ones next in periphero–dorsal sites, and the caudal ones at the caudal tectal end. The terminal arbors are indicated as forked endings and are centred on the tectum. Panels (b) and (c) show the paths of the same ganglion cells after retinal and tectal growth. The terminal arbors (drawn solid in Fig. 11.3) of the three ganglion cells are no longer close to their fascicles, but are instead at their new retinotopic sites close to the centre of the tectum. The earlier positions of the arbors are marked by stippled endings. With considerable growth, as in panel (c), the terminal arbors are far from their previous sites. The previous terminal arbor sites (close to their fascicles) and the current ones are connected by a black line. This is to indicate that the previous and current sites of the terminal arbors are visibly connected by a stretch of axon which links the two. These links, which we called 'extrafascicular axons', should be in the same layer as the terminal arbors (i.e. the synaptic layer) and should indicate the path through which the arbor moved. The tectal axonal path, therefore, should consist of three segments: the fascicular axons, the extrafascicular axons, and the terminal arbor.

Axonal pathways consistent with the concept of shifting

The tripartite morphology of axons became obvious when we traced HRP-labelled axons in tectal whole mounts (Easter and Stuermer 1984; Stuermer 1984). We expected that the length and the orientation of the extrafascicular segments should vary depending on their fascicle of origin and their tectal position. The extrafascicular path between the rostral fascicles and their terminal arbors in the synaptic layer should be long and of rostro–caudal orientation, whereas extrafascicular axons between peripheral fasicles and their terminal arbors should be short and periphero–centrally oriented. These predictions were fulfilled when we traced the routes of HRP-labelled axons in tectal whole mounts (Easter and Stuermer 1984; Stuermer 1984). Figure 11.4. shows two out of many axons which traversed the rostral tectum after they exited from a short rostro–central fascicle to terminate in arbors close to the tectal centre, with an extrafascicular portion travelling rostro–caudally (also see Fig. 11.8 on p. 218). Figure 11.5. illustrates the path of extrafascicular

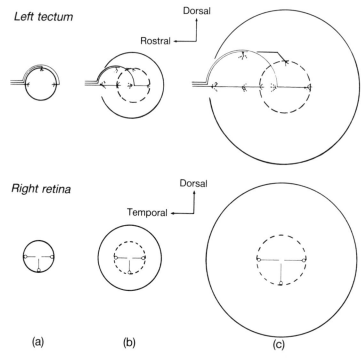

Fig. 11.3. A schematic illustration of the shifting terminals. (a), (b), and (c) show successively older stages in the growth of the retina and tectum. The boundaries of the retina and tectum are indicated as circles. Lower figures: the dashed circles in (b) and (c) mark the boundary of the retina of the earlier stage of development in (a). The three circles indicate representative ganglion cells, a temporal, ventral, and nasal one. Upper figures: the contralateral tectum and the axonal pathways of the three ganglion cells of the lower figure. The fascicle through which their axons enter is initially on the tectal periphery (a), but later becomes enclosed by new tectal tissue. The dashed circle shows the retinotopic termination region of the oldest ganglion cell bodies which lie within the dashed circle in the lower figures. The terminal arbors at the retinotopic sites are sketched as forked endings. The earlier terminal arbor sites are indicated as forked endings with broken lines. The black lines between the fascicular axons (curved lines) and the terminal arbor are the extrafascicular axons which mark the way through which the arbor has shifted. [Reproduced from Easter and Stuermer (1984) by kind permission of the Society for Neuroscience, Bethesda, MD.].

axons between the peripheral fascicle and their peripheral terminal arbors. These extrafascicular segments were short and directed periphero–centrally.

The morphology of the terminal arbors themselves was also quite instructive (Stuermer 1984). Those in the centre of the tectum, i.e. those which must have shifted over considerable distances in the caudal direction, had a typical orientation. Their stem and two major branches (which divided into branchlets) were oriented rostro–caudally, in the direction of the shift. Arbors

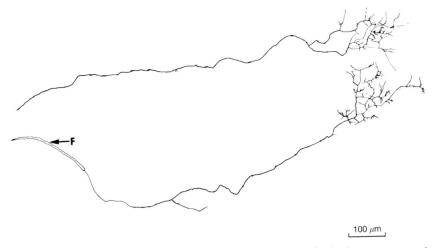

100 μm

Fig. 11.4. A *camera lucida* drawing of two HRP-labelled extrafascicular segments and terminal arbors of retinal axons in the rostral tectum. Note the long caudally orientated axonal paths between their origin in the rostral tectum (to the left) and their terminal arbors close to the tectal centre (to the right). F, fascicle of origin. [Reproduced from Easter and Stuermer (1984) by kind permission of the Society for Neuroscience, Bethesda, MD.]

in the periphery, which had not shifted, had stems, major branches, and branchlets oriented roughly periphero–centrally (see Figs. 11.5. and 11.6).

Further evidence for the shifting of terminal arbors

Another set of experiments with a different approach was strikingly consistent with our view of the shifting of terminal arbors. According to our view any vertical column of tectum at any given site should contain fibres in fascicles in the upper fascicle layer, extrafascicular axons in the synaptic layer, and terminal arbors at their retinotopic sites. All three should be labelled by a vertical penetration with an HRP-coated needle (Easter and Stuermer 1984). In the retina, we would expect to see (1) a labelled patch of retinal ganglion cells in the tectotopic position, labelled through terminals; (2) labelled cells in a portion of a half-annulus, labelled through the fascicular axon; and (3) a row of labelled cells connecting the temporal end of the partial annulus to the terminally labelled patch. This third group derives from extrafascicular axons which once terminated at this site of the HRP application but no longer do so.

The pattern of labelled ganglion cells after one such penetration in rostro–pheripheral tectum is shown in Fig. 11.7. The parent ganglion cells from axons of the injured rostral fasicle in the fasicle layer were found in a partial annulus close to the optic disc (PHA in Fig. 11.7). The parent ganglion cells of the HRP-labelled terminal arbor at this site lay in a cluster in the periphero–temporal retina (CL in Fig. 11.7), tectotopic to the HRP application site, and the ganglion cells from the extrafascicular axons were seen as a link (LC in Fig.

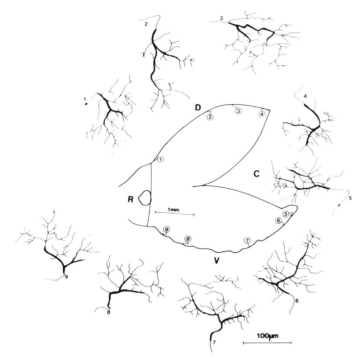

Fig. 11.5. Nine terminal arbors in the peripheral tectum emerging from short, and most from centrally directed, extrafascicular axons. The stem segment of most terminal arbors is centrally orientated (except for numbers 3 and 4). The major branches diverge widely and are often perpendicular to the stem segment (numbers 1 and 6–9). D, dorsal; C, caudal; V, ventral; R, rostral. [Reproduced from Stuermer (1984) by kind permission of the Society for Neuroscience, Bethesda, MD.]

11.7) between the cluster and the partial annulus (PHA in Fig. 11.7). Various parts of the tectum were labelled in this way and the patterns of retrogradely labelled ganglion cells in retina were all consistent with the predictions of our model of the shifting of terminal arbors (Easter and Stuermer 1984).

Summary

During the on-going and geometrically different growth of retina and tectum the retinotopic map is maintained. To account for this finding we believe that the terminal arbors shift. With the continuous arrival of new ganglion cell axons, the old axon arbors abandon the old sites to move on to new retinotopically appropriate sites. This conclusion is supported by a series of experiments using HRP to observe ganglion cell axon morphology.

In the goldfish, the fibres of similar ages are contained within a common fascicle. All of these fascicles are laid down in age-related order, old ones

axons at various stations along their path from the eye to the tectal synaptic layer (for goldfish, see Meyer 1980; Cook 1983; Stuermer and Easter 1984*a*; for amphibians see Fawcett and Gaze 1981; Fujisawa *et al.* 1982; Udin 1978; Taylor and Gaze 1985). Due to constraints in space we cannot do justice to these findings in any detail, but must instead condense the outcome of these investigations to the simplistic statement that regenerating axons never regain the same spatial order as their normal counterparts. This is not to say that the regenerated path is random (Cook 1983), since sorting of fibres occurs at various levels: at the brachial bifurcation (Stuermer and Easter 1984*a*) and in the tectal fascicle layer (Stuermer 1986). However, the precision of the normal order is never achieved, which implies that regenerating fibres have to take novel routes and possibly make more complicated manoeuvres than they do normally to find their retinotopic target sites (Fujisawa *et al.* 1982; Cook 1983; Stuermer 1986; Stuermer, Wizenmann, and Kelber 1986). The following pages will deal with new insights on the navigation of regenerating axons in the tectum and provide a description of their surprisingly complex morphologies during early regeneration.

These experiments also contained some indications that the distribution of the axon terminal endings may not be normal during the early periods of regeneration (Cook 1983; Stuermer and Easter 1984*a*; Schmidt 1985), and recent publications by Meyer, Sakurai, and Schauwecker (1985) and Rankin and Cook (1986) proved this assumption to be right.

The order of terminals early and late during regeneration

Rankin and Cook (1986) assessed the order of axon terminals in early and late regeneration stages by injecting wheat-germ-agglutinin-conjugated HRP (WGA-HRP) (Cook 1983; Stuermer and Easter 1984*a*) at well-defined rostral or caudal tectal sites. WGA-HRP is probably taken up selectively by axonal endings and not by fibres of passage (Cook and Rankin 1984) so that the distribution of the terminal endings at various survival times can be determined by analysing the distribution of the retrogradely labelled ganglion cells in the retina. Since label can be taken up by terminal arbors, growth cones, or other axonal appendages (see below: Stuermer 1986*b*; Stuermer *et al.* 1986), the non-commital term 'axonal endings' was chosen (Rankin and Cook 1986). Indeed, the patterns of ganglion cells in the retina, labelled retrogradely from the WGA-HRP application in the tectum during early regeneration stages, were different from those in normal animals. Early in regeneration the labelled ganglion cells were distributed widely over the retina. At longer survival times, more ganglion cells were labelled in approximately correct quadrants, but still occupied a larger area of the retina than normally. Only at around 70 days did they appear in small clusters at retinotopic sites. These experiments show that a defined population of ganglion cells have their terminal endings distributed widely over the tectum initially, and only gradually condense to occupy appropriate regions (Cook and Rankin 1984; Rankin and Cook 1986).

Meyer *et al.* (1985) also came to the conclusion that the distribution of axon terminals is abnormal early in regeneration. They studied the order of the terminal endings by applying WGA-HRP intra-retinally to small groups of ganglion cells. WGA-HRP is anterogradely transported and accumulates selectively in the terminal endings of the regenerating axons (Meyer *et al.* 1985). These labelled endings were spread widely over large and grossly correct tectal regions in early regeneration, and only gradually became confined into well-defined retinotopically positioned clusters (Meyer *et al.* 1985).

The conclusions from the above experiments were that initially large arbors condense to occupy appropriate territories later on, as envisaged by Schmidt (1985), or that axons deploy their terminals (or parts of them) transiently at ectopic regions and move later to their appropriate sites, or both (Cook and Rankin 1984; Schmidt 1985; Meyer *et al.* 1985; Rankin and Cook 1986). To resolve the case, it is necessary to identify the terminal endings which occupied transiently non-retinotopic regions, but disappear later, and to explore how the axons got to these sites.

Aberrant paths and course corrections of regenerating axons

The experimental protocol

We set out to trace the pathways taken by regenerating axons of defined retinal regional origin at various intervals after optic nerve section, and to investigate their morphologies. For our studies we used HRP to stain the axons as well as the terminal endings (Stuermer 1986; Stuermer *et al.* 1986). Crystals of HRP were applied locally, close to the optic disk, to axons in the retina either dorso–temporally or dorso–nasally (Fig. 11.8). Such HRP applications retrogradely label axons and ganglion cells in a sector comprising between 10 to 20 per cent of the total retinal area. They label anterogradely the axons derived from this retinal sector in the tectum (Stuermer 1984*a*). Similar labelling sites were used in normal animals and regenerates at various intervals after optic nerve section, which allowed us to compare the paths and the morphologies of normal axons with those of regenerates of similar retinal regional origin.

The path of normal dorso–temporal axons

In the normal animal, the fibres of a sector in the dorso–temporal retina take orderly routes which are consistent with our earlier findings (Stuermer and Easter 1984*b*; Stuermer 1984) [Fig. 11.8(a)]. They pass into the tectum through the ventral brachium of the optic tract, and depart from their fascicles in the rostral tectum, following extrafascicular routes of various lengths through the synaptic layer to their retinotopic termination sites. The terminal arbors of the

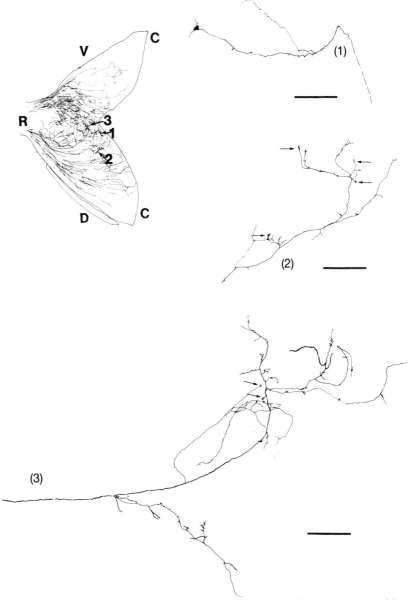

Fig. 11.10. Details of the axons from the tectum shown in Fig. 11.8 (b) at positions indicated in the inset. (1) This axon bears a growth cone and several filopodia and spikes; it dramatically alters its course and runs from the inappropriate caudal tectum back towards the rostral tectum. (2) A widely ramifying axon in the ventro–caudal tectum. The branches bear growth cones (arrows) and filopodia. (3) A widely ramifying axon close to the centre of the tectum. The branches bear numerous filopodia and spikes as well as occasional growth cones (arrows). R, rostral; V, ventral; C, caudal; D, dorsal. Scale bar for all drawings: 100 µm.

from the rostral to the inappropriate caudal tectum, suggesting that these axons may be able to discriminate between more appropriate and inappropriate tectal territories. Some fibres did not make course corrections and to some extent invaded the caudal tectum. With longer regeneration time (see below) these decreased in number. These observations show that misrouted fibres can make changes in orientation during their growth through the tectum. Their corrected paths lead them either directly towards the retinotopic termination region or at least into the more appropriate rostral tectal half.

Morphology of the regenerating axons

Regenerating fibres at regeneration stages of up to three months had appendages typical for actively growing axons, such as simple or multiple growth cones, nests of growth cones, filopodia, and 'spikes' (Stuermer, in prep.). There were axons at various positions in the tectum occupying both the synaptic and the fascicular layer, which were tipped with one leading growth cone. Other axons with growth cones gave rise to spikes and filopodia [Fig. 11.10, axon (1)] and had winding trajectories, typically in the synaptic layer. Yet another group in the synaptic layer had numerous short side branches and one or more growth cones, or even nests of growth cones, on each of these branches. These side branches appeared on stretches of the axon over 800 μm in length (Fig. 11.11.). A further group of axons ramified widely [Fig. 11.11 axons (2) and (3)], typically in a layer just below the fascicle layer, and these ramifications often occurred at ectopic sites far away from the retinotopic regions [Fig. 11.8(b)]. The axons had branches up to 400 μm in length into various directions of the tectum which were studded with growth cones, spikes, and filopodia up to 100 μm long.

Obviously, tectal whole mounts give only static images of growing axons. However, there are reasons to believe that all of these appendages reflect the mechanism of axonal navigation. The branches, including the long ones, may function as 'scouts' which explore the tectal territory, interacting with the local tectal cells and other fibres.

Goldfish axons grown *in vitro* on substrates like laminin or fibronectin bear one or several growth cones, spikes, and filopodia of similar length as those *in vivo*. Time-lapse video recordings of these axons revealed that their appendages are highly mobile elements which alter their shape and their relative positions rapidly as the axons continue to grow (Vielmetter and Stuermer, unpub. obs). How interaction of the axon with the substrate or with the tectal elements is mediated is still unclear.

Axons with growth cones, filopodia, and spikes were still seen in tecta at three months after optic nerve section, although their number decreased with regeneration. For dorso–temporal axons they were usually found in the caudal tectum, i.e. at ectopic sites, indicating that these misrouted axons might still be 'searching' for their appropriate termination region. These features were not detectable in tecta at six and twelve months after optic nerve section.

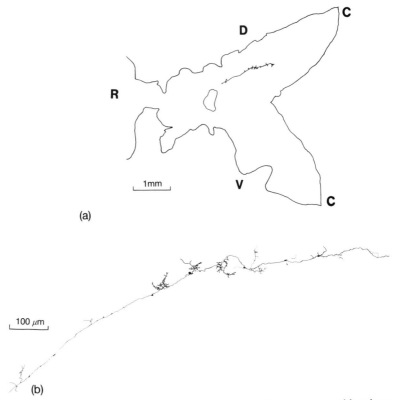

Fig. 11.11. An axon from the dorso–temporal retina in the dorso–rostral hemitectum of another regenerated preparation. This axon bears numerous growth cones on its shaft and short side branches. R, rostral; D, dorsal; V, ventral; C, caudal.

In the late regeneration stages at six and twelve months, the axons had lost most of their side branches and appendages, and ended in a terminal arbor in the appropriate tectal region (Fig. 11.9) (Stuermer 1986). They reached their terminal arbor regions both via normal-like routes and via abnormal routes. The latter exhibited strikingly goal-directed course corrections within the rostral tectum. Only a few of these aberrant axons were found in the most caudal tectum, indicating that most of the wide ramifications seen earlier must have been eliminated.

The path of regenerating dorso–nasal axons
We will not go into detail about the routes of dorso–nasal axons, but will instead highlight a few interesting points. As regenerating dorso–nasal axons course over the dorsal and ventral hemitectum, they preferentially travel along the routes of the previous fascicles, rostral and peripheral ones. Upon departing from rostral fascicles they bend caudally and head into the caudal

tectal half (Stuermer 1986) in a strategy used by normal axons (Stuermer and Easter 1984a). Most dorso–nasal axons remain smooth and unbranched while coursing over the routes of the previous fascicles and begin to exhibit elaborate morphologies, like multiple growth cones, side branches with growth cones, spikes, and filopodia, preferentially in the caudal tectal half. A few exceptions are axons which began to ramify at ectopic sites.

Again, features indicating active axonal growth were present in all tecta of early regeneration stages up to three months, but no longer at nine, ten, and twelve months. In these late regeneration stages, the axons had reached their retinotopic termination region where they ended in terminal arbors (Stuermer 1986a).

CONCLUSIONS

Our experiments led to two major findings:

(1) A substantial number of regenerating axons begin their course through the tectum along highly abnormal routes. During their growth, most of them can correct their course to approach the appropriate retinotopic region.

(2) Growth cones and other growth-related appendages were typically associated with the axons in all tectal regions. They disappeared gradually with regeneration time concurrent with the arrival of axons at their target regions. Growth cones and growth-related appendages were most numerous at times when anatomical mapping experiments with WGA-HRP (Meyer *et al.* 1985; Rankin and Cook 1986) demonstrated widespread terminal endings in the tectum. This strongly suggests that the growth cones, filopodia, and spikes, which were identified in our study as transient axonal endings in early regeneration stages, contribute to a large extent to the diffuseness of the map. We found that the confining of axons to their appropriate target region is accompanied by the loss of growth cones and growth-related appendages, and their disappearance from all tectal regions coincides with the time when mapping experiments by Meyer *et al.* (1985) and Rankin and Cook (1986) revealed a condensation of axon endings into retinotopically grossly correct territories.

Most misrouted axons with either one growth cone at their tips or several growth cones on short side branches had reached their target regions along a direct route or with gradual course corrections. A small number of axons behaved differently. They ramified widely and sent out 'exploratory' branches with growth cones, filopodia, and spikes into various directions of the tectum. These ramifications were no longer present in later regeneration stages. Since there is no evidence for cell death in the retina during optic nerve regeneration in fish, which could account for their elimination (Meyer *et al.* 1985), it is conceivable that these axons maintain those branches which have reached the target region or its vicinity, or they may sprout new branches close to the target region, while branches at ectopic sites are withdrawn or eliminated.

In all tecta, only a small number of axons produced large ramifications. It appears possible, therefore, that they either belong to a subclass of retinal axons (Sur and Sherman 1982) and/or that they represent a particular functional state of some misrouted axons which are unable (for unknown reasons) to perform goal-directed course corrections in the same way as the majority of their regenerating companions. The term 'ramification' was chosen in our study to distinguish the extraordinary branching behaviour of the axons at ectopic regions from tighter terminal arborizations formed by axons at retinotopic regions (Stuermer, in prep.)

In summary, the extent of target-directed course corrections exhibited by the majority of regenerating axons is striking (Stuermer, in prep.). It suggests that the regenerating axons may be sensitive to and respond to some directional cues from the target region.

Our results are meant to address only the question of how grossly correct retinotopic order develops. We do not consider here the further step in development of the retinotopic map, i.e. how this order is tuned into a refined retinotopic map (Schmidt and Edwards 1983; Meyer *et al.* 1985; Rankin and Cook 1986) which must depend on the correlated activity of neighbouring ganglion cell axons (for further information, see Schmidt 1987, this volume).

Further points still need clarification: misrouted axons in goldfish obviously have the capacity to continue to grow and explore the tectum for quite a long time. Concurrently, synaptogenesis occurs, beginning rostrally as early as 15 days after optic nerve section (Schmidt, Edwards, and Stuermer 1983; Stuermer and Easter 1984*a*), reaching its peak at approximately three months (Murray and Edwards 1982). We have no information on whether these early synapses are formed exclusively at retinotopic sites or at random. However, we know that they are functionally active (Schmidt *et al.* 1983). By 34 days, a good number of functionally active synaptic contacts must have been made at retinotopically appropriate sites, since the map assessed electrophysiologically is normal by that time (Schmidt *et al.* 1983).

The obvious questions to emerge are: Which of the axons and which of the axonal appendages described above are involved in forming synaptic connections? Are synaptic connections established only at or near the retinotopically appropriate regions or at ectopic sites as well, as suggested by Rankin and Cook (1986) from their anatomical mapping experiments (see also Schmidt 1985)? Or is the diffuseness of the anatomically assessed map attributable to the transient growth features which may or may not form synapses? The answer to some of these questions might be found using electron microscopy to look at synapse distribution in regenerating tectum, a study which we have recently begun.

ACKNOWLEDGEMENTS

I am most grateful to Mike McKenna for his critical and helpful corrections of the manuscript. Most of the experiments described in the first part of the paper were performed together with Prof. S. S. Easter, Jr., in Ann Arbor, Michigan. The experiments described in the second part of the paper were performed with the excellent technical assistance of A. Wizenmann, A. Kelber, and A. Habring, who were also involved in the laborious work of making the *camera lucida* tracings. I thank R. Groemke-Lutz for her skilful photographical reproductions, and K. Ralinofsky for typing the manuscript.

REFERENCES

Arora, H. L. and Sperry, R. W. (1963). Color discrimination after optic nerve regeneration in the fish Astronotus ocellatus. *Dev. Biol.* **7**, pp. 234–43.

Attardi, D. G. and Sperry, R. W. (1963). Preferential selection of central pathways by regenerating optic fibers. *Exp. Neurol.* **7**, pp. 46–64.

Constantine-Paton, M., Pitts, E. C., and Reh, T. A. (1983). The relationship between retinal axon ingrowth, terminal morphology, and terminal patterning in the optic tectum of the frog. *J. Comp. Neurol.* **218**, pp. 297–313.

Cook, J. E. (1983). Tectal paths of regenerated optic axons in the goldfish: evidence from retrograde labelling with Horseradish Peroxidase. *Exp. Brain Res.* **51**, pp. 533–442.

Cook, J. E. and Rankin, E. C. C. (1984). The use of a lectin-peroxidase conjugate (WGA-HRP) to assess the retinotopic precision of goldfish optic pathway. *Neurosci. Lett.* **48**, pp. 61–6.

Cook, J. E., Rankin, E. C. C., and Stevens, H. P. (1983). A pattern of optic axons in the normal goldfish tectum consistent with the caudal migration of optic terminals during development. *Exp. Brain Res.* **52**, pp. 147–51.

Easter, S. S., Jr. and Stuermer, C. A. (1984). An evaluation of the hypothesis of shifting terminals in goldfish optic tectum. *J. Neurosci.* **4**, pp. 1052–63.

Easter, S. S., Jr., Rusoff, A. C., and Kish, P. E. (1981). The growth and organization of the optic nerve and tract in juvenile and adult goldfish. *J. Neurosci.* **1**, pp. 793–811.

Fawcett, J. W. and Gaze, R. M. (1981). The organization of regenerating axons in the Xenopus optic tract. *Brain Res.* **229**, pp. 487–90.

Fujisawa, H., Tani, N., Watanabe, K., and Ibata, Y. (1982). Branching of regenerating retinal axons and preferential selection of appropriate branches for specific neuronal connection in the newt. *Dev. Biol.* **90**, pp. 43–57.

Gaze, R. M. (1958). The representation of the retina on the optic lobe of the frog. *Q. J. Exp. Physiol.* **43**, pp. 209–14.

Gaze, R. M. (1959). Regeneration of the optic nerve in Xenopus lavis. *Q. J. Exp. Physiol.* **44**, pp. 290–308.

Gaze, R. M. (1960). Regeneration of the optic nerve in amphibia. *Int. Rev. Neurobiol.* **2**, pp. 1–40.

Gaze, R. M. (1970). *The formation of nerve connections.* Academic Press, New York.

12

Motor axon guidance in the developing chick limb

R. VICTORIA STIRLING AND DENNIS SUMMERBELL

Some thirty years ago Paul Weiss summarized our understanding of the control of innervation in the peripheral vertebrate nervous system in an influential book entitled *The analysis of development* (Willier, Weiss, and Hamburger 1955, p. 380). 'Continued experiments in amphibians, and later even more penetratingly in birds, have reiterated an old lesson of biological research: a relation that on first aquaintance appears simple and transparent, when subject to more minute analysis more often than not turns out to be much more complex, if not more obscure, than originally suspected'.

The vertebrates limb is a highly patterned organ. Its nerve supply is a complex branching network which connects the cells in the central nervous system with their targets in the limb. This chapter describes the development of the basic pattern of peripheral innervation of the chick limb and examines the evidence for various mechanisms that may be involved in establishing this pattern. Two aspects will be considered: the gross morphology of the nerve pattern with its characteristic arrangement of branches, and the questions of whether axons make specific choices as they grow towards their targets, and if so, of where these choices are made.

NORMAL DEVELOPMENT OF CHICK LIMB INNERVATION

The pattern in the periphery

The motor axons exit the cord opposite the cranial (anterior) half of the sclerotome of each somite (Keynes and Stern 1985, this volume, Chapter 5). Each ventral root joins the axons from the dorsal root ganglion to form the spinal nerve. The spinal nerves travel medio–ventrally to the myotome through the cranial half-sclerotome to the lateral edge of the somite, then combine together in the flank to form the plexus. They enter the limb bud over a wide front (Roncali 1970; Hollyday 1983), dividing into the main dorsal and ventral nerve trunks as the dorsal and ventral muscle masses begin to differentiate (Bennett, Davey, and Uebel 1980). As the dorsal and ventral muscle masses separate to form individual muscles the main nerve branches are formed. It is easy to forget that at this stage the limb bud is still very small and that the area occupied by the advancing nerves is comparatively large (Fig. 12.1). During the subsequent growth of the limb the nerve pattern gets pulled out, producing distortion (Weiss 1939). Simultaneously there can be complex torsional movements: the triceps, which was initially dorsal, rotates into a more posterior position, while the biceps, which was initially ventral, becomes anterior (Searls 1983). The initial pattern, as seen by silver staining methods at early stages, is radically different from the adult-like pattern seen only two or three days later.

The pattern of axon projections between spinal cord and limb

The vertebrate limb is innervated by several spinal cord segments via the spinal nerves. The distribution of the axons from each spinal nerve can be mapped electrophysiological by stimulating and recording from each root in turn (Landmesser and Morris 1975; Stirling and Summerbell 1977; Pettigrew, Lindeman, and Bennett 1979). These methods have produced conflicting results as to whether there are any transient connections to inappropriate targets early in development. The distribution of axons from each segment can also be mapped anatomically using tracers which are transported orthogradely (from the cell body outwards) along nerve fibres, such as cobalt chloride (Stirling and Summerbell 1979) or the enzyme horseradish peroxidase (HRP) (Landmesser 1978a). Using these methods it is clear that in normal development the distribution of axons from each segment has its adult pattern from the start (Hollyday 1983; Tosney and Landmesser 1985a). Injection of HRP into dorsal root ganglia also shows that the adult distribution of sensory nerves is also present at this time (Scott 1982; Honig 1982).

The spatial arrangement of the motoneurons innervating a single muscle can be mapped following retrograde transport of HRP injected into the muscle (Landmesser 1978a). Each muscle of the limb is innervated by a cranio–caudal elongated cluster of motoneurons located in a characteristic position in the lateral motor column of the spinal cord, otherwise known as the motor pool. The pattern of motor pools is established as soon as the motor axons contact the muscles, with few errors (Landmesser 1978b). Later in development 40 per cent of the motoneurons in the cord die (Hamburger 1975; Laing 1982), with only minor changes in the pattern of motor or sensory projections. The trajectories of motor axons in the limb is well ordered. Axons from motoneurons in the lateral motor horn run in the dorsal sector of the spinal nerves to innervate the dorsal extensor muscles, while those from the medial motor horn travel in the ventral sector to innervate ventral flexor muscles (Figs. 12.2 and 12.3; Summerbell and Stirling 1982). Many authors

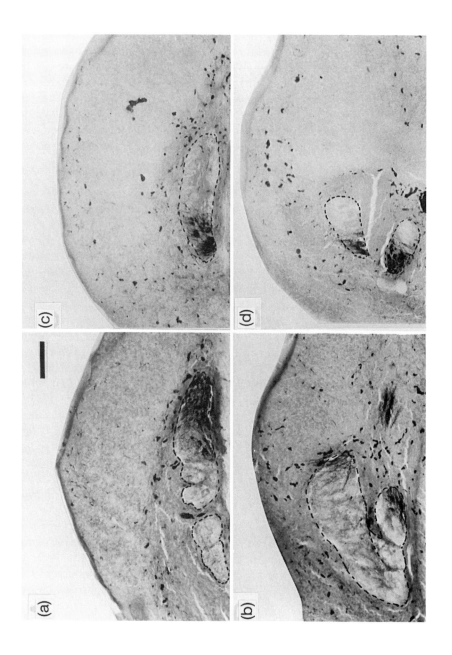

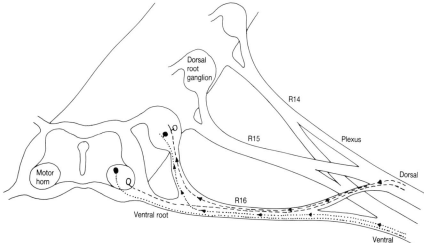

Fig. 12.2. Diagram of the spinal cord and right plexus. Axons from medial motoneurons (solid circles, dotted line) travel ventrally through the plexus and enter the ventral medio–ulnar nerve to reach flexor muscles in the limb. Axons from lateral motoneurons (open circles, dashed line) travel dorsally through the plexus to enter the radial nerve to reach dorsal extensor muscles. The arrangement in the dorsal roots is conjecture. Note that some sensory axons must cross motor axons (arrow) to reach the medio–ulnar nerve (see text).

have pointed out that if neighbouring motor pools connect to neighbouring targets then the trajectory of the axons to these targets is topographically simple (Horder 1978; Lewis 1978; Stirling and Summerbell 1979; Hollyday 1980). Only at the point where the sensory axons from the dorsal ganglia join those in the ventral root do axons obviously cross one another.

Technical limitations

Our understanding of the pattern of innervation has improved due to the development of intracellular tracing methods, but there are still technical limitations. Injected markers may spread into adjacent muscles or away from the site of injection in the cord. It is not possible to ensure that all of the axons

Fig. 12.1. Sections showing the relationship between the ingrowing nerves and the limb bud. Scale bar: 100 μm. (a) Section proximal to the plexus taken at the time the axons reach the elbow following injection of HRP into the ventral cord segments 13/14. (b) Section distal to the plexus from the same specimen. Note the wide front over which the axons enter the limb and also that the labelled axons stay together in the anterior sector through the plexus. (c) Proximal plexus 24 hours later, when the axons reach the wrist, following injection of HRP into the ventral cord at segment 16. (d) Section distal to the plexus from the same specimen. Note that the nerves are much more compact and better defined; labelled axons are confined to the posterior sector.

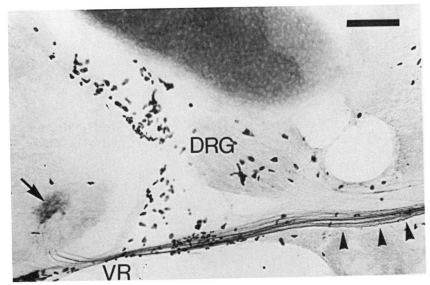

Fig. 12.3. Axons labelled after an injection into the biceps muscle originate from a cluster of cells in the medial motor horn in segment 14 (arrow). The axons leave the cells ventrally, staying ventral in the motor root and in the spinal nerve (arrow heads). The somite which normally supplies myoblasts to the biceps muscle had previously been exchanged for a more caudal somite which normally supplies myoblasts to the triceps muscle. Despite the operation the outgrowth of axons and the innervation pattern of the limb was entirely normal. Scale bar: 100 μm.

from a given injection site or muscle will be filled. The availability of only a single reliable marker can reveal the position of only a single motor pool and cannot show the relationship between different pools. It is therefore not clear whether axons from different pools intermingle in some parts of the tract and later sort out into homogeneous bundles. For example, Hollyday (1983) and Tosney and Landmesser (1985*b*) suggest that the majority of axons 'cross over' one another, especially at the plexus and at nerve branch points, so as to reach their appropriate destinations. Stirling and Summerbell (1985) describe the axons as maintaining cohesion while whole bundles spiral around the nerve to reach the appropriate branch. Progress in resolving this difference of interpretation would be simplified if we had two distinguishable labels that marked different populations of axons.

GUIDANCE CUES IN THE LIMB BUD

Public highways

During innervation of the limb, axons follow a complex route from the neurons in the motor horn and dorsal root ganglia to their targets in the limb.

By the time the definitive nerve pattern is fully formed it consists of tightly defined bundles of axons arranged in a characteristic branching pattern. This has led many authors to suggest that the growing axons must be following some kind of public highway, road, or track to their destinations. Lewis, Al-Ghaith, Swanson and Khan (1983) succinctly describe the tracks as 'public in the sense that they are open to axons from any source, highways in the sense that they constitute a restricted set of permitted routes through the terrain of the limb' (p. 198). However, while this may seem a useful analogy, it should not be interpreted too literally because it may prompt us to search for the wrong kind of cellular mechanism during growth cone migration.

The first problem with the analogy is that we usually examine the pattern at the wrong time. While Theseus sought the Minotaur in the Labyrinth he progressed slowly inwards, trying many wrong turns then retracing his path until eventually he reached his goal. However, the crucial piece of string ultimately traced a direct path apparently making the correct choice at every fork. When we examine the nervous system our silver stain marks the string, but tells us little about Theseus or the behaviour of axonal growth cones.

During initial innervation the appearance is different. When axons first enter the developing limb bud, the width of the advancing axon front is very wide compared to the width of the limb (Fig. 12.1). The earliest branches to muscles are small tufts of axons leaving the nerve (Lewis *et al.* 1983). As development proceeds, the limb bud grows and the nerves are pulled out (Weiss 1939) and 'perineural cells' wrap the axons into tight fascicles (Al-Ghaith and Lewis 1982). The end result is a pattern of tight axon bundles with extended muscle branches. The glia derived from the neural crest may play an important role in the formation of nerve pattern. Following effective ablation of the neural crest, motor nerves do not make the normal pattern within the limb (Hollyday, pers. comm.).

The second problem with the highways analogy concerns the anatomical accuracy of the pattern. The pattern and size of the skeleton is accurately controlled (Summerbell and Wolpert 1973). Even in the normal limb the pattern of nerves is constant only in the sense that axons run predominantly in a proximo–distal direction between other major anatomical features and that there is a fairly constant number of branches. Within these constraints, the position of the branch point and the precise trajectory of the nerve is more or less random even when comparing opposite sides of the same embryo.

In experimentally manipulated limbs the nerve tracks are even more variable. Piatt (1957) working on the axolotl (*Ambystoma*) and Wenger (1951) using chicks both showed that a normal nerve pattern was seen in experimental limbs only when they were grafted in their normal position and orientation and were innervated by their normal nerve source. Narayanan (1964) described the pattern of the segmental nerves to wings grafted with reversed orientation or to ectopic sites. He concluded that nerves formed primary pathways by centrifugal growth 'which is essentially random, within the limitations imposed by the substratum' (p. 59). Hollyday (1981) grafted a supernumerary leg just cranial to the normal leg and found that the innervation pattern was 'largely normal'. Her illustrations show that, while all major branches are present, their positions relative to each other and to other anatomical features are variable. Lewis (1978) grafted a whole limb onto the wrist level of a host embryo, and concluded that the nerve pattern in both host and grafted elbows looked normal. However, his illustrations show fundamental differences between the two. Detailed examination of illustrations of nerve patterns in limbs following spinal cord reversal (Lance-Jones and Landmesser 1981) reveals unique nerves and missing branches. Of course, in all these cases one has access only to the generalization and the chosen illustration. A careful re-examination of our own work showed that it is difficult to find normal nerve patterns in a limb in which there are known errors of projection by motoneurons. In limbs which had been reversed about the dorso–ventral axis, the host ventral nerve moved around the elbow of the grafted reversed wing to innervate its normal targets, including the forearm flexor muscle (Summerbell and Stirling 1982). Another common pattern was an exchange of axons between dorsal and ventral nerves in the forearm. In this case the switch between dorsal and ventral position is far distal to the original plane of reversal. While in proximal regions the axons have made a pattern dictated by the limb tissue and have innervated alien targets, more distally they may correct their trajectory so as to reach appropriate targets (Fig. 12.4). A similar situation was described by Lance-Jones and Landmesser (1980*b*, 1981) in hind limbs innervated by reversed cord segments, where 'occasionally' abnormal nerves connected particular spinal roots with an appropriate target in the limb.

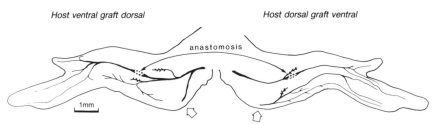

Fig. 12.4. Composite diagram from camera lucida drawings showing dorsal (to the left) and ventral (to the right) nerve patterns taken from several dorso–ventral reversed wings stained with the whole mount Bodian method (Lewis 1978). The host ventral nerve divides into medial and ulnar branches. The ulnar branch travels round the elbow (open arrows) to enter the ventral side of the graft to innervate the ventral forearm flexor appropriately. The medial branch becomes the radial nerve in the graft giving off typical cutaneous branches to the elbow and the forearm extensors; at the arrow there is an anatomosis between the dorsal and ventral nerves in the graft. The host dorsal nerve sends branches to the ventral muscles in the graft before anastomosing with the dorsal nerve in the graft.

These examples suggest that, while axons may be confined to particular positions, in the sense that the early settlers heading West followed the valley bottoms, they do not follow predetermined pathways in the way that we now drive only along the freeway.

Axon navigation

As discussed above, the distances that the first axons have to grow to reach their targets is very small, the width of the entire innervation field is very narrow, and the width of the axon growth front is relatively wide (Fig. 12.1). Nor is each branch of the nerve pattern marked out by a single pioneer axon in the same way that single scouts first establish the route as seen in the developing invertebrate nervous system (Bentley and Keshisnian 1982; Bastiani, Doe, Holfand, and Goodman 1985; Blair and Palka 1985; Durbin this volume, Chapter 1; Blackshaw, this volume, Chapter 2; Bacon, this volume, Chapter 13). Noakes, Bennett, and Davey (1983) serially sectioned the tips of advancing nerves growing into rat diaphragm and described growth cones distributed evenly throughout the length of the nerve with no one growth cone significantly ahead of the others. In the chick limb the distal tip of the nerve is splayed (Summerbell and Stirling 1982) with numerous axons all ending in growth cones (Al-Ghaith and Lewis 1982) so that the nerve tip contacts cells over a wide area of the limb. However, the axons cannot grow anywhere. They are confined to particular positions because, for example, they cannot penetrate cartilage or muscle or the caudal half of the sclerotome (Stern, Sisodiya, and Keynes 1986). There are permissive and non-permissive areas (Tosney and Landmesser 1984). They detour round the ventral margin of the myotome, because they cannot pierce the muscle sheet. They spiral around the humerus to reach the dorsal side, because again they cannot go through cartilage. Finally, they detour around an impermeable barrier, because it is a barrier.

The barrier experiment is important since it suggests that once axons have deviated from their normal route they can return to it. However, we are again faced with an experiment in which the pattern is examined some time after the critical growth processes had occurred. One could imagine that the axons, after passing around the barrier, establish contact with their targets just beyond. Further growth of the limb forces the nerve bundle between barrier and target into a straight line. Alternatively, beyond the barrier there could be two impenetrable areas acting as boundaries to lateral axon growth, subsequent glial activity narrows down the nerve to make it look like a neat narrow 'highway'. It is important to monitor the behaviour of axons and glia as they interact with such barriers before a full interpretation can be made.

Many workers have searched for the clues that axons might follow to their targets. It has been suggested that blood vessels, glia, or extracellular spaces might provide a preferred route for axons (e.g. Singer, Nordländer, and Edgar

1979; Katz, Lasek, and Nauta 1980), but there is no good supporting evidence for this in the limb. Nor are the highways marked out by the myoblasts which precede the axons into the limb. Irradiation of the somites destroys the presumptive myoblasts before they migrate into the limb. However, the gross pattern of nerves within the limb is normal except that short side branches to the muscles may be missing (Lewis, Chevalier, Kieny and Wolpert 1981). Hollyday (pers. com.) has suggested that even the missing muscle branches may be a secondary effect, produced by death of motoneurons that have connected to myoblastless 'muscles'.

There is also to date no direct evidence that extracellular matrix molecules known to be attractive to neurites *in vitro* pave the way for growing axons (Keynes and Stern, 1985, this volume, Chapter 5; Rickmann, Fawcett, and Keynes 1985). For example, the role of neural cell adhesion molecule (NCAM) in providing an adhesion site for axons during development is well documented both *in vivo* (Edelman 1984) and *in vitro* (Rutishauser, Grumet, and Edelman 1983). In the developing chick hind limb it is widely distributed during early stages (Tosney, Watanabe, Landmesser, and Rutishauser 1986), suggesting that it may be important in axon fasiculation and the formation of the neuromuscular junction rather than in the specific guidance of axons.

We have already dealt with the lack of evidence for specific cues acting on early axons as they invade the limb. To return to our Western analogy, the first settlers meander through virgin territory; once the trading post has been established there are clear tracks for later arrivals to follow. Later arriving axons clearly follow their predecessors, and here again glia seem to play an important role; axon growth cones are found between the glial sheath and the existing axons (Al-Ghaith and Lewis 1982).

The evidence for local decision regions

Tosney and Landmesser (1985*b*) distinguish guidance along the major nerve highways from specific localized guidance at 'decision regions'. While we question the idea of highways it is still possible that particular regions such as the plexus are rich in guidance cues which are absent in other regions of the limb. The evidence is derived mainly from experiments in which a topological mismatch is created between motoneurons in the cord and their targets in the limb.

Following antero–posterior reversal of three to four segments of spinal cord (Lance-Jones and Landmesser 1981) the leg develops with a more or less normal pattern of nerves. In some cases, as the axons grow into the limb, they correct their trajectories within the nerve so as to innervate the muscle appropriate to their spatial origin in the cord. Examination of their illustrations shows that in some cases correction takes place in the plexus and in others beyond it (Lance-Jones and Landmesser 1981, Figs. 2 and 5). The ectopic nerves that appear to connect the spinal cord with appropriate target regions in the limb likewise can arise anywhere.

In our experiments, in which the early limb bud is reversed before axons have reached it, we see axons changing course both at the plexus and beyond it, especially in animals where the level of reversal is distal to the plexus (Stirling and Summerbell 1985). When the limb bud is reversed about the dorso–ventral axis, many axons innervate inappropriate muscles (see next section); however the cross-over seen between dorsal and ventral nerves distally (see above and Fig. 12.4) and the displaced nerves suggests that axons can make specific decisions at places where normally there are no branches. The trajectories of motor axons in mirror-image duplications produced by zone of polarizing activity (ZPA) grafts reinforce this conclusion. When the duplication is distal to the plexus, axons from caudal motoneurones change their position in the radial nerve to reach the duplicated muscle [Fig. 11.5(a) and Fig. 11.6(c)]. However, when the duplication is proximal, axons from these motoneurons fail to reach the duplicate of their target muscle [Fig. 12.5(b)]. The difference between the proximal and distal duplications seems to be the presence of a normal plexus. The plexus, therefore, is important in the sense that it is the only place where axons from all three spinal nerves and from medial and lateral regions of the motor horn come close together, but clearly the guidance cues are present throughout the limb and are not restricted to particular regions.

Finally, if we reject the notion of localized 'decision regions', we still need to explain the observation that stimulated this discussion (Tosney and Landmesser 1985*b*, p. 2349). They noted that in the 'decision regions' growth cones are larger and have more complex trajectories. Their operational definition of a muscle nerve decision region was 'a radius of 75 μm around the point where a muscle nerve diverged from a nerve trunk'. The illustration of labelled axons making a course correction at such a decision region is of axons which are travelling along an established nerve. We suggest that the modified behaviour of these growth cones is not a response to localized cues within the limb, but is related to their search for their neighbours within the nerve.

MATCHING OF MOTONEURONS WITH THEIR TARGET MUSCLES

The accuracy of the early motor projection pattern suggests that there may be cellular mechanisms that match motoneurons with specific target muscles in the limb. One way to test this is to alter the topographic relationship between the spinal cord and the limb to see if axons still manage to innervate their appropriate targets. This is equivalent to the classical work of Sperry (1963) on the frog eye and involves either reversing part of the spinal cord, changing the cranio–caudal sequence of the motor pools, or reversing the limb, about either the dorso–ventral or the antero–posterior axis or about both axes. In all

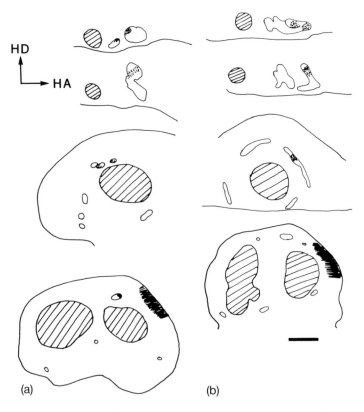

HD
HA

(a)   (b)

Fig. 12.5. Camera lucida drawings of transverse sections of the limb showing the position of axons filled by injection into the anterior duplicated muscle *extensor metacarpi ulnaris* (EMU) in two limbs with antero-posterior mirror-image duplication. Host axes: dorsal upwards and anterior to the right. The sequence of drawings from top to bottom is: proximal to the plexus, at the division into main dorsal and ventral branches, at mid-humerus level, and at the injection site. Scale bar: 200 μm. (a) Level of duplication distal to the shoulder. The plexus is normal: axons in the dorsal sector of the 15th and 16th spinal nerves [from lateral cells in segments 15 and 16 as in Fig. 12.6(c)] appear to change their position in the dorsal radial nerve to reach the duplicated muscle. (b) Level of duplication proximal to the shoulder. The plexus is very abnormal. The spinal nerves never combine and the dorsal nerve is widely spread over the humerus. Injection of the duplicated extensor metacarpi ulnaris muscle labels cells in the lateral horn in segment 14 (i.e. inappropriate); the axons maintain their anterior position in the duplicated limb. The axons from motoneurons in caudal segments are never in a position to reach the duplicated muscle.

such cut-and-paste experiments the operation is performed before the axons have grown into the affected area.

The most consistent evidence that motoneurons connect to their appropriate targets was seen after antero-posterior limb reversal (Stirling and Summerbell 1983, 1985). The motor pools for biceps and triceps muscles (which occupy mutually exclusive positions in the motor horn) were almost always symmetrical on operated and contralateral control sides of single animals [Fig. 12.6(a); Stirling and Summerbell 1985.] When the limb bud was

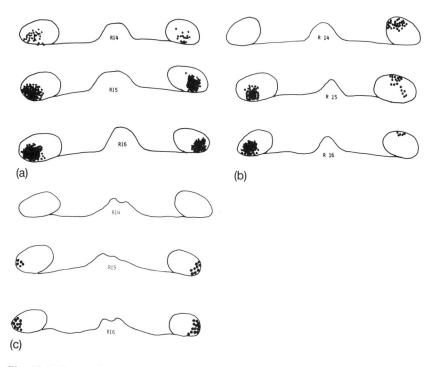

Fig. 12.6. Camera lucida drawings of single 60 μm sections showing the positions of HRP-labelled cells in the motor horn at the level of the 14th, 15th, and 16th spinal roots following injection into symmetrical muscles on unoperated (to the left) and operated (to the right) sides. (a) Antero–posterior limb reversal on the operated side. Triceps muscle injected bilaterally, the position of the labelled cells is symmetrical. (b) Dorso–ventral limb reversal on the operated side. Triceps muscle injected bilaterally, the position of the labelled cells is assymmetrical, position of labelled pool on the operated side characteristic of normal biceps. (c) Antero–posterior duplicated limb on the operated side. Posterior forearm extensor (extensor metacarpi ulnaris) injected on the unoperated side, its anterior duplicate on the operated side. The position of the labelled cells is symmetrical.

reversed about the dorso–ventral axis, injection of a single muscle usually gave asymmetrical labelling (Summerbell and Stirling 1981). For example, injection of the triceps muscle on the operated side always labelled cells asymmetrically [frequently in a position characteristic of its antagonist, the biceps motor pool; Fig. 12.6.(b)]. However, in a minority of muscle injections the labelling was symmetrical showing appropriate innervation. Some muscles, such as *flexor carpi ulnaris*, received appropriate innervation more frequently than others. Whitelaw and Hollyday (1983c) found that in hind limbs reversed at the knee, muscles were innervated inappropriately. By contrast, both Ferguson (1983) and Laing (1984) have found appropriate innervation in dorso–ventrally reversed limbs; we believe this is related to the abnormality of the plexus region. In these experiments the graft is pushed into a hole in the flank of the host embryo while in our experiments the graft is firmly pinned to the host. While the axons penetrate easily into pinned grafts and form a normal looking plexus, when pins are not used, the axons in many cases, do not enter the graft and when they do the plexus is abnormal (Laing, Summerbell and Stirling unpub. obs.).

The interpretation of the results of cord reversal experiments is more difficult since there is no unoperated control side and because the operation is necessarily done at such an early stage that it is difficult to define the region of cord reversed. There is no good control in operated animals, so they must be compared with the normal population. Injection of *sartorius* muscle normally labels cells that are in a more cranial position than those labelled by an injection of *femorotibialis* on the contralateral side. When these two muscles are injected following cranio–caudal reversal of three to four segments of cord the labelled pools are smaller and more diffuse but clearly have the opposite distribution, sartorius being caudal to *femortibialis* (Lance-Jones and Landmesser 1980b). This information about the position of the motor pool can be supplemented with information about the trajectory of the axons by orthograde filling following localized injection of tracer into the cord. In normal animals each cord segment (or spinal nerve) sends axons to predictable nerve branches. Following reversal of three to four segments of cord each segment sends axons to unexpected branches, but in some animals some axons appear to correct their trajectory in the peripheral part of the nerve tract so as to reach appropriate branches (Lance-Jones and Landmesser 1980b). Following reversal of seven to eight segments of spinal cord there was no matching of motoneurons with specific target muscles. Occasionally, however, there were additional ectopic branches that appeared to carry axons to their appropriate muscle (Lance-Jones and Landmesser 1981). The specific connections between motoneurons and their target muscles was also preserved after deletion of cord segments (Lance-Jones and Landmesser 1980a) or deletion of limb segments (Whitelaw and Hollyday 1983a). In these cases the muscles without innervation atrophied later in development and the motoneurons without targets died during the period of cell death.

A supernumerary limb grafted cranial to the normal limb (Hollyday 1981) was innervated by inappropriate segments, but, whatever the orientation, the ventral flexor muscles were always innervated by medial clusters of cells while the extensors were innervated by lateral clusters of cells. Here we may be witnessing another level of specificity. The evidence for some kind of matching of motoneurons and their target muscles in manipulated embryos is good, but axons will functionally innervate alien targets in an orderly fashion and do remain viable beyond the period of cell death (Stirling and Summerbell 1979).

These experiments on specific matching have been confined to an examination of the connections made by motor axons. The projection of sensory cells to their areas of innervation during normal development looks precise from early stages (Scott 1982; Honig 1982). We do not know if sensory cells show the same behaviour when their targets are displaced. In our experiments where limb buds were reversed about both antero–posterior and dorso–ventral axes, both the sensory and motor innervation territories of the spinal nerves were abnormal (Stirling and Summerbell 1979). In antero–posterior duplicated limbs, whereas some caudal motoneurons selectively innervated the duplicated muscle, there was no such evidence of selectivity by sensory axons. This difference in behaviour between motor and sensory axons may reflect the difference in their function.

Possible cues for motoneuron matching

Since muscle branches are absent from muscleless limbs (Lewis *et al.* 1981) and muscle extracts maintain growth and viability of explanted motoneurons (Nurcombe and Bennett 1983), muscles themselves might act as local attractants. Other possible cues may be provided by the somites in a number of ways. Axons may receive their positional identity from the somite as they pass through the cranial half-sclerotome. During development the myoblasts migrate from the somites into the limb, and axons may follow myoblasts from specific segments. The pattern of distribution to the various limb muscles reflects the somitic level of the motoneurons innervating them (Beresford 1983). We have investigated these ideas by reversing, rotating, or exchanging somites in early embryos (Keynes, Stirling, Stern, and Summerbell 1987). In all the operations we performed, both retrograde and orthograde HRP tracing showed the pattern to be the same on operated and unoperated sides (Fig. 12.3). It is unlikely, therefore, that the segmental origin of the myoblasts alone is responsible for the guidance of motor axons. The innervation of duplicated limbs also supports this view, since the anterior duplicated extensor metacarpi ulnaris muscle is probably populated by myoblasts from more cranial rather than from more caudal somites, yet its motor pool lies (as it does on the unoperated side) in the caudal segments.

After destruction of the motor horn, the pattern of sensory nerves is normal except for the absence of muscle branches (Swanson and Lewis 1986), suggesting that motor axons may guide later arriving sensory fibres to the muscle. Localized specific cues may not be required to generate the motor map. Interaction between neighbouring axons and sensitivity to overall polarity cues could also provide adequate guidance cues as has been proposed for the retinotectal projection (Hope, Hammond, and Gaze 1976).

Cell death

Cell death is thought to be a near-ubiquitous phenomenon during the development of the nervous system (Oppenheim 1981b; Lamb 1984). Although it has been proposed that the development of motor pools involves random innervation of muscles followed by death of those cells making inappropriate connections (Pettigrew, Lindeman, and Bennett 1979), this now seems unlikely. If functional contacts are blocked from the time axons first grow into the limb until after the normal period of cell death (e.g. by curare or αBTX), then there is no cell death, but the enlarged pools still show no evidence of errors of projection (Oppenheim 1981a). Indeed the great majority of motoneurons project to the appropriate muscle from the earliest time that connections are made, while the few inappropriate connections are soon eliminated by the end of the phase of cell death (Hollyday 1983; Lance-Jones and Landmesser 1980b; Tosney and Landmesser 1985a). Nor do inappropriate connections necessarily die. Motoneuron pools innervating alien targets in tandem, supernumerary (Whitelaw and Hollyday 1983b), or reversed limbs (Summerbell and Stirling 1981) remain viable. However, motoneuron pools that should have connected to a muscle that has been removed surgically do die (Whitelaw and Hollyday 1983a). It is still possible that cell death plays a minor role through a mechanism involving competition between neuron connected to the same muscle. Mutual reinforcement of near neighbours in the spinal cord promotes survival at the expense of more isolated neurons. The evidence comes from dorso–ventral and antero–posterior limb reversal experiments. In dorso–ventrally reversed limbs many muscles are innervated by inappropriate motoneurons, and the motor horns on unoperated and operated sides are similar in size. However, in antero–posteriorly reversed limbs, where most muscles are innervated by their appropriate pools, the motor horns are reduced in size on the operated side (Stirling and Summerbell 1983). This increased cell death may be related to the fact that initially the motor pools were very diffuse as only some of the axons succeeded in reaching their appropriate targets. Cell death resulted in the development of discrete motor pools innervating muscles in the reversed limb. One must also take into account the role of the development of afferent connections in motoneuron maturation. If both descending tracts and inputs from dorsal root ganglia are removed, there is an increased loss of cells in the motor horn (Okado and Oppenheim 1984). The end result of cell death is the formation of a functionally coherent motor pool of cells with defined afferent and efferent projections creating a reliable motor effector system upon which the animal depends.

CONCLUSIONS

It is fashionable to compare the development of the nervous system in vertebrates to that in insects, for instance, in a recent issue of *Nature* (News and Views section) Taghert and Lichtman (1986) state: 'the stereotyped, precise and cell-specific nature of the axonal guidance (in vertebrates) suggests direct parallels with similar phenomena in insect embryos' (p. 210). The nervous system of insects is said to be simple and precise. Axons grow towards their target by predictable routes. Some of the cells along the route may be particularly important in guiding the axons. If these cells are destroyed the axons halt or grow in the wrong direction. This has led to the concept of 'guidepost' cells (Bastiani *et al.* 1985). While those working on insects may still argue about the details (see Blair and Palka 1985), the simplicity of the system makes it natural to wonder whether analogous mechanisms may play a role in vertebrate limb innervation. Tosney and Landmesser (1985*b*) were greatly influenced by the idea of guideposts in their recent discussion of the 'correction' of axon trajectories in nerves. In insects the nervous system is precisely wired, producing an animal with stereotyped behaviour patterns whose individual success depends on reliability but whose adaptability is limited to genetic variation in its offspring. The vertebrate nervous system is designed for a different kind of life-style: one that will adapt to changing environments within its own lifetime, and whose success depends on the plasticity of its connections. The contrast between automaton and opportunist may be reflected in the way the respective nervous systems develop.

The development of connections between the neurons and their targets does not rely on a single mechanism. We cannot discover which are important by observing the intact animal. Instead, we have to interfere with the system and observe the behaviour of the axons throughout development. The problem is to assess from the results of such experiments which mechanisms might be critical in normal development.

REFERENCES

Al-Ghaith, L. K. and Lewis, J. H. (1982). Pioneer growth cones in virgin mesenchyme: an electron-microscope study in the developing chick wing. *J. Embryol. exp. Morphol.* **68**, pp. 149–60.

Bacon, J. P. (1987). Transplantation of sensory neurons in the insect. In *The making of the nervous system* (eds. J. G. Parnavelas, C. D. Stern, and R. V. Stirling), pp. 248–67. Oxford University Press, Oxford.

244 *Axon guidance in the limb*

Bastiani, M. J., Doe, C. Q., Helfand, S. L., and Goodman, C. S. (1985) Neuronal specificity and growth cone guidance in grasshopper and *Drosophila* embryos. *Trends Neurosci.* **8**, pp. 257–67.

Bennett, M. R., Davey, D. F., and Uebel, K. E. (1980). The growth of segmental nerves from brachial myotomes into the proximal muscles of the chick forelimb during development. *J. Comp. Neurol.* **189**, pp. 335–57.

Bentley, D. and Keshishian, H. (1982). Pioneer neurons and pathways in insect appendages. *Trends Neurosci.* **5**, pp. 354–8.

Beresford, B. (1983). Brachial muscles in the chick embryo: the fate of individual somites. *J. Embryol. exp. Morphol.* **77**, pp. 99–116.

Blackshaw, S. (1987). Cell lineage and the development of identified neurons in the leech. In *The making of the nervous system* (eds. J. G. Parnavelas, C. D. Stern, and R. V. Stirling), pp. 22–51. Oxford University Press, Oxford.

Blair, S. and Palka, J. (1985). Axon guidance in the wing of *Drosophila*. *Trends Neurosci.* **8**, pp. 284–8.

Durbin, R. (1987). Determination of all type in the ventral nervous system of the nematode *Caenorhabditis elegans*. In *The making of the nervous system* (eds. J. G. Parnavelas, C. D. Stern, and R. V. Stirling), pp. 5–21. Oxford University Press, Oxford.

Edelman, G. M. (1984). Modulation of cell adhesion during induction, histogenesis, and perinatal development of the nervous system. *Ann. Rev. Neurosci.* **7**, pp. 339–77.

Ferguson, B. A. (1983). Development of motor innervation of the chick following dorsal–ventral limb bud rotations. *J. Neurosci.* **3**, 1760–72.

Hamburger, V. (1975). Cell death in the development of the lateral motor column of the chick embryo. *J. Comp. Neurol.* **160**, pp. 535–46.

Hollyday, M. (1930). Organisation of motor pools in chick lumbar lateral motor column. *J. Comp. Neurol.* **194**, pp. 143–70.

Hollyday, M. (1981). Rules of motor innervation in chick embryos with supernumerary limbs. *J. Comp. Neurol.* **202**, pp. 439–65.

Hollyday, M. (1983). Development of motor innervation of chick limbs. *Prog. Clin. Med. Res.* **110A**, pp. 183–93.

Honig, M. (1982).The development of sensory projection patterns in embryonic chick hind limb. *J. Physiol. (Lond.)* **330**, pp. 175–202.

Hope, R. A., Hammond, B. J., and Gaze, R. M. (1976). The arrow model: retinotectal specificity and map formation in the goldfish visual system. *Proc. R. Soc. Lond. B.* **194**, pp. 447–66.

Horder, T. J. (1978). Functional adaptability and morphogenetic opportunism the only rules for limb development? *Zoon* **6**, pp. 181–92.

Katz, M. J., Lasek, R. J., and Nauta, H. J. (1980). Ontogeny of substrate pathways and the origin of neural circuit pattern. *Neuroscience.* **5**, pp. 821–83.

Keynes, R. J. and Stern, C. D. (1985). Segmentation and neural development in vertebrates. *Trends Neurosci.* **8**, pp. 220–3.

Keynes, R. J. and Stern, C. D. (1987). The development of neural segmentation in vertebrate embryos. In *The making of the nervous system* (eds. J. G. Parnavelas, C. D. Stern, and R. V. Stirling), pp. 84–100. Oxford University Press, Oxford.

Keynes, R. J., Stirling, R. V., Stern, C. D., and Summerbell, D. C. (1987). The specificity of motor innervation of the chick wing does not depend upon the segmental origin of muscles. *Development* **99**, pp. 565–75.

Laing, N. G. (1982). Motor projection patterns to the hind limb of normal and paralysed chick embryos. *J. Embryol. exp. Morphol.* **72**, pp. 287–93.

Laing, N. G. (1984). Motor innervation of proximally rotated chick embryo wings. *J. Embryol. exp. Morphol.* **83**, pp. 213–23.

Lamb, A. H. (1984). Motoneuron death in the embryo. *CRC Crit. Rev. Clin. Neurobiol.* **1**, pp. 141–79.

Lance-Jones, C. and Landmesser, L. (1980*a*). Motoneuron projection patterns in embryonic chick limbs following partial deletions of the spinal cord. *J. Physiol. (Lond.)* **302**, pp. 559–80.

Lance-Jones, C. and Landmesser, L. (1980*b*). Motoneurone projection patterns in the chick hind limb following early partial reversals of the spinal cord. *J. Physiol. (Lond.)* **302**, pp. 581–602.

Lance-Jones, C. and Landmesser, L. (1981). Pathway selection by embryonic chick motoneurons in an experimentally altered environment. *Proc. R. Soc. Lond. B* **260**, 19–52.

Landmesser, L. (1978*a*). The distribution of motoneurones supplying chick hind limb muscles. *J. Physiol. (Lond.)* **284**, 371–89.

Landmesser, L. (1978*b*). The development of motor projection patterns in the chick hind limb. *J. Physiol. (Lond.)* **284**, pp. 391–414.

Landmesser, L. (1984). The development of specific motor pathways in the chick embryo. *Trends Neurosci.* **7**, pp. 336–9.

Landmesser, L. and Morris, D. G. (1975). The development of functional innervation of the hind limb of the chick embryo. *J. Physiol. (Lond.)* **249**, pp. 301–26.

Lewis, J. (1978). Pathways of axons in the developing chick wing: evidence against chemo-specific guidance. *Zoon* **6**, pp. 175–9.

Lewis, J., Al-Ghaith, L., Swanson, G., and Khan, A. (1983). The control of axon outgrowth in the developing chick wing. *Prog. Clin. Biol. Res.* **110**, pp. 195–205.

Lewis, J., Chevallier, A., Kieny, M., and Wolpert, L. (1981). Muscle nerve branches do not develop in chick wings devoid of muscles. *J. Embryol. exp. Morph.* **64**, pp. 211–32.

Narayanan, C. H. (1964). An experimental analysis of peripheral nerve pattern development in the chick. *J. Exp. Zool.* **156**, pp. 49–60.

Noakes, P. G., Bennett, M. R., and Davey, D. F. (1983). Growth of segmental nerves to the developing rat diaphragm: absence of pioneer axons. *J. Comp. Neurol.* **218**, pp. 365–77.

Nurcombe, V. and Bennett, M. R. (1983). The growth of neurites from explants of brachial spinal cord exposed to different components of wing bud mesenchyme. *J. Comp. Neurol.* **219**, pp. 133–42.

Okado, N. and Oppenheim, R. W. (1984). Cell death of motoneurons in the chick embryo spinal cord and the loss of motoneurons following removal of afferent inputs. *J. Neurosci.* **4**, pp. 1639–52.

Oppenheim, R. W. (1981*a*). Cell death of motoneurons in the chick embryo spinal cord. V. Evidence on the role of cell death and neuromuscular function in the formation of specific connections. *J. Neurosci.* **1**, pp. 141–51.

Oppenheim, R. W. (1981*b*). Neuronal cell death and some related regressive phenomena during neurogenesis: a selective historical review and progress report. In *Studies in developmental neurobiology*, (ed. W. M. Cowan), pp. 74–133. Oxford University Press, Oxford.

Pettigrew, A. G., Lindeman, R., and Bennett, M. R. (1979). Development of the segmental innervation of the chick forelimb. *J. Embryol. exp. Morphol.* **49**, pp. 115–37.

Piatt, J. (1957). Studies on the problem of nerve pattern. II. Innervation of the intact fore-limb by different parts of the central nervous system in *Amblystoma. J. Exp. Zool.* **131**, pp. 173–202.

Rickmann, M., Fawcett, J. W., and Keynes, R. J. (1985). The migration of neural crest cells and the growth of motor axons through the cranial half of the chick somite. *J. Embryol. exp. Morphol.* **90**, pp. 437–55.

Roncali, L. (1970). The brachial plexus and the wing nerve pattern during early development phases in chicken embryos. *Monit. Zool. Ital.* **4**, pp. 81–98.

Rutishauser, U., Grumet, M., and Edelman, G. M. (1983). Neural cell adhesion molecules mediates initial interactions between spinal cord neurons and muscle cells in culture. *J. Cell Biol.* **97**, pp. 145–52.

Scott, S. A. (1982). The development of the segmental pattern of skin sensory innervation in the embryonic chick hind limb. *J. Physiol. (Lond.)* **330**, pp. 203–20.

Searls, R. L. (1983). Shoulder formation, rotation of the wing, and polarity of the wing mesoderm and ectoderm. *Prog. Clin. Med. Res.* **110A**, pp. 165–74.

Singer, M., Norlander, R. H., and Egar, M. (1979). Axonal guidance during embryogenesis and regeneration in the spinal cord of the newt: the blue print hypothesis of neuronal pathway patterning. *J. Comp. Neurol.* **185**, pp. 1–22.

Sperry, R. W. (1963). Chemoaffinity in the orderly growth of nerve fiber patterns and connections. *Proc. Natl. Acad. Sci. USA* **50**, pp. 703–10.

Stern, C. D., Sisodiya, S. M., and Keynes, R. J. (1986). Interactions between neurites and somite cells: inhibition and stimulation of nerve growth in the chick embryo. *J. Embryol. exp. Morphol.* **91**, pp. 209–26.

Stirling, R. V. and Summerbell, D. (1977). The development of functional innervation in the chick wing following truncations and deletions of the proximo–distal axis. *J. Embryol. exp. Morphol.* **41**, pp. 189–207.

Stirling, R. V. and Summerbell, D. (1983). Familiarity breeds contempt: the behaviour of axons in foreign and familiar environments. *Prog. Clin. Med. Res.* **110A**, pp. 217–26.

Stirling, R. V. and Summerbell, D. (1985). The behaviour of growing axons invading developing chick wing buds with dorsoventral or anteroposterior axis reversal. *J. Embryol. exp. Morphol.* **85**, pp. 251–69.

Summerbell, D. and Honig, L. S. (1982). The control of pattern across the antero–posterior axis of the chick limb bud by a unique signalling region. *Amer. Zool.* **22**, pp. 105–16.

Summerbell, D. and Stirling, R. V. (1981). The innervation of dorso–ventrally reversed chick wings: evidence that motor axons do not actively seek out their appropriate targets. *J. Embryol. exp. Morphol.* **61**, pp. 233–47.

Summerbell, D. and Stirling, R. V. (1982). Development of the pattern of peripheral nerves in the chick limb. *Amer. Zool.* **22**, pp. 173–84.

Summerbell, D. and Wolpert, L. (1973). Precision of development in chick limb morphogenesis. *Nature* **224**, pp. 228–9.

Swanson, G. J. and Lewis, J. (1986). Sensory nerve routes in chick wing buds deprived of motor innervation. *J. Embryol. exp. Morphol.* **95**, pp. 37–52

Taghert, P. H. and Lichtman, J. W. (1986). Axon outgrowth in vertebrates. *Nature* **320**, pp. 210–11.

Tosney, K. W. and Landmesser, L. T. (1984). Pattern and specificity of axonal outgrowth following varying degrees of chick limb bud ablation. *J. Neurosci.* **4,** pp. 2518–27.

Tosney, K. W. and Landmesser, L. T. (1985*a*). Specificity of early motoneuron growth cone outgrowth in the chick embryo. *J. Neurosci.* **5,** pp. 2336–44.

Tosney, K. W. and Landmesser, L. T. (1985*b*). Growth cone morphology and trajectory in the lumbosacral region of the chick embryo. *J. Neurosci.* **5,** pp. 2345–58.

Tosney, K. W., Watanabe, M., Landmesser, L., and Rutishauser, U. (1986). The distribution of NCAM in the chick hind limb during axon outgrowth and synaptogenesis. *Dev. Biol.* **114,** pp. 437–52.

Weiss, P. (1939). *Principles of development.* Hafner, New York.

Wenger, E. L. (1951). Determination of structural patterns in the spinal cord of the chick embryo studied by transplantation between brachial and adjacent levels. *J. Exp. Zool.* **116,** pp. 123–64.

Whitelaw, V. and Hollyday, M. (1983*a*). Thigh and calf discrimination in the motor innervation of the chick hindlimb following deletions of limb segments. *J. Neurosci.* **3,** pp. 1199–215.

Whitelaw, V. and Hollyday, M. (1983*b*). Position dependent motor innervation of the chick hindlimb following serial and parallel duplications of limb segments. *J. Neurosci.* **3,** pp. 1216–25.

Whitelaw, V. and Hollyday, M. (1983*c*). Neural pathway constraints in the motor innervation of the chick limb following dorsoventral rotations of distal limb segments. *J. Neurosci.* **3,** pp. 1226–33.

Weiss, P. (1955). Nervous system. In *Analysis of development* (eds B. H. Willier, P. Weiss, and V. Hamburger), pp. 346–401. W. B. Saunders, Philadelphia.

13

Transplantation of sensory neurons in the insect

JONATHAN P. BACON

A fundamental problem in developmental neurobiology is how, in the tangle of the developing nervous system, are neurons able to form specific synaptic connections. Early work on this problem concentrated particularly on the retinotectal system of the frog and of the fish. Observations on the precision with which fibres, regenerating from the cut optic nerve, grow back to the tectum led Sperry (1965) to propose the chemo-affinity hypothesis. In its original formulation, he postulated that each of the cells in the retina acquires some position-specific label which matches up with a complementary label in the tectum. The extreme interpretation of this hypothesis (that each cell acquires a unique label) would impose a considerable load on the finite genome of any animal; consequently many workers in this field today think in terms of a more economical system of gradients of determinants that would give retinal and tectal cells a two-dimensional 'address'. The search for these putative gradients, using both immunology and adhesion assays, has generated much activity; the report (Trisler, Schneider, and Nirenberg 1981) of a gradient in the developing chick retina caused much excitement, but it has not been determined if this gradient is significant in the formation of specific synaptic connections.

Despite our lack of knowledge about the molecules involved in the precise wiring-up of the retinotectal system, work on these preparations is providing a major framework in which to set our ideas about synaptic specificity. Significantly, one of the most exciting recent developments has been to simplify this system by presenting retinal neurons with binary fasciculation choices *in vitro* (Bonhoeffer and Huf 1985). The axons of retinal neurons growing on an ingenious Y maze constructed of axons from different regions of the retina exhibit growth preferences that show some correlations with the ordering of optic nerve fibres.

In a system comprising millions of neurons, this attempt to simplify is a sensible one. Another approach, of course, is to choose a simpler system. The neurons that I will describe in this chapter comprise the mechano–sensory systems of hemimetabolous insects (these do not go through a metamorphosis; instead, they reach the adult stage by moulting through a number of larval instars). Despite the obvious phylogenetic differences, the projection of insect sensory neurons to their central targets bears many similarities to the vertebrate retinotectal system, the essence of which is an array of neurons that are able to assess their peripheral position and then make ordered projections and connections in the central nervous system (CNS).

A number of experimental advantages make the insect nervous system a favourable preparation in which to study how sensory neurons actually form particular projections and connections within the CNS. As already mentioned, one reason is that these systems comprise (relatively) few sensory neurons and interneurons, many of which are identifiable from one individual to another. Another reason is that the development of the sensory neurons is physically separate from that of the CNS; sensory neurons are derived from epidermal cells under the cuticle, in contrast to interneurons and motorneurons which are derived from central neuroblasts. In addition, whereas the CNS has an almost full complement of neurons at the end of embryogenesis, neuroblast division having ceased in all but a few brain centres, sensory neurons continue to be generated from their epidermal precursors throughout the post-embryonic life of the animal. Therefore transplanting pieces of epidermis during post-embryonic development places sensory neurons in altered environments without disruptive surgery to the CNS. Furthermore, since sensory neuron development continues within the transplanted epidermis, the influence of these perturbations can be tested on developing as well as on regenerating sensory neurons.

THE LOCUST WIND-HAIR SYSTEM

My first transplantation attempts, in collaboration with Anderson, used the head wind-hair system of the locust, *Schistocerca gregaria* (Anderson and Bacon 1979; Bacon and Anderson 1985). This system has a number of convenient experimental features. One is that the wind hairs are arranged in well-defined regions on each side of the head. For the present purposes, I shall call these regions *top* (meaning the ipsilateral hairs on top of the head) and *side* (the hairs on the side of the head in front of the compound eye). Each hair is innervated by a single sensory neuron situated beneath the cuticle at the hair's base, and these neurons form arborizations and connections in the CNS as a function of their position on the head [Fig. 13.1(a); Tyrer, Bacon, and Davies 1979; Bacon and Möhl 1983].

This is an ideal system for transplantation. We exchanged cuticle and the underlaying epidermis between *top* and *side* on the head at the second or third instar stage. At the time of transplantation there would typically be only two or three hairs on the patch [Fig. 13.1(b)], though many more would be present when the animal reached the adult stage [Fig. 13.1(c)]. We could identify the graft cuticle at the subsequent instar stages because the patch maintained its pigmentation and approximate shape.

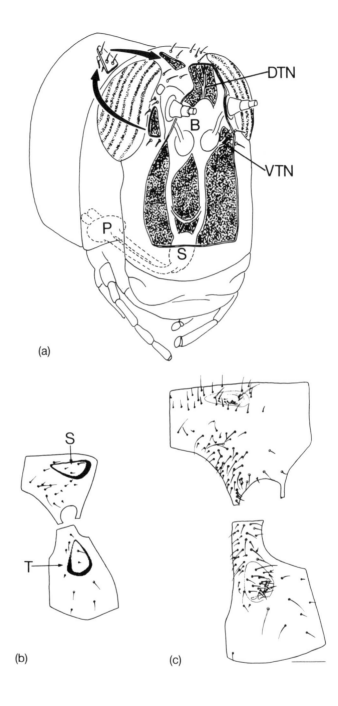

(a)

(b)

(c)

Untransplanted afferents from the *top* region enter the brain via the dorsal tegumentary nerve (DTN) while those from the *side* region use the ventral tegumentary nerve (VTN) [Fig. 13.1(a); Fig. 13.2(a) and (b)]. Both sets of afferents make similar arborizations in the brain but differ markedly in the suboesophageal ganglion [Fig. 13.2(a) and (b)]. Having established this correlation between the position of the sensory neuron on the head and the shape of its afferent projection within the CNS, we transplanted patches of epidermis and cuticle as described before. When the afferent projections from the grafts were cobalt stained in the adults, we found that regenerating axons from hairs present at the time of operation, and newly formed axons from hairs developing after transplantation, enter the CNS by the same nerve as those from the neighbouring undisturbed cuticle; i.e. the VTN in the case of transplants into the *side* region and the DTN in the case of transplants into the *top* region. Despite the fact that the graft axons take an altered trajectory to the CNS, once they enter the CNS they diverge from their neighbouring undisturbed axons and form a pattern of projections which is appropriate to the original location of the graft epidermis and not to its current location [Fig. 13.2(c) and (d)]. The arborizations formed in the CNS are therefore not determined by interactions with the altered environment in which the graft neurons grow, but by an intrinsic property of the epidermis from which they differentiate (Anderson and Bacon 1979).

This experiment also affords one the opportunity to test whether functional connectivity patterns of these sensory neurons are also determined by properties of their epidermis of origin, since afferents from these two wind-hair regions form very different synaptic connections with the tritocerebral commissure giant (TCG) interneuron in the brain (Bacon and Möhl 1983). Unpublished physiological and pharmacological observations suggest that *top* afferents form monosynaptic excitatory cholinergic synapses with the TCG, whereas *side* afferents inhibit the TCG via an unknown number of GABAergic non-spiking interneurons. When the animals with transplants

---

Fig. 13.1. Transplantation experiments in the locust wind-hair system. (a) Semischematic drawing of the locust head. Afferents from hairs on the top of the head fasciculate in the dorsal tegumentary nerve (DTN) and those from the side of the head in the ventral tegumentary nerve (VTN). Both sets of afferents project to the brain (B), the suboesophageal ganglion (S), and the prothoracic ganglion (P). A transplant from the side to the top of the head is shown (Scale bar: 1.5 mm). (b) and (c) Drawings of pieces of the second instar cuticle (b) and adult cuticle (c) from the right side of the animal's head. In this animal, a piece of *top* (T) epidermis and a piece of *side* (S) epidermis were exchanged in the second instar. Shading in (b) indicates the region of clotted haemolymph around the transplants where they were held in place next to the host epidermis. Many hairs develop in the transplants after the operation, though individual hairs present at the time of transplantation are recognized by their location and size in the adult stage (scale bar: 1 mm).

between the *top* and *side* regions became adult, the nature of the central connections made by the afferents from transplanted hairs was examined by intracellular recording from the TCG while these individual hairs or groups of hairs were mechanically stimulated. We found that sensory neurons that regenerate after the transplantation and neurons that develop *de novo* at the ectopic location both form central connections appropriate to their original

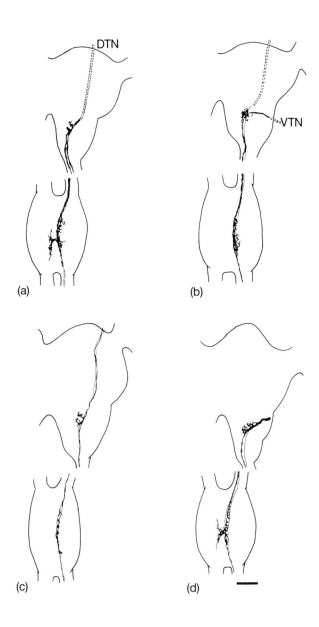

location; i.e. *top* neurons in the transplant excite the TCG though they are entirely surrounded by *side* inhibitory hairs, and transplanted *side* neurons continue to inhibit the TCG though the hairs around them in host tissue provide excitation to the TCG (Bacon and Anderson 1985).

In summary, sensory neurons regenerating or developing *de novo* at ectopic locations as a result of transplantation are forced to take abnormal routes to the CNS. Once there, however, they form projections and functional connections appropriate to the original location of the graft epidermis, and not to their new foreign location. Clearly, the epidermis contains some intrinsic property which determines these features of the neuronal projection, and this commitment is stable in transplanted pieces of epidermis.

A similar result has been reported by transplanting strips of cricket cercal epidermis (a description of the cercus appears in the next section) from one circumferential position on the cercus to another (Walthall and Murphey 1984). However, these results differ from those obtained in the locust in one important way: while no obvious intercalation occurs in the locust experiment when pieces of epidermis of different positional values are closely apposed (French, pers. comm.), in the cricket this close proximity of mismatched positional values throws the epidermal cells into a frenzy of mitoses as they strive to intercalate the missing positional values (French, Bryant, and Bryant 1976; Walthall and Murphey 1986). The fact that intercalation does occur as a result of transplanting tiny pieces of epidermis to foreign locations indicates that some semblance of the original positional address is being maintained in the transplanted patch.

If this is also true in the locust tissue, it follows that these experiments are not a fair test of 'determination' as defined operationally by Slack (1983), since the immediate environment of the regenerating and developing neurons in the patch is not being changed. In order to ask when during their development insect neurons, or their progenitor epidermal cells, become determined to form particular arborizations and connections in the CNS, one would need to transplant single cells to foreign locations; this would be difficult.

Fig. 13.2. Wind-hair afferent arborizations in the CNS. Each panel depicts dorsal views of whole-mount preparations of the right half of the brain (upper drawing) and the whole of the suboesophageal ganglion (lower drawing) following cobalt filling and silver intensification of wind-hair afferents on the right side of the head. (a) *Top* afferent neurons enter the brain via the DTN. Note the contralateral branches in the suboesophageal ganglion. (b) Most *side* neurons enter the brain via the VTN, though a few enter via the DTN. Note the absence of contralateral branches in the suboesophageal ganglion. (c) *Side* neurons transplanted to a *top* position enter the brain via the DTN but continue to produce ipsilateral arborizations in the suboesophageal ganglion. (d) *Top* afferents transplanted to the *side* region of the head form their usual contralateral arborization in the suboesophageal ganglion. Scale bar: 200 μm.

As Anderson and I (1979) were trying to design experiments to test the nature of the positional information being 'read' by developing sensory neurons at the time we originally did these transplantations, we were disappointed that we could not change their fates. The fact, however, that the neurons maintain their original positional characteristics does mean that more interesting experiments can be performed than those described above, in which epidermis was transplanted within the head capsule. By moving the epidermis from one segment to another, one forces the neurons (of known, immutable phenotype) to grow into completely foreign regions of the CNS. Study of sensory neurons challenged in this way may reveal some developmental principles.

Anderson (1981, 1985) has done this. By transplanting patches of head hairs to different locations on the thorax, it was shown that the wind-hair afferents grow into the CNS and arborize in homologous regions of ventral neuropil in whichever thoracic ganglion they enter. The contralateral–ipsilateral distinction between the *top* and *side* afferent arborizations in the suboesophageal ganglion [Fig. 13.2(a) and (b)] is also maintained at ectopic locations.

To investigate the behaviour of insect afferent neurons growing into foreign neuropil with even greater precision than that achieved by Anderson (1981, 1985) demands more of a neuronal system than can be met by the locust wind-hair afferents. The ideal requirements are an array of identified sensory neurons which make different projections and connections within the CNS as a function of their peripheral position, and these cells should be situated beneath a homogeneous area of cuticle sufficiently large to allow easy transplantation. These criteria are probably best met by the cricket cercus—the subject of the next section.

THE CRICKET CERCAL SYSTEM

The cerci are a pair of cone-shaped, hair-covered appendages situated at the rear end of many insects. There are two obvious hair types on the cercus of the cricket, *Acheta domesticus*; the bulbous clavate hairs situated on the proximal medial cercus are gravity sensitive (Murphey 1981; Sakaguchi and Murphey 1983) while the long wind-sensitive filiform hairs are distributed over the entire cercus (Palka, Levine, and Schubiger 1977). I shall concentrate on the filiform hairs in this account. As in the locust head wind-hair system, each hair is innervated by a single neuron. The filiform hair afferents all project to a specialized region of the terminal ganglion called the cercal glomerulus [Fig. 13.3(a) and (b)].

By obtaining physiological recordings from the afferents of the filiform hairs, Murphey and I (Bacon and Murphey 1984) found that at any one circumferential position on the cercus, all the hairs are constrained to vibrate in the same plane and their sensory neurons all have the same directional sensitivity to wind. The majority of hair neurons on the cercus belong to one of four major directionality types. We therefore concentrated our analysis on these. By cobalt staining these sensory neurons at different locations on the cercus, we found that the neurons at any one circumferential position on the cercus all project to the same region of the cercal glomerulus [Fig. 13.3(a)].

There are, however, some hairs at intermediate positions that we deliberately excluded from our study. By careful analysis of these, Walthall and Murphey (1986) have found three more afferent types with directional sensitivity and arborization positions in the glomerulus intermediate between the major types described by Bacon and Murphey (1984). This makes a total of seven different afferent types. It remains to be seen whether further types will be identified or whether positional values around the circumference can only be interpreted in one of seven ways. Another possibility is that there is an infinite number of values which blend into a 'gradient'. Certainly, inspection of Fig. 2 in Palka *et al.* (1977, p. 271) indicates that, at least on the ventral surface of the cercus, the direction of vibration sensitivity appears to change in a gradual fashion.

Our interpretation of these results is that the developing sensory neurons are able to 'read' their position in the periphery and thereby become committed to a certain developmental programme which determines the directional sensitivity of the receptor on the cercus and the location of the sensory neuron's arborization in the CNS. As stated previously, the afferents all terminate in the cercal glomerulus; since the location of each afferent is related to its directionality, it follows that different regions of the glomerulus process wind information from different directions (i.e. the neuropil shows functional demarcation) [Fig. 13.3(a)].

It is in this neuropil that the cercal afferents make connections with a number of large ascending interneurons. The two best studied of these, medial giant interneuron (MGI) and lateral giant interneuron (LGI) (Murphey, Palka, and Hustert 1977), extend from the terminal ganglion [Fig. 13.3(a)] through the thoracic ganglia [Fig. 13.3(c)] to the brain [Fig. 13.3(d)]. They are thought to be involved in escape behaviour. We have studied the dendritic anatomy of these (and other) interneurons in the context of the functionally divided glomerulus in the terminal ganglion, and find a strong correlation between each interneuron's dendritic anatomy and its directional characteristics (Bacon and Murphey 1984). This means that the physiological characteristics of the cercal interneurons can be explained entirely by the location of their dendrites within the sensory array. An elegant confirmation of the idea that different interneuronal branches integrate wind information from different directions is provided by Jacobs and Miller (1985), who managed to micro-dissect some of the interneurons in this system with a fine laser beam after first filling the cell with a fluorescent dye. Burning off individual branches of these interneurons changes their directional characteristics in predictable ways.

The cricket cercal system is therefore understood in considerable detail and it bears many similarities to the retinotectal system, where fibres project into the CNS in an ordered fashion. In this insect system, however, we do not see a one-to-one projection of space into the CNS, as one does in visual and somatosensory systems, since the same wind direction can be sensed by appropriately arranged receptors at different locations on the cercus. This, however, is a minor difference; the major point is that the position of the sensory neuron in the periphery is correlated with its directional sensitivity, with the position of its arborization in the CNS, and with the interneurons with which it forms synapses. This detailed knowledge allows one to interpret the results of perturbation with precision.

TRANSPLANTATION OF THE CRICKET CERCUS TO THE LEG SOCKET

A considerable advantage of working with an appendage, such as the cercus, is that it is relatively easy to transplant it to the vacated socket of another appendage such as the leg or antenna (Fig. 13.4). We transplanted the cercus to the mesothoracic leg stump and found that the cercal (ectopic) afferents grow into the foreign neuropil of the mesothoracic ganglion but do not grow posteriorly towards their normal target in the terminal ganglion. Instead, the ectopic filiform and clavate afferents create an ectopic cercal glomerulus in mesothoracic neuropil (Fig. 13.5). More importantly, this ectopic glomerulus is not tangled and disorganized, but rather exhibits the same functional demarcation as it does in the terminal ganglion. I illustrate this point in Fig. 13.6 using two identified clavate afferents, but the same is also true of the ectopic filiform hair afferent projection. The fact that the same pattern of arborization is recreated in foreign neuropil suggests that the ingrowing ectopic afferents encounter the same landmarks in each of the segmental ganglia (Murphey, Bacon, Sakaguchi, and Johnson 1983).

Another set of landmarks must be repeated in each ganglion since the small bristle (touch-sensitive) hairs on the cercus have afferents which project beneath the cercal glomerulus in the terminal ganglion (Murphey 1985) and this also occurs at the ectopic location [Fig. 13.5(b); Murphey, Bacon, and Johnson 1985].

The ectopic glomerulus created in foreign neuropil does overlap some of the normal interneuronal targets of these fibres as they pass through the thoracic ganglia on their way to the brain [Fig. 13.3(c) and Fig. 13.5]. We were keen to find functional connections between the ectopic afferents and either MGI or LGI because the spatial relationship of the functionally divided afferent projection to these interneurons is different in the mesothoracic compared to the terminal ganglion. If connections had been formed at the ectopic location,

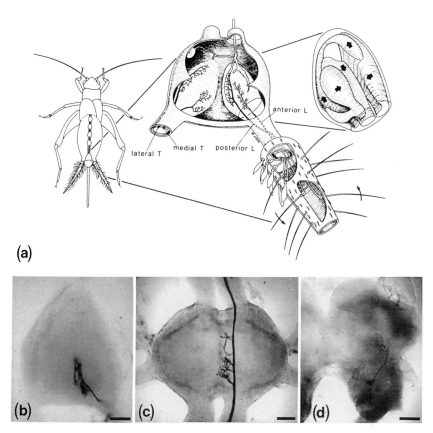

Fig. 13.3. The cercal system of the cricket is understood in considerable anatomical and physiological detail. (a) Left, the pair of hair-covered cerci at the rear end of the animal. Middle, each long filiform hair and bulbous clavate hair is innervated by a single sensory neuron which projects to the cercal glomerulus of the terminal ganglion. Arborizations of the four major filiform afferent types are shown; the optimal wind response of two of these (posterior L and anterior L) are indicated with small arrows. The medial giant interneuron (MGI) is shown in the terminal ganglion. The short bristle hairs on the cercus are touch sensitive; their afferents (not shown in this diagram) project beneath the cercal glomerulus to the anterior ventral region of the terminal ganglion [called the bristle neuropil by Murphey (1985)]. Right, space-filling model of one glomerulus indicates the target area for each type of afferent and thus the directionality of that region of neuropil (arrows). (After Bacon and Murphey 1984.) (b) Cobalt fill of a posterior L afferent in the terminal ganglion. Scale bar: 100 μm. (c) MGI produces short branches in the mesothoracic ganglion as it passes through the thorax on its way to the brain. Scale bar: 100 μm. (d) The lateral gaint interneuron in the protocerebrum of the brain. Scale bar: 200 μm.

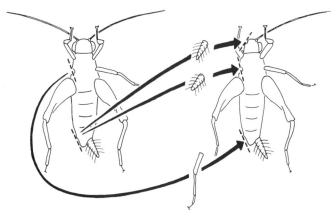

Fig. 13.4. The transplant operations performed in this study. The cercus is transplanted from the donor to the ipsilateral vacated leg or antennal socket of the recipient animal; a leg is transplanted to the ipsilateral cercal socket.

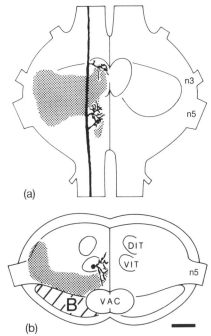

Fig. 13.5. The ectopic cercal glomerulus in the intermediate neuropil of the mesothoracic ganglion (stippled) in plan view (a) and transverse section (b) contains afferents of the filiform and clavate hairs. The short bristle hairs on the ectopic cercus project ventrally to the bristle neuropil (striped, B). LGI's ascending axon and branches are also shown. n3 n5, third and fifth peripheral nerves; VAC, ventral association centre; DIT, dorsal intermediate tract; VIT, ventral intermediate tract. Scale bar: 100 μm.

therefore, measuring the new directional selectivity of these interneurons in response to ectopic input would have provided a neat test of the idea that these anatomical relationships are the determinants of directional selectivity. However, careful intracellular recording in both MGI and LGI in the thoracic ganglia revealed no evidence of synaptic connectivity from the ectopic cercal afferents. It would appear that these afferent fibres cannot recognize their normal targets at a foreign location.

The ectopic afferents, however, did form some functional connections as has been reported by Edwards and Sahota (1967). By probing the connectives near the mesothoracic ganglion with hexamminecobalt chloride filled electrodes, we were able to locate and stain a number of interneurons that were excited when the ectopic cercus was touched or stimulated with wind (Murphey *et al.* 1983, 1985). The cell shown in Fig. 13.7(a) responds to touching the ectopic cercus. This stimulus would particularly activate the bristle hair afferents which project to the ventral region of the ganglion [Fig.

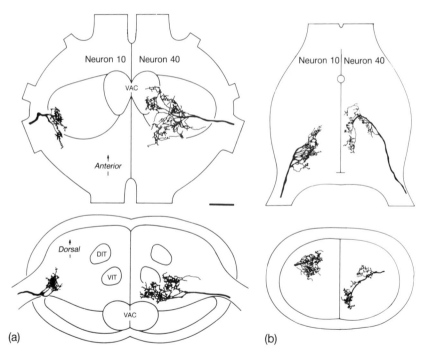

Fig. 13.6. Identified clavate hair neurons make similar projections at ectopic and normal locations. (a) Mesothoracic ganglion and (b) terminal ganglion in plan view (top) and transverse section (bottom). Neuron 10 arborizes laterally in both ganglia whereas neuron 40 does so nearer the midline. VAC, ventral association centre; DIT, dorsal intermediate tract; VIT, ventral intermediate tract. Scale bar: 100 μm. [Reproduced from Murphey (1983) by kind permission of Springer-Verlag, Berlin.]

13.5(b)] and this interneuron does arborize predominantly in ventral neuropil (Murphey *et al.* 1985). Some of the normal inputs to this interneuron are the afferents from the large tibial thread hairs [Fig. 13.7(b)] which also project to ventral neuropil (Johnson and Murphey 1985).

One expectation of transplanting sensory afferents to other segments might be that the cells would form functional synaptic connections with segmental homologues of their normal targets, or with their normal targets if these are capable of receiving synaptic input in each ganglion. We have been unable to stain the cell body of the interneuron shown in Fig. 13.7(a). However, Murphey (1985) has identified at least one interneuron originating in the terminal ganglion with similar characteristics (touch sensitive, input in more than one ganglion); it is possible that the cell in Fig. 13.7(a) is either the same as that already identified by Murphey, or is one of its segmental homologues.

The interneurons identified anatomically all received input from the ectopic bristle projection and indeed have arborizations in the most ventral region of neuropil [marked B in Fig. 13.5(b)]. We did not identify any cells responding to sound stimulation which would unequivocally stimulate some of the filiform afferents, or to gravity stimuli which would stimulate the clavate afferents. Both of these afferent types project into the ectopic glomerulus in intermediate neuropil and none of the stained interneurons that received ectopic input arborized in this region.

Such probing, however, is unlikely to produce a complete catalogue of all the neurons receiving synaptic input from the ectopic afferents. A different strategy might be to record from previously identified neurons known to arborize in regions invaded by ectopic afferents. A cercal transplant to the prothoracic leg socket, for example, would force the ectopic filiform afferents

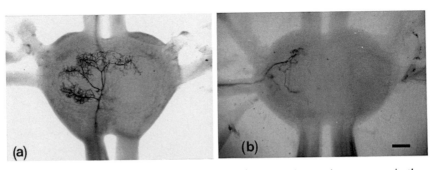

(a)   (b)

Fig. 13.7. Ectopic cercal afferents make functional connections to interneurons in the thoracic ganglia. (a) Cobalt stain of an interneuron in the prothoracic ganglion that is excited by stroking the ectopic cercus situated on the mesothorax. This cell has identical arborizations in each of the thoracic and abdominal ganglia and receives sensory information from many segments of the body. (b) Afferent fibre from one of the large tibial thread hairs on the mesothoracic leg. This is one of the cells that provides the normal input to the cell shown in (a). Scale bar: 100 μm.

to arborize in acoustic (intermediate) neuropil, and the formation of functional connections with the large identified acoustic interneurons (Wohlers and Huber 1978) could then be tested.

TRANSPLANTATION OF THE CRICKET LEG TO THE CERCAL SOCKET

The reciprocal experiment, transplanting a leg to the cercal socket, has also been performed in the cricket at the fifth instar stage of development. After allowing the ectopic sensory afferents to grow into the CNS, the leg bristle hair neurons were cobalt stained and found to project beneath the cercal glomerulus to the anterior bristle neuropil in the terminal ganglion (Murphey 1985; Murphey *et al.* 1985). This demonstrates the equivalence of the cercal bristle hairs and the bristle hairs of the leg. We have not attempted to test the physiological connections made by the leg hair afferents projecting to the terminal ganglion.

TRANSPLANTATION OF THE LOCUST CERCUS TO THE ANTENNAL SOCKET

It is also relatively easy to transplant the cercus to the antennal socket. We have performed this experiment on the locust, *Locusta migratoria*. We had good reasons for choosing this animal; although we know somewhat less about its cercal afferent projection than about the cricket's, our knowledge of normal sensory projections to the locust brain is more extensive, and a number of putative target interneurons in areas likely to be invaded by the ectopic afferents have already been described (Bacon and Tyrer 1978; Williams 1975).

By performing the transplant at the third instar stage and cobalt filling single afferent neurons when the animals became adult, we find that the ectopic cercal afferents enter the brain, not via the remnants of the severed antennal nerve, but via a small-diameter nerve in the vicinity of the ventral tegumentary nerve. The neurons arborize in a well-defined region of the dorsal deutocerebral neuropil [Fig. 13.8(a)] which is known to be occupied by head wind-hair afferents (Fig. 13.2). We find no obvious differences between afferent projections from different regions of the ectopic cercus. This area is also innervated by afferents from the campaniform sensilla at the base of the flagellum (Gewecke 1979), but not by the chemoreceptors of the flagellum which arborize in the ventral deutocerebrum. A few ectopic hair afferents do project further towards the suboesophageal ganglion but we have been unable to follow the fibres that far.

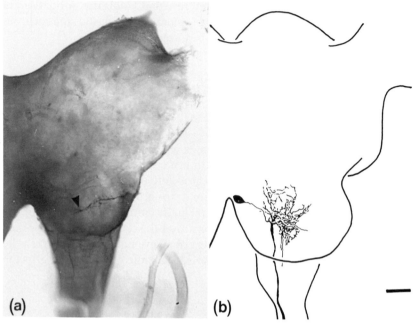

Fig. 13.8. Ectopic cercal projection to the brain. (a) Cobalt-filled afferent from a single filiform hair on the ectopic cercus projects to the dorsal deutocerebrum of the brain. The arrow marks the brain region occupied by the wind-hair afferents. (b) The TCG interneuron arborizes in this same region of neuropil. It receives excitatory and inhibitory input from the wind-hair afferents (Bacon and Möhl 1983) and inhibitory input from the ectopic cercal afferents. Scale bar: 100 μm.

Since these fibres arborize in exactly the neuropilar region occupied by the wind-hair afferents, we began our search for possible target neurons by recording in the cell bodies of identified wind-sensitive interneurons. At least two of these receive input from the ectopic cercus.

The tritocerebral commissure giant (TCG) interneuron [Fig 13.8(b); Bacon and Möhl 1983) is inhibited when the ectopic cercus is touched lightly, though wind stimulation of the cercus has no effect. In contrast, the cell shown in Fig. 13.9(a) [provisionally called lobula giant 2 (LG2)] is excited by wind stimulation delivered to the ectopic cercus [Fig. 13.9(b)]. This cell has an extremely complex anatomy and is multimodal, receiving input from both hair regions, the ipsilateral antenna and compound eye, and from ascending fibres.

Thus the afferents from the ectopic cercus make inhibitory functional connections with the TCG and excitatory connections with LG2. In both cases, the sign of the synaptic connection received by the interneuron from the

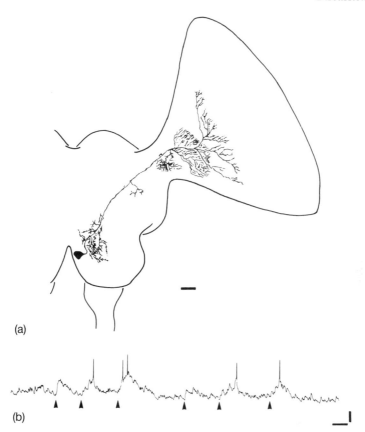

(a)

(b)

Fig. 13.9. LG2 interneuron receives excitatory input from the ectopic cercus. (a) Drawing of the cell in plan view. Scale bar: 100 μm. (b) Intracellular recording in LG2 while delivering wind puffs to the ectopic cercus (arrows) produces barrages of EPSPs, some resulting in spikes. Scale bars: horizontal 200 ms; vertical, 5 mV.

ectopic afferents is the same as that normally received from *side* wind-hair afferents. It appears that cercal afferents and *side* wind-hair afferents are specified to form similar connections in the CNS.

DISCUSSION

Transplanting insect epidermis from one location to another is an excellent way of challenging sensory neurons with foreign environments. Having established that the phenotype of these sensory neurons is maintained at ectopic locations, these experiments reveal, with high precision, two important kinds of developmental parsimony. The first is that the arborizations made by the same sensory neuron, in its normal or ectopic location, point out equivalent regions of neuropil in the repeated segmental ganglia. The second is that by forcing the sensory neurons to grow into foreign neuropil, where they are unable to reach their normal targets, the cells form synaptic connections with other interneurons. The key issue is to find out why this occurs. The minimum statement that can be made here is that since some interneurons become partially denervated as a result of removing the leg or the antenna, they may become receptive to other neuronal input as has been described in some vertebrate systems (e.g. Courtney and Roper 1976). This may not be a good model for specific synaptogenesis in development. If the process by which ectopic afferents form synaptic connections is rather unspecific, the problem may be compounded by the fact that the transmitter substance at the first order synapses in many insect mechano–sensory systems appears to be ACh (Sattelle 1980). This would mean that transmitter–receptor compatibility would not present a barrier to promiscuous synapse formation.

A bolder interpretation of our data is that interneurons in different ganglia of the CNS, in being able to accept synaptic input from the same identified afferents, share some common features of surface label and that these labels would not be shared by neurons unable to receive that synaptic input. The specificity of synaptic connections in normal development is not compromised because these cells are only allowed to connect as a result of the transplantation. The task, of course, is to find these labels. We are attempting to construct catalogues of cells that receive common sensory input as a result of transplantation experiments. It might prove possible to use these sets of identified cells as 'search images' for antibody staining to antigens important in the cell–cell recognition process.

It remains to be seen whether a transplanted sensory neuron will form synapses with the segmental homologues of its normal target interneurons when introduced at an ectopic location. This would be an intriguing result, especially in the light of Zipser and McKay's (1981) report of antibodies that stain all segmental homologues of some identified neurons in the leech CNS.

The transplantation method is an excellent way to provide neurons with new neighbours and to test their compatibility in terms of synaptic connectivity. However, the method does suffer the inherent disadvantage that a sensory neuron, specified, for instance, to grow into ventral neuropil, will do so regardless of whichever ganglion it finds itself in; this prevents one from testing the cell's ability to connect to dorsal cells beyond the reach of its arborizations (Fig. 13.10), and means that all possible combinations of cell–cell connectivity cannot be tested.

At present, we are attempting to circumvent this problem by using the technique of neuron culture, growing identified neurons next to each other in a dish and then testing for functional connections. By plucking cells out of the anatomical constraints of the CNS, we can begin to control all the parameters of the cell's environment, including the identity of its neighbours.

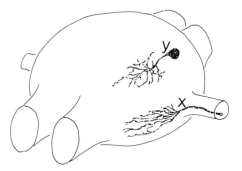

Fig. 13.10. Limitations of the transplantation technique. Sensory neuron X arborizes in ventral neuropil in whichever ganglion it enters. Its ability to form direct functional synapses with interneuron Y, which arborizes in dorsal neuropil, cannot be tested.

Neuronal transplantation is undoubtedly a powerful technique that has provided major insights into the way the insect CNS is constructed. However, used in isolation it has probably been stretched to the limits of innovation, and further work will only extend the catalogue of possible synaptic permutations. We believe that these experiments should be executed in conjunction with the kinds of *in vitro* and immunological investigations outlined. Such a combined approach ought to provide fresh insights into the problem of cell–cell recognition and the development of specific synaptic connections.

ACKNOWLEDGMENTS

I wish to thank Will Fuller and Kevin Thompson for their help in the preparation of this manuscript.

REFERENCES

Anderson, H. (1981). Projections from sensory neurons developing at ectopic sites in insects. *J. Embryol. exp. Morphol. (Suppl.)* **65,** pp. 209–24.
Anderson, H. (1985). The development of projections and connections from transplanted locust sensory neurons. *J. Embryol. exp. Morphol.* **85,** pp. 207–24.
Anderson, H. and Bacon, J. (1979). Developmental determination of neuronal projection patterns from wind-sensitive hairs in the locust, *Schistocerca gregaria*. *Dev. Biol.* **72,** pp. 364–73.
Bacon, J. and Anderson, H. (1985). Developmental determination of central connections of sensory neurones from wind-sensitive hairs in the locust, *Schistocerca gregaria*. *J. Exp. Biol.* **114,** pp. 679–83.

Bacon, J. and Möhl, B. (1983). The tritocerebral commissure giant (TCG) wind-sensitive interneurone in the locust. 1. Its activity in straight flight. *J. Comp. Physiol.* **150**, pp. 439–52.

Bacon, J. P. and Murphey, R. K. (1984) Receptive fields of cricket giant interneurones are related to their dendritic structure. *J. Physiol. (Lond.)* **352**, pp. 601–23.

Bacon, J. and Tyrer, N. M. (1978). The tritocerebral giant (TCG): a bimodal interneurone in the locust, *Schistocerca gregaria. J. Comp. Physiol.* **126**, pp. 317–25.

Bonhoeffer, F. and Huf, J. (1985). Position dependent properties of retinal axons and their growth cones. *Nature* **315**, pp. 409–10.

Courtney, K. and Roper, S. (1976). Sprouting and synapses after partial denervation of frog cardiac ganglion. *Nature* **259**, pp. 317–9.

Edwards, J. and Sahota, T. S. (1967). Regeneration of a sensory system: the formation of central connections by normal and transplanted cerci of the house cricket *Acheta domesticus. J. Exp. Zool.* **166**, pp. 387–95.

French, V., Bryant, P. J., and Bryant, S. V. (1976). Pattern regulation in epimorphic fields. *Science*, **183**, pp. 969–81.

Gewecke, M. (1979). Central projection of antennal afferents for the flight motor in *Locusta migratoria* (Orthoptera: Acrididae). *Entomologia Generalis* **5**, pp. 317–20.

Jacobs, G. A. and Miller, J. P. (1985). Functional properties of individual neuronal branches isolated *in situ* by laser photoinactivation. *Science* **228**, pp. 344–8.

Johnson, S. E. and Murphey, R. K. (1985). The afferent projection of mesothoracic bristle hairs in the cricket, *Acheta domesticus. J. Comp. Physiol A,* **156**, pp. 369–79.

Murphey, R. K. (1981). The structure and development of a somatotopic map in crickets: The cercal afferent projection. *Dev. Biol.* **88**, pp. 236–46.

Murphey, R. K. (1983). Maps in the insect nervous system, their implications for synaptic connectivity and target location in the real world. In *Neuroethology and behavioural physiology* (eds. F. Huber and H. Markl), pp. 176–88. Springer-Verlag, Berlin.

Murphey, R. K. (1985). A second cricket cercal sensory system; bristle hairs and the interneurons they activate. *J. Comp. Physiol. A.* **156**, pp. 357–67.

Murphey, R. K., Bacon, J. P., and Johnson, S. E. (1985). Ectopic neurons and the organization of insect sensory systems. *J. Comp. Physiol. A.* **156**, pp. 381–9.

Murphey, R. K., Palka, J., and Hustert, R. (1977). The cercus-to-giant interneuron system of crickets. II. Response characteristics of two giant interneurons. *J. Comp. Physiol.* **119**, pp. 285–300.

Murphey, R. K., Bacon, J. P., Sakaguchi, D. S., and Johnson, S. E. (1983). Transplantation of cricket sensory neurons to ectopic locations: arborizations and synaptic connections. *J. Neurosci.* **3**, pp. 659–72.

Palka, J., Levine, R., and Schubiger, M. (1977). The cercus-to-giant interneurone system of crickets. I. Some attributes of the sensory cells. *J. Comp. Physiol.* **119**, pp. 267–83.

Sakaguchi, D. S. and Murphey, R. K. (1983). The equilibrium detecting system of the cricket: physiology and morphology of an identified interneuron. *J. Comp. Physiol.* **150**, pp. 141–52.

Sattelle, D. B. (1980). Acetylcholine receptors of insects. *Adv. Insect Physiol.* **15**, pp. 215–315.

Slack, J. M. W. (1983). *From egg to embryo.* Cambridge University Press, Cambridge.

Sperry, R. W. (1965). Embryogenesis of behavioural nerve nets. In *Organogenesis* (eds. R. L. Dehaan and H. Ursprung), pp. 161–71, Holt, Rinehart and Winston, New York.

Trisler, C. D., Schneider, M. D., and Nirenberg, M. (1981). A topographic gradient of molecules in retina can be used to identify neuron position. *Proc. Natl. Acad. Sci. USA.* **78**, pp. 2145–9.

Tyrer, N. M., Bacon, J. P., and Davies, C. A. (1979). Sensory projections from the wind-sensitive head hairs of the locust *Schistocerca gregaria:* distribution in the CNS. *Cell Tissue Res.* **203**, pp. 79–92.

Walthall, W. W. and Murphey, R. K. (1984). Rules for neural development revealed by chimaeric sensory systems in crickets. *Nature* **311**, pp. 57–9.

Walthall, W. W. and Murphey, R. K. (1986). Positional information, compartments, and the cercal sensory system of crickets. *Dev. Biol.* **113**, pp. 182–200.

Williams, J. D. L. (1975). Anatomical studies on the insect central nervous system: a ground plan of the mid-brain and an introduction to the central complex in the locust, *Schistocerca gregaria* (Orthoptera). *J. Zool.* **176**, pp. 67–86.

Wohlers, D. and Huber, F. (1978). Intracellular recording and staining of cricket auditory interneurones in *Gryllus campestris* (L.) and *Gryllus bimaculatus* (de Geer). *J. Comp. Physiol.* **127**, pp. 11–28.

Zipser, B. and McKay, R. (1981). Monoclonal antibodies distinguish identifiable neurones in the leech. *Nature* **289**, pp. 549–54.

14

Astrocyte heterogeneity in the vertebrate central nervous system

ROBERT H. MILLER

Early studies on the organization and development of macroglial cells, were based primarily on morphological techniques such as Golgi impregnation (Cajal 1913; Stensaas and Stensaas 1968). More recently, a combination of electron microscopy, autoradiography, and immunofluorescence has been used to investigate glial cell development in specific regions of the vertebrate central nervous system (CNS) (Skoff, Price, and Stocks 1976a, 1976b; Fulcrand and Privat 1977).

Studies with Golgi impregnation led early workers to propose two major classes of macroglial cells: oligodendroglia and astroglia. While the role of oligodendroglia in the formation of CNS myelin is now well established (Bunge 1968; Peters and Vaughn 1970; Somjen and Trachtenberg 1979), the functions of astroglia are less well-defined. Two morphologically distinct types of astrocytes can be recognized in the vertebrate CNS (Peters, Palay, and Webster 1976): *protoplasmic astrocytes*, found mainly in grey matter, with sheet-like processes containing few fibrils (Weigert 1895) that appear to wrap around neuronal elements, and *fibrous astrocytes*, with their cell bodies located in white matter and characterized by a large number of stellate processes packed with fibrils (Weigert 1895). This early classification has been confirmed by electron microscopy, which revealed additional differences between the two types of astrocytes (Peters *et al.* 1976). The fibrils that characterize fibrous astrocytes were found to be 10 nm intermediate filaments (Mori and Leblond 1969) composed mainly of glial fibrillary acidic protein (GFAP; Schachner, Hedley-White, Hsu, Schoonmaker, and Bignami 1977). The outline of fibrous astrocytes was found to be comparatively regular, while that of protoplasmic astrocytes is irregular. Other ultrastructural criteria, such as the number of microtubules, have also been used to characterize these two types of astrocyte (Peters *et al.* 1976).

GLIAL CELL DEVELOPMENT IN THE RAT OPTIC NERVE

The optic nerve has been used extensively to study glial cell development. It contains no neuronal cell bodies, the majority of the cells being either astrocytes or oligodendrocytes. The ganglion cell axons that run through the nerve are unbranched, and, in the rat, the majority are myelinated. These aspects, combined with the comparative accessibility and long length of the nerve, make it an ideal system for studying a variety of phenomena, including axonal transport (Brady, Tytell, Heriot, and Lasek 1981), gliogenesis (Skoff *et al.* 1976*a*, 1976*b*) and myelinogenesis (Skoff, Toland, and Nast 1980; Waxman and Black 1984).

Light and electron microscopic studies of the developing nerve have shown that astrocytes begin to develop a few days before birth, while oligodendrocytes do not appear until the first post-natal week (Vaughn 1969; Kuwabara 1974; Skoff *et al.* 1976*a*, 1967*b*). It has been suggested from autoradiographic experiments that, by the end of the first post-natal week, most of the astrocytes in the rat optic nerve have appeared, while the majority of oligodendrocytes develop in the second and third post-natal week (Skoff *et al.* 1976*a*, 1976*b*; Valat, Privat, and Fulchrand 1983). These studies have added to our understanding of the sequence of glial cell development in the optic nerve, but failed to determine the lineage relationships between the different cell types because it is difficult to recognize immature cell types by their morphology alone. There are two different views on the origin of glial cells: the first is that astrocytes and oligodendrocytes develop from different precursor cells in the neonatal optic nerve (Skoff *et al.* 1976*a*, 1976*b*). The second is that the two cell types develop from a common glioblast present in the neonatal nerve (Privat, Valat, and Fulcrand 1981).

Two assumptions have been made in these studies: that the neuroglia of the mature optic nerve develop from the cells of the optic stalk, rather than by migration of cells from the diencephalon or retina (Vaughn 1969), and that the astrocytes of mature nerve are a homogeneous population of white-matter (fibrous) astrocytes. Recent work, using a combination of cell-type-specific markers and tissue culture, has provided evidence for two subpopulations of astrocytes in the nerve, suggesting that the second assumption may be an oversimplification.

IN VITRO EVIDENCE FOR TWO MACROGLIAL CELL LINEAGES IN THE OPTIC NERVE

In cultures of developing optic nerve, three types of macroglial cells can be recognized on the basis of their morphology, their response to growth factors, and their ability to stain with cell-type-specific antibodies. Oligodendrocytes can be distinguished using antibodies to galactocerebroside (Raff, Mirsky, Fields, Lisak, Dorfmann, Silberberg, Gregson, Liebowitz, and Kennedy 1978), the major glycolipid in myelin. Astrocytes can be identified with antibodies to GFAP (Bignami, Eng, Dahl, and Uyeda 1972), the major protein in glial intermediate filaments. Two subpopulations of GFAP-positive

(GFAP+) astrocytes can be distinguished *in vitro*; they are referred to as type-1 and type-2 (Raff, Abney, Cohen, Lindsay, and Noble 1983). Most type-1 astrocytes have a fibroblast morphology (Fig. 14.1) and are labelled by an antibody that reacts with a cell surface antigen (rat neural antigen-2, Ran-2) (Bartlett, Noble, Pruss, Raff, Rattray, and Williams 1981), but the majority do not label with monoclonal antibody F4-A2B5 (Eisenbarth, Walsh and Nirenberg 1979) or tetanus toxin, both of which are thought to bind specific gangliosides (van Heyningen 1963; Eisenbarth *et al.* 1979). Type-1 astrocytes proliferate in response to epidermal growth factor (EGF) and extracts of bovine pituitary gland. In contrast, most type-2 astrocytes have a process-bearing morphology, and label with A2B5 antibody and tetanus toxin, but not with Ran-2 antibody (Fig. 14.1). These cells are not stimulated to proliferate by EGF or pituitary extract. There is no evidence that either type of astrocyte can spontaneously change into the other in culture.

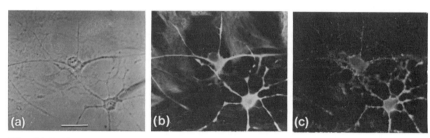

Fig. 14.1. Two types of astrocytes in culture. (a) Phase contrast; (b) anti-GFAP, followed by goat anti-rabbit-fluorescein, and (c) A2B5, followed by goat anti-mouse-rhodamine. Note the two process bearing type-2 astrocytes stain with antibodies to GFAP (b) and with the mononclonal antibody A2B5 (c), while the flat type-1 astrocytes stain with antibodies to GFAP (b), but not with A2B5. Scale bar: 25 μm.

The two types of astrocyte develop in culture from two different precursor cells (Raff *et al.* 1984*a, b*). (Fig. 14.2). Type-1 astrocytes develop from a cell that has the antigenic phenotype Ran-2+ and GFAP−, while type-2 astrocytes develop from a bipotential A2B5+, GFAP− progenitor cell. This bipotential progenitor cell differentiates into a type-2 astrocyte if cultured in the presence of 10 per cent fetal calf serum (FCS) or into an oligodendrocyte if cultured in serum-free medium (Raff, Miller, and Noble 1983*b*). For this reason, this precursor cell is called an oligodendrocyte-type-2-astrocyte (O-2A) progenitor.

IN VIVO EVIDENCE FOR TWO MACROGLIAL LINEAGES IN THE RAT OPTIC NERVE

Cells with phenotypes corresponding to type-1 and -2 astrocytes can be

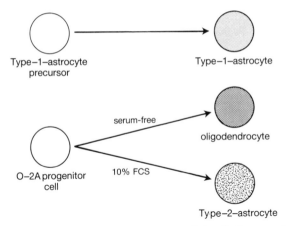

Fig. 14.2. Schematic representation of the two glial cell lineages in cultures of developing rat optic nerve. Note that a type-1 astrocyte precursor gives rise to only type-1 astrocytes, while the O-2A progenitor gives rise to oligodendrocytes if cultured in the abscence of serum, and a type-2 astrocyte if cultured in the presence of 10 per cent serum.

distinguished in the intact nerve with the antibody A2B5 on semi-thin frozen sections of adult or developing optic nerve (Miller and Raff 1984). These are found in different locations in the nerve. The majority of type-1 astrocytes (A2B5−, GFAP+) are found at the periphery of the nerve and contribute to the glial limiting membrane, while most of the type-2 astrocytes (A2B5+, GFAP+) are found in the interior of the nerve (Miller and Raff 1984), suggesting that the two types of astrocyte seen in culture exist *in vivo*. Type-1 astrocytes are found as early as embryonic day 15 (E15), while oligodendro-cytes do not appear until the first post-natal week, and type-2 astrocytes are not present either in sections of optic nerve or in suspension until the second post-natal week (Miller, David, Patel, Abney, and Raff 1985). Quantitative analysis of the cell types, combined with autoradiographic studies in the developing nerve, suggest that the appearance of type-2 astrocytes is not the result of a conversion of type-1 astrocytes, but represents the differentiation of a progenitor cell *in vivo* (Miller *et al.* 1985).

FUNCTIONAL SIGNIFICANCE OF TWO TYPES OF ASTROCYTE IN THE OPTIC NERVE

Type-1 astrocytes

The functional significance of the two types of astrocyte in the optic nerve is not clearly understood. However, an important property of astrocytes is their ability to form a glial scar in response to a CNS lesion (Maxwell and Kruger 1965; Vaughn and Pease 1970). A number of observations suggest that glial scars in white matter are formed mainly by type-1 astrocytes. In a study designed to examine the influence of axons on glial cell development, we have found that transection of the neonatal rat optic nerve has little effect on the number of type-1 astrocytes that develop subsequently, but there is a massive reduction in the number of oligodendrocytes and type-2 astrocytes in the nerve stump (David, Miller, Patel, and Raff 1984). This suggests that there is a period in development when intact axons are required for the subsequent elaboration of a full complement of the O-2A glial cell lineage in the optic nerve.

In the light of these observations, we have examined the phenotype of astrocytes that formed a glial scar following both enucleation and a stab wound to the corpus callosum in the adult rat (Miller, Abney, David, ffrench-Constant, Lindsay, Patel, Stone, and Raff 1986). Although the majority of the astrocytes in semi-thin frozen sections of normal adult corpus callosum had an antigenic phenotype similar to the type-2 astrocytes in the optic nerve (A2B5+, GFAP+), following a stab wound most of the reactive astrocytes that were released by dissociation eight days later had a type-1 phenotype (A2B5−, GFAP+). Moreover, frozen sections made 20 weeks after the lesion showed that most of the astrocytes in the region of the wound were type-1.

Similar results were obtained in the adult optic nerve: in the first week following enucleation both type-1 and type-2 astrocytes incorporated ^{3}H-thymidine. However, in frozen sections made 20 weeks after enucleation the majority of the astrocytes had type-1 phenotype (Miller *et al.* 1986). Furthermore, only half the normal number of astrocytes remained in the nerve. While it is possible that type-2 astrocytes become A2B5− following nerve transection and contribute to the formation of the glial scar, a simpler interpretation of these observations is that the glial scar is composed mostly of type-1 astrocytes, and that the decrease in the number of astrocytes seen following transection of the optic nerve is mainly a result of the death of type-2 astrocytes (Miller *et al.* 1986).

Type-2 astrocytes

Recent evidence suggests that the astrocyte processes that contribute to the structure of the nodes of Ranvier in the rat optic nerve are derived from type-2 astrocytes. Morphological studies in the optic nerve and spinal cord have demonstrated that astrocyte processes encircle the exposed axolemma at nodes of Ranvier in the CNS (Hildebrand 1971; Hildebrand and Waxman 1984; Raine 1984; Waxman and Black 1984). In semi-thin and ultra-thin frozen sections of adult rat optic nerve it has been shown that the J1 cell adhesion glycoprotein (Kruse, Keilhauer, Faissner, Timpl, and Schachner 1985) is concentrated on and around these perinodal astrocyte processes and on fine longitudinal glial processes elsewhere in the nerve; large glial processes, in contrast, are not labelled (ffrench-Constant, Miller, Kruse, Schachner, and Raff 1986).

In cultures of perinatal optic nerve the majority of type-2 astrocytes, oligodendrocytes, and their progenitor cells were stained with anti-NSP-4 monoclonal antibody (Rougon, Hirsch, Hirn, Guenet, and Goridis 1983), which recognizes a number of glycoproteins, including J1. Sections of optic nerve bind anti-NSP-4 in an identical pattern to anti-J1 antiserum. However, very few cells with type-1 astrocyte phenotype were stained in such cultures (ffrench-Constant and Raff 1981). Since all perinodal astrocyte processes in the nerve appear to be J1 + and NSP-4 +, it seems likely that they are derived primarily from type-2 astrocytes. It has been proposed that the O-2A cell lineage gives rise to cells specialized in the production of myelin sheaths and nodes of Ranvier in the CNS. This may explain why type-2 astrocytes are related more closely to oligodendrocytes than to type-1 astrocytes (ffrench-Constant and Raff 1986).

Morphological differences in the astrocytes of the rat optic nerve

There may be morphological differences between type-1 and -2 astrocytes in the adult optic nerve. This is based on two lines of evidence. First, labelling with A2B5 and anti-GFAP shows that the majority of the type-1 astrocytes are associated with the pial surface of the nerve, while the majority of the type-2 astrocytes are found in the interior of the nerve. Second, it can be inferred from studies with J1 and NSP-4 antibodies *in vitro* that the labelled perinodal and fine longitudinal astrocyte processes in the nerve are derived from type-2 astrocytes, while the unlabelled radial processes come from type-1 astrocytes. Based on these observations, we would expect that those cells at the pial surface (type-1) should mostly have radial processes and few longitudinal processes, while those astrocytes in the centre of the nerve (type-2) should have mainly fine longitudinal processes. However, conventional light and electron microscopy of the optic nerve and staining with antibodies to GFAP and A2B5 failed to reveal any significant difference in the morphology of the astrocytes in the nerve.

Recently, by combining a modified Golgi procedure with semi-thin longitudinal sections through the optic nerve, we found an orthogonal pattern of astrocyte processes in the nerve (Fig. 14.3). Most of the processes of astrocytes associated with the pial surface of the nerve run radially through the nerve [Fig. 14.3(a) and (b)] and appear to be largely unbranched, with no fine longitudinal processes. In contrast, at the centre of the nerve there are astrocytes with short radial processes and long slender processes that run longitudinally among the myelinated axons [Fig. 14.3(a) and (b)]. These findings support our idea that those cells with radial processes which contact

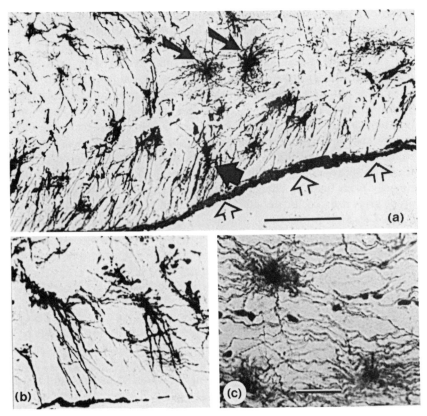

Fig. 14.3. Golgi visualization of two morphologically distinct types of astrocyte in the adult rat optic nerve. Note the orthogonal array of astrocyte process in the nerve. Those cells at the pial surface [open arrows in (a)] appear to have primarily radial processes [see large filled in arrow in (a), enlarged in (b)], and may represent type-1 astrocytes, while those cells in the centre of the nerve have primarily fine longitudinal process [small filled-in arrows in (a), and enlarged in (c)] and may represent type-2 astrocytes. Scale bar: 100 μm in (a); 25 μm in (b) and (c).

the pial surface represent type-1 astrocytes, while those with fine longitudinal processes, found in the centre of the nerve, represent type-2 astrocytes.

Not only are there different astrocyte subpopulations in any one region of the optic nerve, but different regions of the nerve contain astrocytes with different morphological characteristics. Skoff, Knapp, and Bartlett (1986) have shown that labelling with antibodies against GFAP reveals differences in the organization of the astrocytes at the chiasm and, more strikingly, behind the eye, at the lamina cribosa. The significance of these differences is unclear. The existence of morphological variations in the glia along a single fibre tract suggests that axons are not responsible for the observed variation in glial cell structure; rather that it represents intrinsic differences in the glia themselves (Skoff *et al.* 1986).

Do type-1 and type-2 astrocytes represent protoplasmic and fibrous astrocytes?

Initially, we considered the possibility that, in cultures of developing optic nerve, type-1 astrocytes represent protoplasmic astrocytes because they appear to be morphologically and serologically identical to the predominant astrocyte cell type seen in culture and in sections of CNS grey matter. Type-2 astrocytes, by contrast, were suggested to represent fibrous astrocytes because they are mainly found in sections of, and cultures derived from, white matter (Raff *et al.* 1983*a*; Miller and Raff 1984). However, our more recent work (Miller *et al.* 1986) suggests that it may not be justifiable to define astrocyte heterogeneity in the optic nerve by using the fibrous/protoplasmic distinction. In the original definition of grey matter protoplasmic astrocytes (Peters *et al.* 1976), these cells were said to contain few intermediate filaments. However, type-1 astrocytes found in the myelinated rat optic nerve appear to contain a considerable number of intermediate filaments, although they stain less intensely with antibodies to GFAP. Also, although the majority of astrocytes in white matter glial scars contain a large number of glial filaments, and therefore have been referred to as fibrous astrocytes (Vaughn and Pease 1970), they have type-1 astrocyte phenotype. It is clear, therefore, that type-1 astrocytes are capable of expressing large amounts of glial filaments under certain conditions such as cell culture and in response to a lesion *in vivo* (Bignami and Dahl 1976). The density of glial filaments in the cytoplasm is therefore an unreliable indicator of the origin of the cell. It seems likely that there are more subclasses of astrocytes still to be identified (Schachner 1982); for this reason, a numerical classification may prove to be more useful.

GLIAL DEVELOPMENT IN OTHER REGIONS OF THE CNS

Studies of the organization of glial cells have been conducted during normal development and following an experimental lesion in the spinal cord of a number of animals, including chick (Fujita 1965), primate (Choi 1981; Choi and Kim 1985), mouse (Barrett, Donati, and Guth 1984), and rat (Liuzzi and Miller 1987). These studies have provided evidence that within the spinal cord there is glial cell heterogeneity, as in the optic nerve.

In the rat spinal cord, Golgi impregnation and staining with anti-GFAP antibodies suggests that, while there appears to be a single type of astrocyte in grey matter, there are at least two forms of GFAP+ astrocytes in white matter. Cells with the morphology of classical fibrous astrocytes can be found scattered among the myelinated axons. These cells stain strongly with antibodies against GFAP, suggesting that they contain a large number of intermediate filaments. In addition, there are astrocytes in this region that have a pronounced radial orientation and span the white matter. Characteristically, the radial cells appear to contact the pial surface of the spinal cord, although their cell body may be located deep in the white matter of the cord giving them a bipolar appearance (Liuzzi and Miller 1987).

In the mouse spinal cord, cells with this radial morphology are seen with GFAP labelling only after a rostral lesion has been made to the spinal cord (Barrett *et al.* 1984). It has been proposed that the appearance of these cells results from the considerable hypertrophy of their processes in response to the lesion.

At present the immunological markers used to define glial cell lineages in the optic nerve of the rat have not been tested rigorously in other regions of the CNS. However, by analogy with the optic nerve, where it has been suggested that reactive gliosis is a property mainly restricted to type-1 astrocytes (Miller *et al.* 1986), the radially oriented astrocytes of the spinal cord may be equivalent to the type-1 astrocytes of the optic nerve. Consistent with this hypothesis is the observation that these cells appear early in development both in the optic nerve and in the spinal cord, and that they maintain an interaction with the pial surface in both locations.

In a recent study, Hajos and Basco (1984) have proposed that radial glial-derived cells have a common morphology, and that all of them contact a surface of the brain. They suggest that in the CNS there are two populations of astrocytes: those in the deep neuropil, and those that contact the pial surface. The functions of the two types of astrocytes may be different: those in the neuropil may have the functions usually ascribed to astrocytes, while surface glia may be involved in the transport of material between brain fluid spaces. According to this classification, the radially oriented cells of the rat spinal cord would represent the surface contact glia, like the type-1 astrocytes of the optic nerve, while the free astrocytes of the spinal cord would correspond to the type-2 astrocytes of the optic nerve.

ASTROCYTES IN THE AMPHIBIAN SPINAL CORD

There is now strong evidence for heterogeneity among astrocytes of the mammalian CNS. Is there similar astrocytic diversity in other vertebrates? In general, the higher an animal is in the phylogenetic tree, the greater the number and variety of cell types in its nervous system. Therefore, in a less complex nervous system such astrocytic heterogeneity may be less likely to occur.

Using a combination of horseradish peroxidase filling and GFAP immunofluorescence, we found only a single type of astrocyte in the frog spinal cord, whose processes appear to be regionally specialized (Miller and Liuzzi 1986). These astrocytes retain both their radial orientation and their contact with the pial surface throughout the life of the animal. The morphology and biochemical characteristics of the astrocyte processes are different in the grey- and white-matter regions of the cord. In grey matter, a large number of fine lateral branches leave the primary process, and appear to wrap neurons, while in white matter there is little lateral branching of the primary process.

Staining of transverse frozen sections of spinal cord with antibodies against GFAP suggested that glial filaments are located mainly in those regions of the radial glial processes that span the white matter. This observation was confirmed by electron microscopy, which showed that there are few intermediate filaments in grey matter, as compared to white matter (Miller and Liuzzi 1986).

As is the case in axons, there is no protein synthetic machinery in the processes of astrocytes. However, unlike neurons, where intermediate filaments are synthesized in the cell body and transported down the length of the axon in the form of long polymers (Lasek, Garner, and Brady 1984), it seems that, in the glial cell, intermediate filament polymerization must occur, at least in part, along the length of the cell process. The correlation between the location of intermediate filaments and white-matter tracts suggests that the astrocyte may be responding to the neural environment by expressing GFAP-reactivity. It is interesting that one of the differences between white-matter (fibrous) astrocytes and protoplasmic astrocytes in mammals is that the former contain more glial filaments in their cytoplasm (Peters *et al.* 1976; Ludwin, Kosek and Eng 1976). It seems plausible that this difference reflects the location of the astrocyte rather than some intrinsic cellular property.

The functional significance of astrocyte heterogeneity in the mammalian spinal cord is unclear. It has been suggested that astrocytes of the grey matter are involved in the isolation of receptive surfaces (Peters and Palay 1965; Peters *et al.* 1976), while white-matter astrocytes may have a structural role in myelinated tracts (Hildebrand 1971). In the frog spinal cord it may be that the single type of astrocyte combines the functions as well as the properties of mammalian grey- and white-matter astrocytes through the regional specialization of its processes.

CONCLUSIONS

There is now good evidence that cells classified as astrocytes are considerably more diverse than had previously been recognized. Their proposed functional diversity could indicate that the heading 'astrocytes' encompasses a variety of different cell types. Specific functions have yet to be correlated with known populations of astrocytes, which will not be a simple task.

The best evidence for different lineal origins of the different types of astrocytes comes from work on the optic nerve, and from *in vitro* experiments, where it has been possible to manipulate the cell populations and their fluid environment. It is clear that cellular location and morphology alone are unreliable criteria for defining different glial cell lineages. Observations on the astrocytes of the frog spinal cord show that the morphological and some of the biochemical characteristics used to distinguish between different subpopulations of astrocytes in the vertebrate CNS may be consequences of the neural environment of the glial cell.

Since oligodendrocytes or their precursors are capable of migrating long distances in the adult CNS (Lachapelle, Gumpel, Baulac, Jacque, Duc, and Baumann 1983; Gumpel, Lachapelle, Jacque, and Baumann 1985); the same may be true for astrocytes or astrocyte precursors. In this case the final expression of the characteristics of the glial cell in the CNS would be a result both of its intrinsic properties and of the environment in which it is located. A variety of new cell-type-specific markers and further *in vitro* experiments will be required to determine the contributions of each of these factors to glial cell development.

ACKNOWLEDGMENTS

I wish to thank M. C. Raff and C. ffrench-Constant for their helpful comments, and R. J. Lasek for many stimulating discussions.

REFERENCES

Barrett, C. P., Donati, E. J., and Guth, L. (1984). Differences between adult and neonatal rats in their astroglial response to spinal injury. *Exp. Neurol.* **84,** pp. 374–84.

Bartlett, P. F., Noble, M. D., Pruss, R. M., Raff, M. C., Rattray, S., and Williams, C. A. (1981). Rat neural antigen-2 (Ran-2): a cell surface antigen on astrocytes, ependymal cells, Muller cells and Leptomenginges defined by a monoclonal antibody. *Brain Res.* **204,** pp. 339–51.

Bignami, A. and Dahl, D. (1976). The astrocyte response to stabbing. Immunofluorescence studies with antibodies to astrocyte specific protein (GFA) in mammalian and submammalian vertebrates. *Neuropathol. Appl. Neurobiol.* **2,** pp. 99–110.

Bignami, A., Eng, L. F., Dahl, D., and Uyeda, C. T. (1972). Localisation of the glial fibrillary acidic protein in astrocytes by immunofluorescence. *Brain Res.* **43,** pp. 429–35.

Brady, S. T., Tytell, M., Heriot, K., and Lasek, R. J. (1981). Axonal transport of calmodulin: a physiological approach to long term associations between proteins. *J. Cell Biol.* **89,** pp. 607–14.

Bunge, R. P. (1968). Glial cells and the central myelin sheath. *Physiol. Rev.* **48,** pp. 197–251.

Cajal, S. R. (1913). Sobre un nuevo método de impregnación de la neuroglía y sus resultados en los centros nerviosos del hombre y animales. *Trab. Lab. Invest. Biol. Univ. Madr.* **11,** pp. 219–37.

Choi, B. H. (1981). Radial glia of developing human fetal spinal cord—Golgi, immunohistochemical and electron microscopic study. *Dev. Brain Res.* **1,** pp. 249–67.

Choi, B. H. and Kim, R. C. (1985). Expression of glial fibrillary acid protein by immature oligodendroglia and its implications. *J. Neuroimmunol.* **8,** pp. 215–35.

David, S., Miller, R. H., Patel, R., and Raff, M. C. (1984). Effects of neonatal transection on glial development in the rat optic nerve: evidence that the oligodendrocyte-type-2 astrocyte cell lineage depends on axons for its survival. *J. Neurocytol.* **13,** pp. 961–74.

Eisenbarth, G. S., Walsh, F. S., and Nirenberg, M. (1979). Monoclonal antibody to a plasma membrane antigen of neurons. *Proc. Natl. Acad. Sci. USA* **79,** pp. 4913–17.

ffrench-Constant, C., Miller, R. H., Kruse, J., Schachner, M., and Raff, M. C. (1986). Molecular specialization of the astrocyte processes at nodes of Ranvier in rat optic nerve. *J. Cell Biol.* **102,** pp. 844–52.

ffrench-Constant, C. and Raff, M. C. (1986). Evidence that the oligodendrocyte-type-2-astrocyte cell lineage is specialized for myelination. *Nature* **323,** pp. 335–8.

Fujita, S. (1965). An autoradiographic study on the origin and fate of the subpial glioblasts in the embryonic chick spinal cord. *J. Comp. Neurol.* **124,** pp. 51–60.

Fulcrand, J. and Privat, A. (1977). Neuroglial reactions secondary to Wallerian degeneration in the optic nerve of the postnatal rat: ultrastructural and quantitative study. *J. Comp. Neurol.* **176,** pp. 189–224.

Gumpel, M., Lachapelle, F., Jacque, C., and Baumann, N. (1985). Central nervous tissue transplantation into mouse brain: differentiation of myelin from transplanted oligodendrocytes. In *Neural grafting in the mammalian CNS* (eds. A. Björklund and U. Stenevi), pp. 151–8. Elsevier, Amsterdam.

Hajós, F. and Bascó, E. (1984). The surface-contact glia. *Advances in Anat. Embryo. and Cell Biol.* **84,** pp. 1–79.

Hildebrand, C. (1971). Ultrastructural and light microscope studies of the nodal region in large myelinated fibres of adult cat spinal cord white matter. *Acta. Physiol. Scand. Suppl.* **363–370,** pp. 43–50.

Hildebrand, C. and Waxman, S. G. (1984). Postnatal differentiation of rat optic fibres: electron microscope observations on the development of nodes of Ranvier and axoglial relations. *J. Comp. Neurol* **224,** pp. 25–37.

Kruse, J., Keilhauer, G., Faissner, A., Timpl, R., and Schachner, M. (1985). The J1 glycoprotein—a novel nervous system cell adhesion molecule of the L2/HNK-1 family. *Nature* **316,** pp. 146–8.

Kuwabara, T. (1974). Development of the optic nerve of the rat. *Invest. Opthalmol.* **13,** pp. 732–45.

Lachapelle, F., Gumpel, M., Baulac, M., Jacque, C., Duc, P., and Bauumann, N. (1983). Transplantation of CNS fragments into the brain of shiverer mutant mice: extensive myelinatin by implanted oligodendrocytes. *Dev. Neurosci.* **6,** pp. 325–34.

Lasek, R. J., Garner, J., and Brady, S. T. (1984), Axonal transport of the cytoplasmic matrix. *J. Cell Biol.* **99,** pp. 212–22.

Liuzzi, F. J. and Miller, R. H. (1987). Radially oriented astrocytes in the adult rat spinal cord. *Brain Res.* **403,** pp. 385–8.

Ludwin, S. K., Kosek, J. C., and Eng, L. F. (1976). The topographic distribution of S-100 and GFA proteins in the adult brain: an immunohistochemical study using horseradish peroxidase labelled antibodies. *J. Comp. Neurol.* **165**, pp. 197–208.

Maxwell, D. S. and Kruger, L. (1965). The fine structure of astrocytes in the cerebral cortex and their response to focal injury produced by heavy ionizing particles. *J. Cell Biol.* **25**, pp. 141–57.

Miller, R. H. and Liuzzi, F. J. (1986). Regional specialization of the radial glial cells of the adult frog spinal cord. *J. Neurocytol.* **15**, pp. 187–96.

Miller, R. H. and Raff, M. C. (1984). Fibrous and protoplasmic astrocytes are biochemically and developmentally distinct. *J. Neurosci.* **4**, pp. 585–92.

Miller, R. H., David, S., Patel, R., Abney, E. R., and Raff, M. C. (1985). A quantitative immunohistochemical study of macroglial cell development in the rat optic nerve: in vivo evidence for two distinct astrocyte lineages. *Dev. Biol.* **111**, pp. 35–41.

Miller, R. H., Abney, E. R., David, S., ffrench-Constant, C., Lindsay, R., Patel, R., Stone, J., and Raff, M. C. (1986). Is reactive gliosis a property of a distinct subpopulation of astrocytes. *J. Neurosci.* **6**, pp. 22–9.

Mori, S. and Leblond, C. P. (1969). Electron microscopic features and proliferation of astrocytes in the corpus callosum of the rat. *J. Comp. Neurol.* **137**, pp. 197–205.

Peters, A. and Palay, S. L. (1965). An electron microscope study of the distribution and patterns of astroglial processes in the central nervous system. *J. Anat.* **99**, p. 419.

Peters, A. and Vaughn, J. E. (1970). Morphology and development of the myelin sheath. In *Myelination* (eds. A. N. Davison and A. Peters), pp. 3–79. Charles C. Thomas, Springfield, Ill..

Peters, A., Palay, S. L., and Webster, H. deF. (1976). *The fine structure of the nervous system: The neurons and supporting cells*, pp. 223–48. W. B. Saunders, Philadelphia, PA.

Privat, A., Valat, J., and Fulcrand, J (1981). Proliferation of neuroglial cell lines in the degenerating optic nerve of young rats. An autoradiographic study. *J. Neuropathol. Exp. Neurol.* **40**, pp. 46–60.

Raff, M. C., Mirsky, R., Fields, K. L., Lisak, R. P., Dorfmann, S. H., Silberberg, D. H, Gregson, N. A., Liebowitz, S., and Kennedy, M. (1978). Galactocerebroside: a specific cell surface antigenic marker for oligodendrocytes in culture. *Nature* **274**, pp. 813–16.

Raff, M. C., Abney, E. R., Cohen, J., Lindsay, R., and Noble, M. (1983*a*). Two types of astrocytes in cultures of developing rat white matter: differences in morphology, surface gangliosides and growth characteristics. *J. Neurosci.* **3**, pp. 1289–300.

Raff, M. C., Miller, R. H., and Noble, M. (1983*b*). A glial progenitor cell that develops in vitro into an astrocyte or an oligodendrocyte depending on the culture medium. *Nature* **303**, pp. 390–6.

Raff, M. C., Williams, B. P., and Miller, R. H. (1984). The in vitro differentiation of a bipotential glial progenitor cell. *EMBO J.* **3**, pp. 1857–64.

Raine, C. S. (1984). On the association between perinodal astroyte process and the node of Ranvier in the central nervous system *J. Neurocytol.* **13**, pp. 21–7.

Rougon, G., Hirsch, M. R., Hirn, M., Guenet, J. L., an Goridis, C. (1983). Monoclonal antibody to neural cell surface protein. Identification of a glycoprotein family of restricted cellular localization. *Neuroscience.* **10**, pp. 511–20.

Schachner, M. (1982). Immunological analysis of cellular heterogeneity in the cerebellum. In *Neuroimmunology* (ed. J. Brockes), pp. 215–50, Plenum Press, New York.

Schachner, M., Hedley-White, E. T., Hsu, D. W., Schoonmaker, G., and Bignami, A. (1977). Ultrastructural localization of glial fibrillary acid protein in mouse cerebellum by immuno-peroxidase labelling. *J. Cell Biol.* **75,** pp. 67–73.

Skoff, R. P., Knapp, P. E., Bartlett, W. P. (1986). Astrocytic diversity in the optic nerve: a cytoarchitectural study. In: *Astrocytes* vol. 1. (ed Fedoroff and Vernadakis), pp. 269–91. Academic Press, New York.

Skoff, R. P., Price, D., and Stocks, A. (1976a). Electron microscopic autoradiographic studies of gliogensis in rat optic nerve. 1. Cell proliferation. *J. Comp. Neurol.* **169,** pp. 291–312.

Skoff, R. P., Price, D., and Stocks, A. (1976b). Electron microscopic autoradiographic studies of gliogensis in rat optic nerve. 2. Time of origin. *J. Comp. Neurol.* **169,** pp. 313–33.

Skoff, R. P., Toland, D., and Nast, E. (1980). Pattern of myelination and the distribution of neruroglial cells along the developing optic system of the rat and rabbit. *J. Comp. Neurol.* **191,** pp. 237–53.

Somjen, G. G. and Trachtenberg, M. (1979). Neuroglia as generator of extracellular current. In *Origin of cerebral field potentials* (eds. E. J. Spackman and H. Caspers), pp. Thieme, Stuttgart.

Stensaas, L. J., and Stensaas, S.S. (1968). Astrocytic neuroglial cells: oligodendrocytes and microgliacytes in the spinal cord of the toad. I. Light microscopy. *Z. Zellforsch.* **86,** pp. 184–213.

Valat, J., Privat, A., and Fulcrand, J. (1983). Multiplication and differentiation of glial cells in the optic nerve of the postnatal rat. *Anat. Embryol.* **167,** pp, 335–46.

Van Heyningen, W. E. (1963). The fixation of tetanus toxin, strychnine, serotonin and other substances by gangliosides. *J. Gen. Microbiol.* **31,** pp. 375–87.

Vaughn, J. E. (1969). An electron microscopic analysis of gliogensis in rat optic nerve. *Z. Zellforsch.* **94,** pp. 293–324.

Vaughn, J. E. and Pease, D. C. (1970). Electron microscopic studies of Wallerian degeneration in rat optic nerves 2. Astrocytes, oligodendrocytes and adventitial cells. *J. Comp. Neurol.* **140,** pp. 207–26.

Waxman, S. G., and Black, J. A. (1984). Freeze fracture ultrastructure of the perinodal astrocyte and associated glial junctions. *Brain Res.* **308,** pp. 77–87.

Weigert, F. (1895). *Beitrage zur Kenntnis der normalen menschlichen Neuroglia.* Weisbrod, Frankfurt am Main.

15

Roles of glia and neural crest cells in creating axon pathways and boundaries in the vertebrate central and peripheral nervous systems

M. R. POSTON, J. FREDIEU, P. R. CARNEY, AND J. SILVER

The mechanisms that guide axons to their targets in the developing vertebrate nervous system have been sought for over a century. Since every answer to a question about axonal guidance usually gives rise to several new questions, there is some truth in the paradox that the more we learn about axonal guidance, the less we appear to know (see Preface).

Over the years a great deal of progress has been made. Improved techniques, both *in vivo* and *in vitro*, have led to many new and intriguing observations which, in turn, have led to the development and testing of interesting hypotheses and theories. Two of the most important of these are the *chemo-affinity hypothesis* and the *contact guidance theory*. The chemo-affinity hypothesis (Sperry 1944) proposes that growing axons are guided by a chemical matching system between *specific* axons and their appropriate pathways and targets. The contact guidance theory (Weiss 1955) proposes that growing axons, in particular their tips, or growth cones, are guided by contact with surrounding structures that are geometrically organized. A detailed comparison of the two is beyond the scope of this chapter (for reviews, see Hankin and Silver 1986).

The aim of this chapter is to examine the role of neuroectodermally-derived tissues or structures in the formation of axon pathways and boundaries. An axon pathway is a region of tissue which serves as a substrate along which axons can grow *en route* to their targets. An axon boundary is a region of tissue immediately adjacent to a pathway but which fails to serve as a substrate for axon growth. Few, if any, axons will be present in a boundary region, while in the nearby pathway numerous axons will be present. Evidence for contact guidance may be sought through comparative observations of the physical nature of pathway and boundary regions in relation to the position of growth cones. As we shall see, molecular differences between pathways and boundaries may also exist, which will affect axonal growth.

This chapter is divided into several related sections. In the first section, the roles of primitive glia in the formation of a major axon pathway, the corpus callosum, are discussed. Then, an axon boundary structure between the optic and olfactory tracts, the glial knot, is briefly described. In the next section, the emphasis shifts to the possible roles of neural crest and crest-like cells in pathway and boundary formation. The development of the distal and proximal auditory pathways from placodal (otic) crest and the possible role of trunk neural crest in motor root and sensory root formation in the spinal cord are described. Then, the possible role of the neural crest in the formation of an axon refractory boundary along the length of the dorsal seam of the neural tube is discussed. Finally, we present data from recent studies which describe the dorsal midline region of the embryonic day 6 (E6) chick tectum. In this region, cells exhibiting several neural crest-like characteristics may play simultaneous roles in forming an ectopic, transient, peripheral axon pathway while indirectly forming a boundary separating the two tectal lobes.

THE ROLE OF GLIA IN THE FORMATION OF AXON PATHWAYS AND BOUNDARIES

The glial sling

In mammals (excluding certain monotremes and marsupials), the corpus callosum comprises a continuous and massive sheet of cortical commissural axons which connect the two cerebral, or telencephalic, hemispheres (Sidman, Angevine, and Taber-Pierce 1971, pp. 29–35). The dorsal connection by these commissural axons occurs across the longitudinal (interhemispheric) fissure which, during early stages of embryonic development, completely separates the paired telencephalic vesicles (the presumptive cerebral hemispheres). An important question, which until a few years ago was unresolved, is: Does a non-neuronal structure exist which directs the growth of these axons across the fissure, thereby forming the corpus callosum?

To answer this question, Silver, Lorenz, Wahlston, and Coughlin (1982), using serial sections and three-dimensional computer reconstruction, studied the time and location of emergence of pioneering callosal fibres to form the commissure between the cerebral hemispheres in mice. They also examined embryos at pre-axonal stages to determine the nature and configuration of the terrain through which the first callosal fibres grow. Silver and his colleagues found that, on E15, a population of glial cells begins to migrate medially from the subventricular zones of both lateral ventricles, through the fused walls of the dorsal septum, and to the midline below the longitudinal fissure (Silver *et al.* 1982, Figs. 2 and 14). These cells then unite via many *puncta adherentia* to form a bridge-like structure, the 'glial sling'. The accumulation of cells forming the sling, while spanning the lateral ventricles, becomes more densely packed on E16. The glial sling, positioned well rostral (approximately 200 μm) to the lamina terminalis, is thus formed before the pioneering callosal fibres first cross the midline on E17. The earliest wave of callosal fibres travels in a compact bundle immediately below the longitudinal fissure and above, but not among, the cells of the glial sling [Silver *et al.* 1982, Figs. 4(c) and 4(d)]. As more fibres add to the compact bundle (now the corpus callosum), on E18–19 and post-natal stages, they do so along the subventricular surface, of which the sling is a part (Hankin and Silver 1986). This preferential growth by new callosal fibres nearer the sling results in a displacement of older callosal fibres dorsally, away from the sling. However, from E18 onward, the glial sling degenerates and its resident cells are consumed by macrophages. Therefore the glial sling is a transient structure in the mouse embryo, being present from E15 to post-natal day 2 (P2).

To provide direct evidence that the transient glial sling provides guidance cues to the callosal fibres, Silver *et al.* (1982) surgically lesioned the sling on E15–16, before the arrival at the midline of callosal fibers on E17. Performed *in utero*, the operation involved cutting the sling with a microneedle passed down and along the longitudinal fissure. This type of lesion consistently produces acallosal individuals in which the callosal fibres, instead of crossing the midline into the contralateral hemispheres, whirl into very large neuromas (or tangles of axons) adjacent to the longitudinal fissure and rostral to the hippocampus (Silver *et al.* 1982, Figs. 8 and 9). These neuromas are also observed in a genetically acallosal mutant strain of mice in which the sling fails to form. Since the neuromas observed in the artificially produced acallosal mice and those in the genetically acallosal mice are morphologically indistinguishable, Silver and his colleagues concluded that the glial sling does provide guidance cues to callosal fibres crossing the cerebral midline.

Interestingly, in the surgically-produced acallosal mice, the callosal axons maintain a potential to grow across the longitudinal fissure post-natally if they are presented with a properly aligned, glia-coated substrate spanning the two hemispheres. Silver and Ogawa (1983) found that when a piece of cellulose membrane filter (cut to a shape resembling that of the normal glial sling) is properly inserted into the forebrain of such surgically-generated acallosal mice, some of the fibres within the neuromas will exit and cross the midline via the implanted filter (Silver and Ogawa, 1983, Fig. 1). The implant becomes coated with glial cells (astrocytes) which have migrated medially from the subventricular zone, the same location that gives rise to the cells that form the glial sling. Shortly after these astrocytes invest the implant and attach to it by extending processes into the pores of the filter, callosal axons extend from the neuromas onto the astrocytes and cross to the contralateral hemisphere (Smith, Miller, and Silver 1985; Smith, Miller, and Silver 1986). However, the ability of these glial cells to promote axon growth across the glial-coated implant is limited. A critical period exists in that only glial cells from younger (embryonic and early postnatal) animals are able to promote axon growth. In older animals (after P10), astrocytes migrate onto the implant but instead form scars. Callosal fibres subsequently fail to use them (and the implant below) to cross the midline, with the result that the callosum does not reform (Smith *et al.* 1986).

The cells of the glial sling were originally thought to consist only of a population of stellate glia (Silver *et al.* 1985). However, recent anti-GFAP (glial fibrillary acidic protein) staining of the corresponding glial sling region in the cat embryo (Silver *et al.* 1985) indicates that a subpopulation of radial glia is also present. A highly ordered pattern of GFAP staining, in many ways resembling a scaffold, can be seen beneath and among the callosal fibers. The long filamentous nature of the staining pattern suggests the presence of long processes characteristic of radial glia. Particular types of radially arranged glia are believed to direct orderly neuronal migrations (Rakic 1971; Rakic and Sidman 1973), but their role in axon growth is less well documented. It is also possible that the radially organized cells in the cat glial sling direct the medial migration of glia to the midline, where they coalesce to form the dense portion of the sling. These cells, sitting on their radial glial scaffolding, may, in concert, provide guidance cues to the oncoming callosal fibres. The sling, in addition to providing a contralateral directive, may also prevent callosal fibres from continuing ventrally to enter the septum. The dense clustering of sling cells eliminates (or at least greatly reduces) the extracellular space necessary for growth cone movement (Silver and Robb 1979). Thus the sling not only serves as a pathway in that the rostrally located callosal fibres grow medially along its upper surface, but it also can be thought of as a glial-derived, axon-refractory boundary.

The glial knot

A second glial-derived, axon refractory boundary is present at the optic chiasm of mice and chicken embryos. This structure, the 'glial knot', is a region of specialized neuroepithelium at the diencephalic–telencephalic junction, immediately rostral to where optic fibres will travel in the chiasm. The knot was first described in the mouse embryo (Silver 1984) and has now also been observed and described more fully in the chick embryo (Poston, Rutishauser, and Silver 1985; Silver, Poston, and Rutishauser 1987).

When optic axons from the retinal ganglion cells in the eye first arrive at the developing optic chiasm they are presented with four potential avenues via continuous sheets of neuroepithelium. Two of these, one on either side of the midline, are the optic tracts leading to the optic or tectal lobes. A third is the contralateral optic nerve leading to the other eye. The fourth potential avenue lies rostrally, across the diencephalic–telencephalic junction and into the olfactory region of the basal telencephalon. Optic axons grow preferentially along the first two avenues and transiently along the third (McLoon and Lund 1982; O'Leary, Gerfen, and Cowan 1983), but rarely, if ever, along the fourth avenue and into the olfactory pathways (Pickard and Silverman 1981). Conversely, olfactory axons grow caudally in the olfactory tracts but rarely, if ever, cross the diencephalic–telencephalic junction to enter the optic chiasm (Källen 1954). The basic segregation of optic and olfactory projections suggested the presence of an axon refractory boundary at the diencephalic–telencephalic junction. While studying this region in E2–5 chick embryos, we observed several cellular, molecular, and developmental peculiarities, which we have attributed to the glial knot.

Comparisons of the neuroepithelium where axons do and do not grow at the diencephalic–telencephalic junction indicate striking morphological differences. Axon-rich regions (the optic and olfactory tracts) on either side of the rostral border of the chiasm possess wide marginal zones which contain long radial processes. These neuroepithelial processes are separated by wide extracellular spaces, filled with matrix. Axons grow preferentially through these spaces (Silver and Robb 1979) adhering to the radial processes and their pial end-feet (Silver and Rutishauser 1984). Conversely, at the rostral border of the chiasm the marginal zone is eliminated by a dense, interwoven cluster of cells, the glial knot. The knot cells lack long radial processes and have cell bodies located near the glial limitans. Therefore, the extracellular spaces and radial processes through and along which axons prefer to grow are absent, or at least greatly reduced at the knot. Interestingly, these differences in the cellular terrains of the knot and the optic and olfactory tracts are discernible at preaxonal stages; that is, before the arrival of optic axons at the chiasm in late-E3 chick embryos.

The knot also differs from the optic and olfactory tracts at the molecular level, particularly with regard to the neural cell adhesion molecule, NCAM (Rutishauser, Thiery, Brackenbury, and Edelman 1978; Rutishauser 1984). NCAM, which facilitates axon fasciculation and axon–glia interactions, is just detectable on the support cells within the presumptive chiasm and the optic and olfactory tracts at, or slightly before, the time when pioneering optic fibres first arrive at the chiasm late on E3. During the following two days, the amount of NCAM revealed by indirect antibody staining in the chiasm and tracts is greatly increased. The increased amount of NCAM is probably due both to the continual addition of axons and to increased expression of NCAM by support cells. Thus a molecule that promotes axonal growth is present exactly in the regions where it will be needed, and, at least for the optic system, a preformed pathway of NCAM exists (Silver and Rutishauser 1984).

Conversely, the cells of the presumptive knot region do not appear to express NCAM either pre-axonally or after the arrival of fibres in the chiasm and caudal olfactory tract. This complete absence persists across the floor of the diencephalic–telencephalic junction and distinguishes the knot from the chiasm and tract regions. If both optic and olfactory axons were unable to cross this zone, which may have reduced adhesivity aside from the morphological constraints mentioned above, they would remain separated. The lack of NCAM at the knot suggests that the control of its expression plays an important role in axonal guidance at the diencephalic–telencephalic junction.

What events trigger the knot region to become an axon boundary, as opposed to an axon pathway? We have observed very extensive necrosis in the presumptive knot region on E2/3 but little or none in the presumptive chiasm or presumptive optic and olfactory tracts (Poston *et al.* 1985). This zone of death, the suboptic death centre, was first described by Ernst (1926), who suggested that it might serve a morphogenetic function by causing (or being caused by) the ventral and forward shift of the eyes. Källen (1965) proposed instead that the cells were genetically predestined to die. He removed the eye rudiments and still observed the massive degeneration along the floor of the diencephalic–telencephalic junction. We have observed that the density of the cells in the knot on days E4–5 increases as the amount of cell death decreases. It is tempting to speculate that the massive cell death that occurs pre-axonally at the diencephalic–telencephalic junction may trigger, in some way, the formation of the dense, disorganized, and NCAM-free cluster of cells we have called the knot. Regardless of the possible role of cell death in the creation of the knot, this glial structure appears to function as an axon boundary which separates the developing optic and olfactory systems in the chick embryo.

THE ROLE OF NEURAL CREST AND CREST-LIKE CELLS IN THE FORMATION OF AXON PATHWAYS AND BOUNDARIES

The developing auditory nerve in the mouse embryo: the role of preformed crest pathways

Carney and Silver (1983) have described the developing distal auditory pathway in the mouse embryo. In the E9·5 embryo an accumulation of cells forms between the developing otocyst and the auditory (VIII) ganglion just rostral to it (Carney and Silver 1983, Fig. 2). Because of its distinctive shape the cell accumulation has been called the 'funnel'. Laterally, its narrowest portion lies near the rostro–lateral wall of the otocyst and its wider portion near the VIII ganglion. The funnel cells probably represent otic neural crest, migrating away from the developing otocyst before the peripheral auditory fibres from the VIII ganglion project to the otocyst on E11·5. It was determined that the distal auditory axons grow along the cells within the limits of the funnel (Carney and Silver 1983). It was proposed that the funnel cells, by providing an adhesive substrate favourable to the distal auditory axons, could influence their growth and directionality toward the otocyst. By providing a favourable substrate for axonal guidance in the manner predicted by the contact guidance theory, these otic crest cells, which form the funnel, serve as an axon pathway much the way that the subependymal cells of the glial sling do.

The part of the 'funnel' first described by Carney and Silver (1983) only connected the VIII ganglion with the otocyst. It was not determined how central fibres of the VIII ganglion were directed to the brain or how they gained access to the central nervous system (CNS) through the basal lamina. Here we describe a recently discovered continuation of the funnel structure between the VIII ganglion and the hindbrain [Fig. 15.1(a) and (c)], which also forms pre-axonally.

In the E9·5 mouse embryo, otic crest begin to migrate medially away from the otocyst toward the presumptive VIII ganglion and the hindbrain. Some of these cells are presumptive auditory neuroblasts and will collect in the VIII ganglion primordium (Altman and Bayer 1982). Others contribute to the lateral portion of the funnel located between the otocyst and the VIII ganglion (Carney and Silver 1983). Still others migrate medially beyond the VIII ganglion and accumulate into a funnel-shaped structure with a wide end medial to the VIII ganglion and a narrow end inserted into the hindbrain [Fig. 15.1(a)]. This structure is formed pre-axonally, before central fibres project out of the VIII ganglion on E10·5/11·5. Some of the funnel cells actually invade the parenchyma of the hindbrain [note the cell just within the hindbrain in Fig. 15.1(c)] and therefore, presumably, disrupt the basal lamina. Electron microscope investigations have verified the basal lamina disruption (not shown). This breakdown of the basal lamina may be necessary to allow the central auditory fibres easy access to the hindbrain. Where funnel cells abut the hindbrain, neuroepithelial processes penetrate outward through the basal lamina and form contacts with the funnel cells.

As the pioneer central axons emerge from the VIII ganglion on E10·5 and extend medially toward the hindbrain, they grow within the cellular limits of the medial portion of the funnel. Also growing along the funnel cells, the facial

---

Fig. 15.1. (a) 1 μm plastic, near-coronal section through the head of an E9.5 mouse embryo. In this section the developing otocyst (OT), the auditory (VIII) and facial (VII) cranial ganglia, and part of the hindbrain (H) can be seen. Note the accumulation of cells, called the medial funnel (MF), between the VIII ganglion and the H (scale bar = 50 μm). (b) Higher magnification of the outer edge of the OT [open arrow in (a)] near the VIII ganglion. Note the epitheloid cell (arrow) which is exiting the OT opposite the beginning of the lateral funnel (LF), an accumulation of crest-like cells between the OT and the VIII ganglion which guides peripherally projecting axons from the VIII ganglion to the OT (scale bar = 20 μm). (c) Higher magnification of the narrowed region [solid arrow in (a)] of the medial funnel near the H. The cells of the funnel (arrow) extend right to the surface of the H and in this E9.5 embryo form a pre-axonal pathway for the centrally projecting axons from the VIII ganglion (scale bar = 30 μm). (d) 1 μm plastic, near-coronal section through the head of an E11 mouse embryo. The medial funnel is not as evident as in the E9.5 embryo [see (a)], but some of its cells have become associated with the axons projecting from the VIII ganglion into the H along the developing eight cranial nerve (arrow) (scale bar = 50 μm.)

axons (from the VII ganglion) join with the central auditory axons to form a single bundle that reaches the hindbrain by E11.5 [Fig. 15.1(d)]. By this time the funnel is no longer apparent. It appears that some of its cells become aligned along the axons (Fig. 15.2) and have begun to wrap processes around

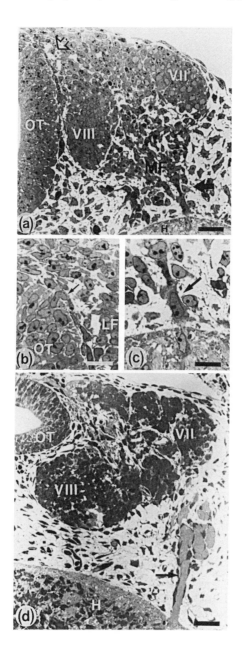

them (not shown). Thus, after the axons have contacted the crest cells within the funnel, the crest cells begin to express the characteristics of Schwann cells. However, the basal lamina surrounding the Schwann cell–axon units does not appear for several more days.

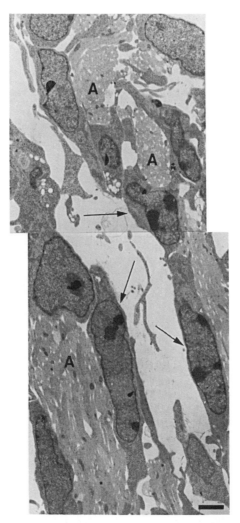

Fig. 15.2. Electron micrograph of the CN VIII of an E11 mouse embryo similar to the one seen in Fig. 15.1 (d). Note that the remaining medial funnel cells (arrows) are alligned along the axons (A); these cells, presumptive Schwann cells, also send out processes which wrap around the axons (not shown) (scale bar = 1·5 μm.)

HNK-1 staining of the developing auditory system in E2 chicken embryos

To determine if the funnel cells were truly a 'crest' population we used polyclonal antibodies to an antigen recognized by a monoclonal antibody, HNK-1. Many cells are HNK-1-positive (Tucker, Aoyama, Lipinski, Tursz, and Thiery 1984), but in young embryos HNK-1 labels trunk neural crest cells and can help distinguish them from adjacent mesenchymal tissues (Fig. 15.3). This has been advantageous in the numerous determinations of migratory routes (throughout the mesenchymal compartments of the embryo) taken by trunk and cephalic crest (e.g. see Rickmann, Fawcett, and Keynes 1985; Bronner-Fraser 1985). Since HNK-1 antibodies were generated in mice, we wanted to determine if a 'crest' pathway similar to that in the mouse existed for the VIII nerve in an avian species, where HNK-1 antibodies are selective. In E2 chick embryos, embryonic stage 12 in Hamburger and Hamilton 1951, a pre-axonal stage for VIII ganglion axons, HNK-1-positive, 'otic crest' cells appear to migrate out of the otocyst (which shows a differential pattern of HNK-1 staining) to form a cellular structure between the otocyst, the VIII ganglion, and the auditory region of the hindbrain (Fig. 15.4). This structure, morphologically similar to the funnel described in the mouse, contains a contiguous chain of HNK-1-positive cells which together extend from the

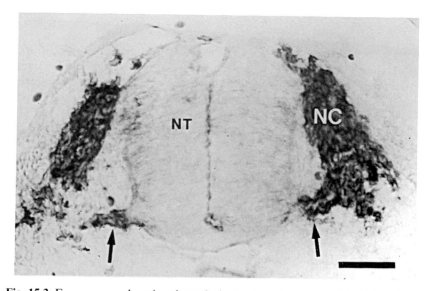

Fig. 15.3. Frozen coronal section through the trunk region of an E2.5 chick embryo, stained with HNK-1 antibody. Neural crest cells (NC) on either side of the neural tube (NT) are distinctly stained. Note the absence of staining at the dorsal midline region of the NT. Arrows indicate presumptive Schwann cells at the ventral motor roots (scale bar = 50 μm.)

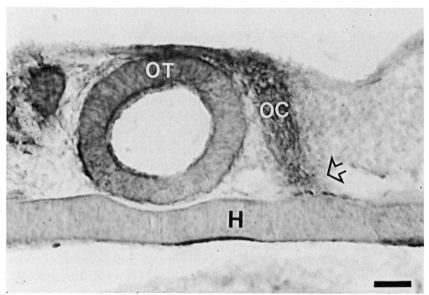

Fig. 15.4. Frozen coronal section through the otocyst (OT) of an E2 chick embryo. The section was stained with HNK-1 antibody and shows HNK-1 positive otic crest cells (OC) which have migrated out of the OT even to the hindbrain (H). The open arrow indicates where a similar region (on a section of a different E2 embryo) is magnified in Fig. 15.5 (scale bar = 40 μm.)

rostro–lateral aspect of the otocyst all the way to the hindbrain. In addition, a few HNK-1-positive cells get through the basal lamina and can be found within the parenchyma of the hindbrain, but never deeper than the marginal zone (Fig. 15.5). Based on the morphological observations of the funnel in the mouse embryo (Carney and Silver 1983) and its HNK-1 positivity in the E2 chicken embryo (present results), there is evidence to suggest that the funnel is formed from the aggregation of otic crest cells which migrate from the otocyst. In turn, the funnel functions as a preformed pathway for the distal auditory axons to reach the otocyst and for the proximal auditory axons to reach the hindbrain.

The possible role of crest in motor and sensory root formation

If otic crest cells play a role in the formation of the auditory nerve, could neural crest cells play a similar role in the formation of motor and sensory roots? This question has been the focus of many studies and much debate (see Hughes 1968). Harrison (1924), for example, grafted two frog embryos together after having removed their neural crest. Two weeks later he observed the state of development of their nervous systems. The embryos lacked both dorsal root ganglia and Schwann cells surrounding the proximal motor

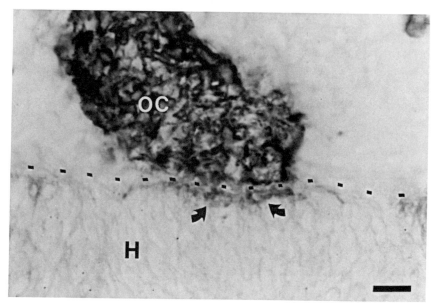

Fig. 15.5. Frozen coronal section of an E2 chick embryo (a pre-axonal stage for the VIII ganglion) that shows HNK-1-positive otic crest cells (OC) which have migrated to the hindbrain (H). Note that some of the HNK-1-positive OC (arrows) have actually crossed the outer surface (dotted line) of the H and have migrated into it (scale bar = 12 μm.)

nerves. These motor nerves, however, were innervating their normal targets peripherally. Harrison concluded that Schwann cells, a derivative of trunk neural crest, did not play a role in the guidance of these fibres. On the other hand, Yntema (1943) removed the crest from the axolotl, *Amblystoma punctatum*, and found that deficient motor innervation of the limbs occurred. He concluded that sheath cells (Schwann cells) were necessary for the motor fibres to reach their targets and establish a complete distribution. Recently, similar results have been reported in chick embryos (Carpenter and Hollyday 1986). Rickmann *et al.* (1985) have removed trunk crest from young chick embryos and observed the growth of motor axons through the anterior halves of the somites. The rationale was that if crest guided the motor axons through the rostral half of the somite, their ablation would prevent such guidance. Their results indicated, however, that the motor axons could grow through the somite without the crest present, although this growth was slower than in normal embryos with intact crest. Based on these results, it was concluded that crest cells are not a prerequisite for motor axon outgrowth, although they might still facilitate that growth. The role of neural crest in the formation of motor (and probably sensory as well) root pathways therefore still needs to be resolved.

THE POSSIBLE ROLE OF CREST IN THE FORMATION OF AN AXON REFRACTORY BOUNDARY ALONG THE DORSAL SEAM OF THE NEURAL TUBE

Just as is the case for axon pathways, the role of crest in the formation of axon boundaries is also unclear. No specific example of crest cells actually blocking axonal growth (as the knot apparently does at the optic chiasm) has been reported.

Crest cells migrate from the dorsal lips or from the newly fused dorsum of the neural tube to start their migration throughout the embryo. The dorsal seam of the neural tube results from the fusion of the neuroepithelium from which crest cells have migrated. Except for very specialized dorsal commissures, the dorsal seam does not have axons growing from one side to the other. This is in contrast to the ventral part of the neural tube which is highly commissurized (particularly in the spinal cord). Cajal (1960) (also see Holley 1982) observed aberrant motor fibres which would grow dorsally in the spinal cord and then exit in the sensory spinal root. These fibres never grow medially across the dorsal seam and into the contralateral side of the spinal cord. Likewise, commissural fibres usually grow ventrally, rarely dorsally to exit in the dorsal root and never across the dorsal midline. Why is the dorsal seam so refractory to axonal growth? Does the neural crest somehow change the dorsal seam, essentially making it an axon boundary region?

THE DORSAL MIDLINE REGION OF THE E6 CHICKEN TECTUM, WHERE CREST-LIKE CELLS MAY CAUSE THE FORMATION OF BOTH A PATHWAY AND A BOUNDARY REGION

The separation of the tectal lobes and its functional significance

If, as was suggested above, much of the dorsal seam of the neural tube acts as an axon refractory boundary, then the dorsal seam at the midline of the mesencephalon might also be predicted to act as one. In chickens, the dorsal half of the mesencephalon develops into the tectal lobes, which receive primary visual information from the eyes. In the adult fowl, most of the optic fibres from one eye extend down the optic nerve, cross the midline at the optic chiasm, enter the contralateral optic tract, and proceed to innervate the contralateral tectal lobe (Goldberg 1974; Rager 1980). Under normal circumstances the optic fibres never re-cross the midline to innervate the ipsilateral tectal lobe. This separation of input has functional and behavioural significance by preventing improper visual input to reflex centers located in the tectal efferent system. For example, input to the tectum from the wrong eye causes abnormal eye- and head-turning away from visual stimuli (Schneider, Jhaveri, Edwards, and So 1985).

Such incorrect tectal input can be obtained in post-natal hamsters by surgically removing the superficial layers of one side of the superior colliculus, the mammalian equivalent of the tectum (Schneider 1973). When the optic axons arrive at the colliculus, their normal contralateral target has been removed. However, the axons find a new target by growing, via a 'necrotic' tissue bridge (So 1979), across the midline and into the ipsilateral colliculus. These 'misplaced' axons compete with the correct axons (those appropriate for the undamaged side) for terminal fields in the medial aspects of the remaining colliculus and form functional synapses. Thus an abnormal projection to the 'wrong' side of the tectum occurs, and maladaptive behaviour can result (Schneider *et al.* 1985).

These collicular lesion experiments have shown that optic fibres have the potential at least, when given the opportunity under abnormal circumstances, to cross the midline and innervate the wrong side of the brain. However, these fibres do not fulfil this potential in the normal embryo. This suggests the presence of a boundary, or the absence of a necessary pathway, at the region connecting the tectal lobes during development. If the tectal midline does function as a boundary, then what are the cellular and molecular mechanisms by which the boundary is created?

In the adult fowl the optic lobes are well separated by the tenuous roof of the Sylvian aqueduct. However, in the E6 chick when the optic fibres first arrive at the mesencephalon, the optic lobes are contiguous across the midline via a short stretch of neuroepithelium. This region gradually lengthens as the optic lobes begin rotating laterally away from each other on E7 (Goldberg 1974; Rogers 1960). Thus, in the embryo, optic fibres have only a short potential avenue of growth that could lead them astray across the tectal midline and into the wrong side of the brain. However, under normal circumstances they rarely, if ever, make this pathway error. We were interested in this region and wished to determine if it had characteristics in common with the pathways and boundaries previously discussed.

Background on the innervation of the tectum by optic fibres

When optic fibres arrive at the medial walls of the tectal hemispheres on E6, the tectum has a distinct shape resembling the upper half of a short cylinder which has a long invagination running lengthwise down its dorsal half. The cylinder corresponds to the mesencephalon of the developing brain, and its dorsal half, including the longitudinal invagination, to the tectum (the ventral half of the cylinder represents the presumptive tegmentum). That region of tectal neuroepithelium which connects the ventral most aspects of the walls of the invagination will be referred to as the tectal midline, and it can be seen below the asterisk in Fig 15.6(a). Figures 15.6–15.14 are either light or electron micrographs of coronal sections (some immuno-stained) through that region.

Optic fibres, arriving from the optic tracts, reach the ventral and lateral aspects of the anterior part of the tectal hemipheres on E5–6 (Goldberg 1974). Using anti-NCAM antibodies as a crude assay for nerve fibres, axons can also be seen throughout the medial walls of the anterior optic lobes at E6 [Fig. 15.6(a)]. Quickly thereafter, the fibres grow in both lateral-to-medial and rostral-to-caudal directions over the entire surface of the tectum. By E12 the entire tectum is innervated by retinal ganglion cell axons (De Long and Coulombre 1965). The optic fibres are located superficially in the marginal zone (Silver and Rutishauser 1984) in close proximity to the deeper tectal efferent fibres [arrow in Fig. 15.6(a)]. At this stage some of the fibres grow a short distance into, but do not cross, the tectal midline [Fig. 15.6(b), dark staining].

Gaps in the glial limitans at the tectal midline

A concentrated solution of horseradish peroxidase (HRP) injected into the tectal mesenchyme between the tectal lobes [see Fig. 15.6(a)] preferentially adheres to the glial limitans of the neuroepithelium, thereby distinctly marking the division between neuroepithelial and mesenchymal tissues (Fig. 15.7). The HRP-stained glial limitans could be seen in light or electron micrographs. Interestingly, this 'enhancement' of the glial limitans by HRP was most prominent along the surface of the tectal midline, while the glial limitans of the medial tectal walls was emphasized much less.

At E6 many discontinuities were present in the glial limitans of the tectal midline [Fig. 15.7(a), and Fig. 10(b), later]. The gaps varied in diameter from approximately 0·5 mm to several microns and generally involved the complete absence of the basal lamina and a drastic disruption of the marginal end-feet. Careful examination of the glial limitans, both with and without the injection of HRP, indicated that the gaps occurred almost exclusively at the tectal midline region and not along the medial walls of the optic lobes. The gaps in the glial limitans were often observed in association with two other phenomena, the crossing of the glial limitans by either axons or large-bodied cells.

Projection of axons across the glial limitans into the mesenchyme

At E6, axons often appeared to exit the neuroepithelium through the gaps into the overlying mesenchyme. Often whole fascicles could be seen extending across the glial limitans [Fig. 15.7(a) and (b), and Fig. 15.8(a) and (c)]. Growth cones were found along the neuroepithelial end-feet within the tectal midline and frequently near the gaps [Fig. 15.8(b)].

Although transmission electron microscopy indicated that the structures

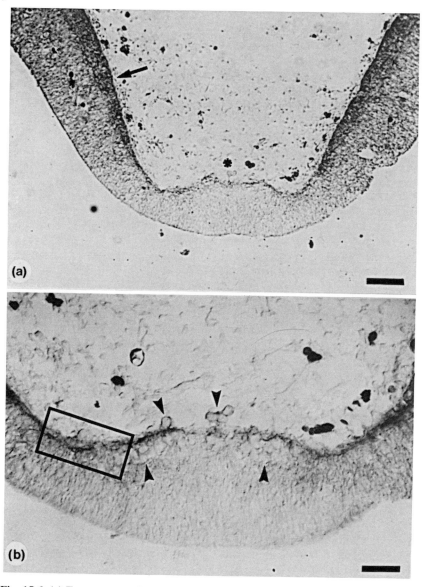

Fig. 15.6. (a) Frozen coronal section of the anterior tectum of an E6 chicken embryo stained for NCAM. The arrow indicates the marginal zone containing both optic fibres (superficial) and tectal efferent fibers (deep); the asterisk indicates the approximate region above which in some E5 embryos a concentrated solution of horseradish peroxidase was injected into mesenchyme dorsal to the tectal midline (which is just below the asterisk) (scale bar = 75 µm). (b) Higher magnification of a similar section stained for NCAM. The box approximately corresponds to the regions shown in Figs. 15.8(d) and 15.9. The arrowheads indicate large, NCAM-negative cells inside and outside of the neuroepithelium, with NCAM-positive, axon-like structures in close association to them (scale bar = 50 µm).

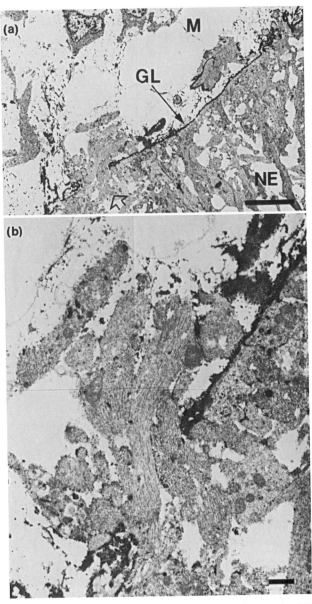

Fig. 15.7. (a) Electron micrograph of a coronal section at the tectal midline of an E6 embryo. Note the gap or discontinuity (lower left) in the glial limitans (GL) at the outer surface of the neuroepithelium (NE). The GL was preferentially adhered to by HRP (dark material) injected into the mesenchyme (M) on E5 [see Fig. 15.6(a)]. Open arrow points to the area shown in higher magnification in (b) (scale bar = 5 μm). (b) Higher magnification of the gap in the GL through which axon-like structures appear to exit the NE (scale bar = 1·0 μm).

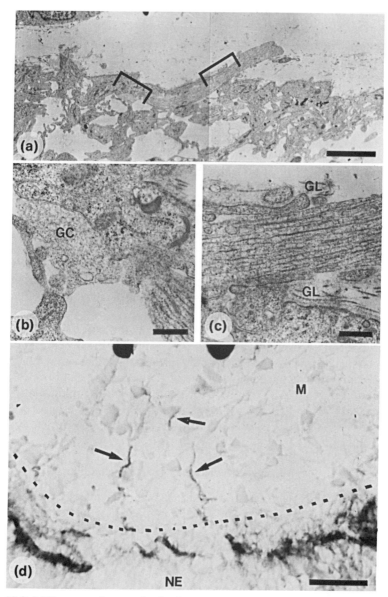

Fig. 15.8. (a)Electron micrograph of a single axon-like structure projecting across the glial limitans (GL) and into the mesenchyme at the tectal midline of an E6 embryo (scale bar=5 μm). (b) Higher magnification of area below the left bracket in (a) showing a possible growth cone (GC) in the marginal zone (scale bar=0·6 μm). (c) Higher magnification of area below right bracket in (a) showing an axon-like structure projecting through the GL (scale bar=0·6 μm). (d) Frozen section corresponding to the boxed area in Fig. 15.6. (b). The section was stained with an antibody directed against the 8D9 antigen that is present on axon fibre pathways. Note the thin, 8D9-positive structures (arrows) in the mesenchyme (M) as well as more numerous ones within the neuroepithelium (NE), the outer edge of which is indicated by a dotted line (scale bar=25 μm).

projecting across the glial limitans were rich in microtubules, a hallmark of axons [Fig. 15.8(c)], immunohistochemical evidence was also needed for further verification. Coronal sections of the tecta of E6 chicken embryos were obtained and stained with 8D9 antibody, which is expressed only by axons (Vance Lemmon, pers. com.). Structures positive for 8D9 were readily observed within the neuroepithelium both at the medial tectal walls and at the tectal midline. Fortuitous sections also showed the presence of very thin, 8D9-positive structures in the mesenchyme [Fig. 15.8(d) and Fig. 15.9]. These structures were sometimes quite distant from the glial limitans [Fig. 15.8(d)], but usually they were located within 50–100 µm of the brain (Fig. 15.9). Whether these 8D9-positive structures were optic axons or tectal efferents, or, more likely, both, has not yet been determined conclusively. However, the 8D9-positive structures in the mesenchyme appeared to be contiguous with both superficial (optic) and deeper (tectal efferent) axons within the ventro–medial walls of the optic lobes. Also, preliminary studies of specimens injected into the right eye with HRP indicate that some of the axons exiting the midline tectal neuroepithelium into the overlying mesenchyme may, indeed, be optic axons (not shown).

Further immuno–histochemical evidence that the structures exiting the neuroepithelium through gaps in the glial limitans were axons came from sections stained for NCAM. Once again, fortuitous sections showed NCAM-positive structures immediately outside of the neuroepithelium which were contiguous with NCAM-positive axons within the neuroepithelium. Some sections showed axons which projected across the glial limitans in association with large NCAM-negative cells in the mesenchyme [Fig. 15.6(b), left arrow in mesenchyme].

Large HNK-1-positive, crest-like cells may cross the glial limitans

Besides axons, large cells were observed to span the glial limitans exclusively at the tectal midine. These cells were sometimes found in isolation [Fig. 15.10(a)

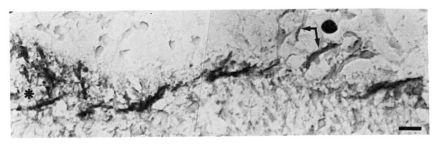

Fig. 15.9. Frozen section corresponding to the boxed area in Fig. 15.6.(b). The section was stained for the presence of axons with 8D9 antibody. Note the contiguity of the labelled axon-like structures both within the walls of the tectal hemisphere (∗) and outside of the neuroepithelium (arrows) (scale bar = 20 µm).

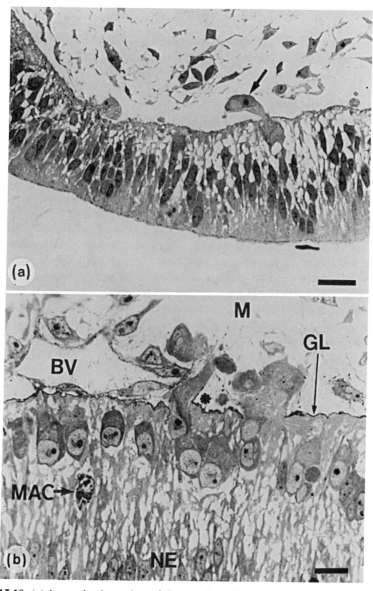

Fig. 15.10. (a) 1 μm plastic section of the tectal midline of an E6 chick embryo. The section, stained with toluidine blue, shows three large cells, two immediately outside the neuroepithelium and one within it. Note that one of the cells in the mesenchyme (arrow) has a process which crosses the glial limitans and apposes the large cell within the neuroepithelium (scale bar = 20 μm). (b) 1 μm plastic section of the midline tectum of an E6 embryo which had received an injection of HRP into the mesenchyme (M) between the optic lobes on E5. The glial limitans (GL) is emphasized by the HRP, and discontinuities where large cells are crossing it can be readily seen. Note the almost linear arrangement of large cells immediately within the neuroepithelium and their size compared with the other neuroepithelial cells (NE). MAC, macrophage which has ingested HRP; BV, blood vessel (scale bar = 30 μm).

and (b), left side] or, more often, in clusters [Fig. 15.10(b), right side]. Whether this represents cell migration into or out of the tectum, has not yet been determined. Some cells in the mesenchyme had processes which looked as if they grew into the neuroepithelium and forced the glial limitans inward [Fig. 15.13(a) and 15.13(b), later]. Other cells within the margin of the neuroepithelium had processes which forced the glial limitans outward into the mesenchyme and, in addition, had mis-shapen nuclei which suggested migration toward the mesenchyme (Fig. 15.10(b), asterisk). A similar distortion of nuclei has been reported in 'mesenchymal' cells escaping from the mouse embryonic trigeminal placode (Nichols 1986). Placodal cells, which enter the mesenchyme and subsequently aggregate and differentiate into the neurons of the trigeminal (X or Gausserian) cranial sensory ganglion, first develop processes which penetrate the placodal basal lamina. The leading edges of cell nuclei then 'squeeze' into these processes as the cells migrate away from the placode. At the E6 chick tectal midline, similarly mis-shapen nuclei were observed in processes which penetrated the basal lamina, suggesting migration across it. Regardless of the direction of that migration, it was evident that large cells were migrating through gaps in the glial limitans.

The migration of these large cells into or out of the neuroepithelium raised the possibility that they might be some derivative of the neural crest, a highly migratory and pluripotential population of cells (Horstadius 1950; Weston 1970; Le Douarin 1980, 1986; Erickson 1986). Frozen sections stained with HNK-1 antibody indicated that many of the large migratory cells were indeed HNK-1-positive. These HNK-1-positive cells were found either alone or clustered all along the glial limitans of the tectal midline, but rarely along the tectal walls. Thus HNK-1-positive cells at the tectal midline colocalized with emigrating axons and gaps in the basal lamina. The HNK-1-positive cells could be found immediately within the neuroepithelium [Fig. 15.11(a, c)] or immediately outside the glial limitans in the mesenchyme [Fig. 11(b)]. Often the cells in the mesenchyme had HNK-1-positive processes which projected into the midline neuroepithelium [arrows in Fig. 11(b)]. Occasionally an HNK-1-positive cell with an unusual process was observed some distance from the neuroepithelium in the mesenchyme [Fig. 15.12(a, b)].

Aetiological consideration of the large HNK-1-positive cells of the tectal midline: are they neural crest or crest-derived cells?

That the large cells observed at the tectal midline are HNK-1-positive is not conclusive evidence that they are in fact neural crest or crest-derived cells. Other cell types express the HNK-1 antigen, and the epitope recognized by the HNK-1 antibody is present on other cell surface molecules such as NCAM, L1, myelin-associated glycoprotein, and others. Although before E3 migrating crest cells are more dramatically stained by HNK-1 than probably any other embryonic cell, after E3 other cell types, particularly neuroepithelial cells, begin to progressively express the HNK-1 antigen on their cell surfaces (Tucker *et al.* 1984). This would explain the HNK-1 staining of much of the neuroepithelium of the medial walls of the tectal lobes (see below). None the less, the intense HNK-1 staining of the large midline cells compared to that of the well characterized neural crest and the precise localization of these cells with cells proposed by others to be neural crest based on generation and chimaeric studies (see below), at the very least suggest the *possibility* that they could be neural crest or crest-derived cells.

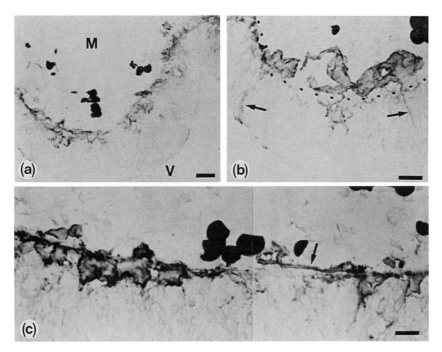

Fig. 15.11. (a) Frozen section of an E6 chick tectal midline, stained with HNK-1 antibody. HNK-1-positive cells are located immediately within the glial limitans. The intensely stained structures in the mesenchyme (M) are red blood cells which have an endogenous peroxidase. V, ventricle (scale bar = 25 µm). (b) Another coronal section stained for HNK-1. Note the large HNK-1-positive cells just outside of the glial limitans (dotted line) and the one within it. Also note the cell processes (arrows) extending into the neuroepithelium from HNK-1-positive cells in the mesenchyme (scale bar = 15 µm). (c) Frozen section stained with the HNK-1 antibody showing HNK-1-positive cells immediately within the glial limitans at the tectal midline. Some of the cells send long processes (arrow) out of the neuroepithelium into the mesenchyme (scale bar = 20 µm).

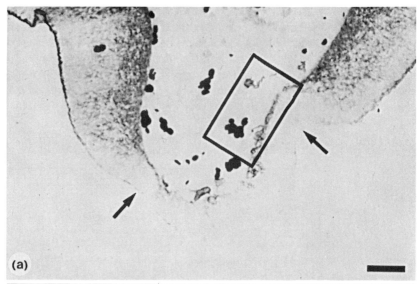

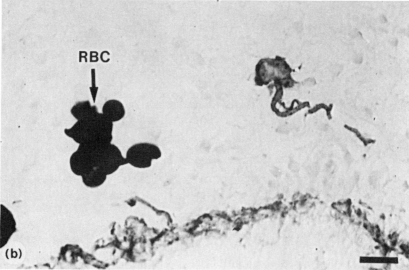

Fig. 15.12. (a) Coronal section of an E6 embryo stained with HNK-1. The tectal midline region consists of the neuroepithelium between the arrows. Note that, except for the superficial regions near the glial limitans, this midline neuroepithelium is negative for HNK-1. However, more laterally (on the medial walls of the optic lobes) HNK-1 reactivity is more widespread in the neuroepithelium but still more concentrated at the margin [compared to the NCAM reactivity of the same region as seen in Figure 15.6(a)] (scale bar = 50 μm). (b) Higher magnification of the boxed area in (a). Note the large HNK-1-positive cell and its unusual HNK-1-positive process in the mesenchyme. RBC, red blood cells (scale bar = 20 μm).

HNK-1 and NCAM reactivities in the tectal medial walls and the tectal midline

As would be expected from the above, the marginal and mantle zones of the medial tectal walls were also HNK-1-positive at E6. At the tectal midline, however, all of the HNK-1-positive reactivity could be attributed entirely to the large cells described above; the rest of the tectal midline neuroepithelium was HNK-1-negative [Fig. 15.12(a)]. This was similar to the dorsal seam of the neural tube being HNK-1-negative while crest cells were migrating away (Fig. 15.3). Whether the dorsal seam remains HNK-1-negative from E2 through E6 was not determined. A continual HNK-1-negativity (with the exception of the large cells) at the dorsal tectal seam would be very interesting and could play a role in the events occurring in this region.

The NCAM reactivity of the medial tectal walls was similar to that for HNK-1: widespread throughout the neuroepithelium but most concentrated at the margin where optic and tectal efferent fibres were present [Fig. 15.6(a)]. However, the NCAM reactivity of the tectal midline was different than that for HNK-1 in one way. The large cells found migrating across the glial limitans were HNK-1-positive but NCAM-negative [Fig. 15.6(b) arrows in neuroepithelium]. This observation is consistent with the large cells being migrating crest cells, since these cells do not express NCAM (Thiery, Duband, Rutishauser, and Edelman 1982). The remainder of the neuroepithelium of the tectal midline region was also NCAM-negative [Fig. 15.6(a)]. Thus, whereas the tectal walls and the neuroepithelial cells of the tectal midline each have similar reactivities with HNK-1 and against NCAM (i.e. positive for both antigens or negative for both antigens, respectively), the large cells of the tectal midline region have different reactivities for antibodies against these two antigens.

The mesencephalic nucleus of the trigeminal nerve and its embryonic origin from neural crest

Although the tectal midline is not a site for the crossing of optic fibres from one lobe to the other, it is the site for the formation of a unique sensory nucleus within the CNS. The mesencephalic nucleus of the trigeminal nerve (MNTN), present in all jawed vertebrates, is associated with proprioception of the lower jaw musculature (Piatt 1945). It consists mainly of unipolar sensory neurons arranged in a linear sheet (Weinberg 1928). Morphologically and functionally, these MNTN neurons are comparable to those found in the dorsal root ganglia of the spinal cord and the sensory ganglia of the cranial nerves. In the adult chick, the MNTN neurons are divided into a lateral group within the stratum griseum periventriculare of the optic lobes (a deep tectal layer near the ependyma), and a medial group located in the roof of the Sylvian aqueduct (Narayanan and Narayanan 1978). Each group extends from the posterior commissure rostrally to the decussation of the trochlear nerve (cranial neuron

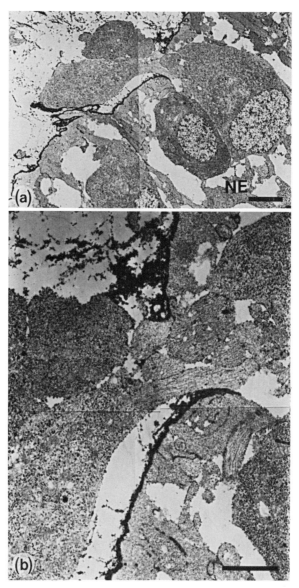

Fig. 15.13. (a) Electron micrograph of the midline tectum of an E6 chick embryo which had HRP injected into the mesenchyme between the optic lobes on E5. Note the large cells (corresponding to the HNK-1-positive cells seen in frozen sections) within the neuroepithelium (NE) and the parts of two cells just outside of the HRP-labelled glial limitans [compare with Fig. 15.10(b)] (scale bar = 5 μm). (b) Higher magnification of the gap in the glial limitans seen in (a). Note the deflection of the glial limitans into the neuroepithelium by an axon-like structure full of microtubules extending from one of the large cells in the mesenchyme (scale bar = 2·5 μm).

IV) caudally (Weinberg 1928). Hiscock and Straznicky (1986) have investigated the formation of the axonal projections of MNTN neurons by injecting HRP into the jaw-closing muscles of E6–15 and post-hatched chicken embryos. By observing the numbers and the first appearance of HRP-labelled MNTN neurons, they determined that the outgrowth of MNTN processes to their peripheral targets occurred between E10–14; outgrowth via central processes, which exclusively terminated in the trigeminal motor nucleus, began on E13. Therefore, the formation of the MNTN occurs early in the ontogeny of the chick embryo.

However, the embryonic origin of the cells within the MNTN was unresolved for many years after its initial anatomical characterization in the chick (Weinberg 1928). Recently, studies of the generation times of MNTN neurons (Rogers and Cowan 1973), as well as quail–duck chimeric transplantation experiments (Narayanan and Narayanan 1978), have provided strong but somewhat circumstantial evidence that the MNTN neurons are derived from mesencephalic crest. Rogers and Cowan (1973), using injections of ^{3}H-thymidine into chick embryonic blastoderm between E2–5, determined that the entire population of MNTN neurons was generated during E3–4. Previous autoradiographic studies on the development of the optic tectum (La Vail and Cowan 1971) had indicated that the stratum griseum periventriculare (within which the lateral MNTN neurons are located in the adult) is generated during E4–6 from the tectal neuroepithelium. Because of this difference in generation times, Rogers and Cowan (1973) suggested that the earlier generation of the MNTN neurons was indirect evidence of their origin from neural crest or the neural folds. Besides several other interesting observations, they also observed labelled cells present in the mesenchymal tissue immediately overlying the roof of the Sylvian aqueduct that were identical in appearance to those of the medial MNTN neurons within the glial limitans. As Rogers and Cowan (1973) pointed out, if the MNTN is partially or completely derived from the neural crest, then the observed cells outside the glial limitans might be presumptive MNTN neurons which, having initially migrated away with other crest cells, had somehow reversed their direction to migrate back to the CNS. Once having crossed the glial limitans, these cells might then differentiate into the MNTN neurons.

Further support that this was indeed occurring was provided by the crest transplantation experiments of Narayanan and Narayanan (1978). They unilaterally transplanted quail mesencephalic crest in place of duck mesencephalic crest and, after several days of further development, observed the locations of the quail cells in the host (duck) mesencephalon. Quail cells, easily distinguishable from duck cells because of their condensed heterochromatin, were found midway in the roof of the Sylvian aqueduct, extending laterally into the tectal lobes, particularly in the stratum griseum periventriculare. Quail cells were found clustered on both sides of the glial limitans, similar to the way the HNK-1-positive cells we observed were clustered at the E6 chick tectal midline. The generation studies and the crest chimeric transplantation experiments both provided evidence that the MNTN was derived from neural crest. Could the HNK-1-positive cells we observed at the tectal midline be the presumptive sensory neurons of the MNTN?

Ultrastructural characterization of the large cells of the tectal midline: do they constitute the mesencephalic nucleus of the trigeminal nerve?

In 1 μm plastic sections the large cells just within the glial limitans along the tectal midline appear to be linearly arranged [Fig. 15.10(b)]. They are very large, some reaching a diameter of 40 μm or more. Since the tectal midline, as we have been describing it here, is the future roof of the Sylvian aqueduct in the chick embryo (Weinberg 1928), it is probable that these large, linearly arranged cells are in fact the presumptive sensory neurons of the MNTN. The cells, in electron micrographs, do resemble neurons. They have pale nuclei, and several of them, whether outside of the neuroepithelium [Fig. 15.13(a) and (b)] or inside of it (Fig. 15.14), possess neurites. It is possible that some of these neurites may also exit the neuroepithelium through gaps in the glial limitans. That these cells have, by E6, begun to produce neurites is a reasonable assumption, since by E10 the peripheral processes of MNTN neurons have begun reaching their targets, the jaw-closing muscles (Hiscock and Straznicky 1986).

Hypothesis

Neural crest cells, or cells exhibiting several characteristics of crest, may migrate across the glial limitans at the midline of the tectum between the tectal lobes (the future roof of the Sylvian aqueduct). In doing so, these cells, destined to become the neurons of the MNTN, grossly disrupt the marginal zone and create gaps in the overlying glial limitans. Itinerant axons, some of which may be optic axons from the eyes, grow into the midline but are shunted out into the surrounding mesenchyme. Since this ectopic, 'peripheral' pathway into the mesenchyme is not found in the adult, the misrouted axons, whether optic, tectal efferent, or proprioceptive (from the MNTN), must either retract back into the tectal neuroepithelium where more appropriate targets are available or die and be phagocytosed. In either case, the axons essentially are prevented from traversing a potential avenue, the midline tectal neuroepithelium. In this way, the neural crest cells which proportedly become the neurons of the MNTN act indirectly to form an axon boundary between the two tectal lobes. If, as preliminary data suggests, some of these misrouted axons are optic fibres, then this unique combination of events may have functional and behavioural significance by preventing the wrong visual input from reaching the wrong tectal lobe.

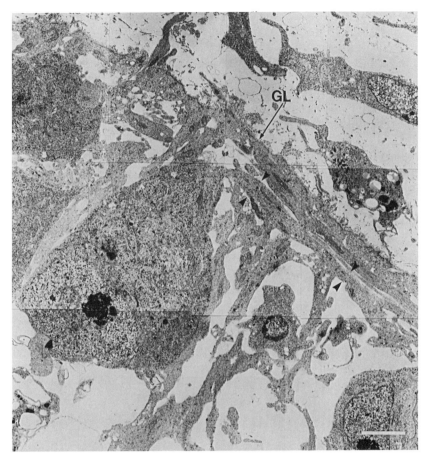

Fig. 15.14. Electron micrograph of a large cell just within the glial limitans (GL). Note that the cell has a long axon-like structure (indicated by arrow-heads) which courses laterally just within the neuroepithelium (scale bar = 3·0 μm).

CONCLUSIONS

In this chapter we have discussed how two types of neuroectodermally-derived cells, glia and neural crest cells, may play roles in the formation of axon pathways and boundaries and thus influence axonal guidance. We have concentrated, in some detail, on four structures, the 'sling', 'knot', 'funnel', and 'tectal midline'. In general, these non-neuronal structures have several characteristics in common, and yet are different in several ways also. All four are specialized tissues which, either physically or molecularly, or both, can provide guidance cues to axons. They are, to some extent, oriented at a gross level which may provide physical cues to axons. They are generally preformed; that is, present before the arrival of the axons they might guide. The structures also differ in their locations, their configurations, and their mechanisms of guidance. For example, the sling and the funnel form aggregations of cells along which callosal and auditory axons respectively will grow. The knot and the 'crest' at the tectal midline disrupt the marginal zones in their respective regions, but they do it in different ways. The knot forms a narrow rod of densely clustered cells through which axons will not pass. The 'crest' at the tectal midline perforates the marginal zone, which subsequently allows axons to be misrouted away from a potential avenue of growth. Although the mechanisms of forming axon boundaries are different, the end result is the same. These similarities and differences between glial and crest structures which play a role in pathway and boundary formation will no doubt be an area of future research in the attempt to understand axonal guidance better.

ACKNOWLEDGEMENTS

We would like to thank Drs Storey Landis, Urs Rutishauser, and Vance Lemmon for their generous gifts of the HNK-1, NCAM, and 8D9 antibodies, respectively. We would also like to thank Catherine Doller for her excellent technical assistance. This research was supported by grants to J. Silver from the National Eye Institute, the Spinal Cord Society, and the National Science Foundation.

REFERENCES

Altman, J. and Bayer, S. A. (1982). Development of the cranial nerve ganglia and related nuclei in the rat. *Adv. Anat. Embryol. Cell Biol.* **74**, pp. 39–46.

Bronner-Fraser, M. (1985). Alterations in neural crest migration by a monoclonal antibody that affects cell adhesion. *J. Cell Biol.* **101**, pp. 610–7.

Cajal, S. R. (1960). *Studies in vertebrate neurogenesis* (translated by L. Guth). Charles Thomas, Springfield, IL.

Carney, P. R. and Silver, J. (1983). Studies on cell migration and axon guidance in the developing distal auditory system of the mouse. *J. Comp. Neurol.* **215**, pp. 359–69.

Carpenter, E. M. and Hollyday, M. (1986). Defective innervation of chick limbs in the absence of presumptive Schwann cells. *Neurosci. Abstr.* **12**, p. 1210.

De Long, G. R. and Coulombre, A. J. (1965). Development of the retinotectal topographic projection in the chick embryo. *Exp. Neurol.* **13**, pp. 351–63.

Erickson, C. (1986). Morphogenesis of the neural crest. In *Development biology, a comprehensile synthesis: Vol. 2., The cellular basis of morphogenesis* (ed. L. W. Browder), pp. 481–543. Plenum Press, New York.

Ernst, M. (1926). Uber untergang von Zellen wahrend der normalen Entwicklung bei wirbeltieren. *Z. ges Anat: J. Z. Anat. Entw-Gesch.* **19**, pp. 228–62.

Goldberg, S. (1974). Studies on the mechanics of development of the visual pathways in the chick embryo. *Dev. Biol.* **36,** pp. 24–43.

Hamburger, V. and Hamilton, H. L. (1951). A series of normal stages in the development of the chick embryo. *J. Morphol.* **88,** pp. 49–92.

Hankin, M. H. and Silver, J. (1986). Mechanisms of axonal guidance: the problem of intersecting fiber systems. In *Developmental biology, a comprehensive synthesis: Vol. 2, The cellular basis of morphogenesis* (ed. L. W. Browder), pp. 565–604. Plenum Press, New York.

Harrison, R. G. (1924). Neuroblast versus sheath cell in the development of peripheral nerves. *J. Comp. Neurol.* **37,** pp. 123–205.

Hiscock, J. and Straznicky, C. (1986). The formation of axonal projections of the mesencephalic trigeminal neurones in chick embryos. *J. Embryol. exp. Morphol.* **93,** pp. 281–90.

Holley, J. A. (1982). Early development of the circumferential axonal pathway in mouse and chick spinal cord. *J. Comp. Neurol.* **205,** pp. 371–82.

Hörstadius, S. (1950). *The neural crest: its properties and derivatives in the light of experimental research.* Oxford University Press, London.

Hughes, A. F. W. (1968). *Aspects of neural ontogeny.* Logos Press, London.

Källen, B. (1954). The embryology of the telencephalic fibre systems in the mouse. *J. Embryol. exp. Morphol.* **2,** pp. 87–100.

Källen, B. (1965). Degeneration and regeneration in the vertebrate CNS during embryogenesis. *Prog. Brain Res.* **14,** pp. 77–96.

La Vail, J. and Cowan, W. M. (1971). The development of the chick optic tectum. I. Normal morphology and cytoarchitectonic development. *Brain Res.* **28,** pp. 391–419.

Le Douarin, N. M. (1980). The ontogeny of the neural crest in avian embryo chimaeras. *Nature* **286,** pp. 663–9.

Le Douarin, N. M. (1986). Cell line segregation during peripheral nervous system ontogeny. *Science* **231,** pp. 1515–22.

McLoon, S. C. and Lund, R. D. (1982). Transient retinofugal pathways in the developing chick. *Exp. Brain Res.* **45,** pp. 277–84.

Narayanan, C. H. and Narayanan, Y. (1978). Determination of the embryonic origin of the mesencephalic nucleus of the trigeminal nerve in birds. *J. Embryol. exp. Morphol.* **43,** pp. 85–105.

Nichols, D. (1986). Mesenchyme formation from the trigeminal placodes of the mouse embryo. *Am. J. Anat.* **176,** pp. 19–31.

O'Leary, D. D. M., Gerfen, C. R. and Cowan, W. M. (1983). The development and restriction of the ipsilateral retinofugal projection in the chick. *Dev. Brain Res.* **10,** pp. 93–109.

Piatt, J. (1945). Origin of mesencephalic V root cells in Amblystoma. *J. Comp. Neurol.* **82,** pp. 35–53.

Pickard, G. E. and Silverman, A. J. (1981). Direct retinal projections to the hypothalamus, piriform cortex, and optic nuclei in the golden hamster as demonstrated by a sensitive anterograde HRP technique. *J. Comp. Neurol.* **196,** pp. 155–72.

Poston, M., Rutishauser, U., and Silver, J. (1985). Physical and molecular factors that influence axonal guidance at the developing optic chiasm. *Neurosci. Abstr.* **11,** p. 584.

Rager, G. H. (1980). Development of the retinotectal projection in the chicken. *Adv. Embryol. Cell Biol.* **63**, pp. 1–92.

Rakic, P. (1971). Neuron–glia relationships during granule cell migrations in developing cerebellar cortex. A Golgi and electron microscopic study in *Macacus rhesus. J. Comp. Neurol.* **141**, pp. 283–312.

Rakic, P. and Sidman, R. L. (1973). Organization of cerebellar cortex secondary to deficit of granule cells in Weaver mutant mice. *J. Comp. Neurol.* **152**, pp. 133–62.

Rickman, M., Fawcett, J. W., and Keynes, R. J. (1985). The migration of neural crest and the growth of motor axons through the rostral half of the chick somite. *J. Embryol. exp. Morphol.* **90**, pp. 437–55.

Rogers, K. T. (1960). Studies on the chick brain of biochemical differentiation related to morphological differentiation. I. Morphological development. *J. Exp. Zool.* **144**, pp. 77–87.

Rogers, L. A. and Cowan, W. M. (1973). The development of the mesencephalic nucleus of the trigeminal nerve in the chick. *J. Comp. Neurol.* **147**, pp. 291–320.

Rutishauser, U. (1984). Molecular and biological properties of a neural cell adhesion molecule. *Cold Spring Harbor Symp. Quant. Biol.* **48**, pp. 501–14.

Rutishauser, U., Thiery, J.-P., Brackenbury, B., and Edelman, G. M. (1978). Adhesion among neural cells of the chick embryo. III. Relationship of the surface molecule CAM to cell adhesion and the development of histotypic patterns. *J. Cell Biol.* **79**, pp. 371–81.

Schneider, G. E. (1973). Early lesions of superior colliculus: factors affecting the formation of abnormal retinal projections. *Brain Behav. Evol.* **8**, pp. 73–109.

Schneider, G. E., Jhaveri, S., Edwards, M. A., and So, K. -F. (1985). Regeneration, re-routing, and redistribution of axons after early lesions: changes with age, and functional impact. In *Recent achievements in restorative neurology 1: Upper motor neuron functions and disfunctions* (eds. Eccles, Dimitrijevic) pp. 291–310. Publishers S. Karger, Basel, Switzerland.

Sidman, R. L., Angevine, J. B., and Taber-Pierce, E. (1971). *Atlas of the mouse brain and spinal cord.* Harvard University Press, Harvard, MA.

Silver, J. (1984). Studies on the factors that govern directionality of axonal growth in the embryonic optic nerve and at the chiasm of mice. *J, Comp. Neurol.* **223**, pp. 238–51.

Silver, J. and Ogawa, M. Y. (1983). Postnatally induced formation of the corpus collusum in acallosal mice on glial-coated cellulose bridges. *Science* **220**, pp. 1067–9.

Silver J. and Robb, R. M. (1979). Studies on the development of the eye cup and optic nerve in normal mice and in mutants with congenital optic nerve aplasia. *Dev. Biol.* **68**, pp. 175–90.

Silver, J. and Rutishauser, U. (1984). Guidance of optic axons in vivo by a preformed adhesive pathway on neuroepithelial endfeet. *Dev. Biol.* **106**, pp. 485–99.

Silver, J., Poston, M., and Rutishauser, U. (1987). Axon pathway boundaries in the developing brain. I. Cellular and molecular determinants that separate the optic and olfactory projections. *J. Neurosci.* **7**, pp. 2264–72.

Silver, J., Lorenz, S. E., Wahlsten, S., and Coughlin, J. (1982). Axonal guidance during development of the great cerebral commissures: descriptive and experimental studies, in vivo, on the role of preformed glial pathways. *J. Comp. Neurol.* **210**, pp. 10–29.

Silver, J., Smith, G. M., Miller, R. H., and Levitt, P. R. (1985). The immature astrocyte: its role during normal CNS axon tract development and its ability to reduce scar formation when transplanted into the brains of adults. *Neurosci. Abstr.* **11,** p. 334.

Smith, G. M., Miller, R. H., and Silver, J. (1985). Changes in glial reactivity to implantation of nitrocellulose bridges into acallosal animals at various ages and the effect on regenerating callosal axons. *Neurosci. Abstr.* **11,** p. 255

Smith, G. M., Miller, R. H., and Silver, J. (1986). The changing role of forebrain astrocytes during development, regenerative failure, and induced regeneration upon transplantation. *J. Comp. Neurol.* **251,** pp. 23–43.

So, K. -F. (1979). Development of abnormal recrossing retinotectal projections after superior colliculus lesions in newborn Syrian hamsters. *J. Comp. Neurol.* **186,** pp. 241–58.

Sperry, R. W. (1944). Optic nerve regeneration with return of vision in anurans. *J. Neurophysiol.* **7,** pp. 57–9.

Sperry, R. W. (1963). Chemoaffinity in the orderly growth of nerve fiber patterns and connections. *Proc. Natl. Acad. Sci. USA* **30,** pp. 703–10.

Thiery, J. -P., Duband, J. -L., Rutishauser, U., and Edelman, G. M. (1982). Cell adhesion molecules in early chick embryogenesis. *Proc. Natl. Acad. Sci. USA* **79,** pp. 6737–41.

Tucker, G. C., Aoyama, H., Lipinski, M., Tursz, T., and Thiery, J. -P. (1984). Identical reactivity of monoclonal antibodies HNK-1 and NC-1: conservation in vertebrates on cells derived from neural primordium and on some leukocytes. *Cell Differ.* **14,** pp. 223–30.

Weinberg, E. (1928). The mesencephalic root of the fifth nerve: a comparative anatomical study. *J. Comp. Neurol.* **46,** pp. 249–405.

Weiss, P. A. (1955). Nervous system (neurogenesis). In *Analysis of development* (eds. B. H. Willier, P. Weiss and V. Hamburger), pp. 346–401. W. B. Saunders, Philadelphia. PA.

Weston, J. A. (1970). The migration and differentiation of neural crest cells. *Ad. Morphogen.* **8,** pp. 41–114.

Yntema, C. L. (1943). Deficient efferent innervation of the extremities following removal of neural crest in Amblystoma. *J. Exp. Zoology.* **94,** pp. 319–49.

PART IV

Sharpening the pattern

Introduction

A unique feature of the nervous system is that the details of the connections made between different structures are of vital importance to the organism. If the specificity of nerve connections were to be dictated entirely by the genome, axons should never make wrong connections. However, it is thought that at least some axons occasionally do make mistakes. These mistakes might be rectified in a number of different ways. One way is to remove the offending neurons by cell death. Another is the selective withdrawal of specific branches. A third, which may be more common during earlier development while the nervous system is more plastic, is the stabilization of some connections at the expense of others.

How does the embryo identify the neurons that make incorrect connections and discriminate between correctly and incorrectly connected axons and dendrites? One mechanism might depend upon the activity of the neuron and of the target organ. To use an extreme example, neurons that fail to connect to any target could die, perhaps as a result of failure of non-innervated targets to secrete some trophic factor necessary for the survival of the innervating neuron. Neurons that make inappropriate connections might also die, although it is more difficult to envisage how the inappropriate connections might be identified. There may be very sophisticated mechanisms to rank synapses according to the degree of correctness in relation to their neighbours or other factors. These synapses could then be either eliminated or stabilized following a more or less precise hierarchy of connective appropriateness. If this is true, there must be mechanisms able to *quantify* the correctness of individual synaptic connections. It is not yet known whether such mechanisms exist.

This section examines these mechanisms, and raises the question of how the correct connections are favoured over those less suitable. The idea of a hierarchy of potential connections is linked closely to the concept of *competition*, a theme that recurs throughout this section: during development, neuronal processes may compete for synaptic connections to the target.

16

Loss of axonal projections in the development of the mammalian brain

GIORGIO M. INNOCENTI

'In the early observations on the outgrowth and termination of nerve fibers it appeared that different fiber types must be guided to their respective end organs and other connection sites by selective chemical or electrical forces. . .' 'These selectivity concepts later came under attack. . .' 'At the height of this antiselectivity movement I was led'. . . 'to postulate again in 1939 a form of chemical selectivity in nerve growth even more extreme in some respects than in the earlier proposals.'. . . 'It is apparent from the results that not only the synaptic terminals, but also in these fishes the route by which the growing optic fibers reach those terminals, is selectively determined, presumably on the basis of similar or identical chemoaffinity factors' (Sperry 1963, pp. 703 and 706).

The quotations above illustrate an interesting ambiguity in what remains the leading hypothesis on the mechanisms responsible for the formation of neural connections. The process whereby in development a neuron comes to establish permanent contacts with its target can be broken down into at least the following steps: axonal growth, target recognition, synaptogenesis, synaptic maintenance or stabilization. It is, however, unclear whether, at each of these steps, chemical affinity and in particular affinity for the same factor determines what an axon will do and, therefore, the adult pattern of connections. In recent years, though, attention has been paid to systems in which the topography established by axonal growth, although selective in some respects, is very dissimilar from the adult one. The latter emerges from neuronal death, elimination of long axons, or restriction of terminal arbors. These phenomena are part of a broader class of development events often collectively referred to as developmental exuberance or regressive developmental events. Developmental exuberance includes also the overproduction and elimination of neurons, dendrites, spines, and synapses and the transitory expression of chemical properties. Elimination of syllables in song-learning birds (Marler and Peters 1982) and even certain brain malformations may belong to this group of phenomena. Here we will focus mainly on the overproduction and elimination of long axonal pathways, although some of the considerations in the last section may apply more widely.

it appears probable that a general signal, possibly a hormone, may simultaneously induce the elimination of the transitory axons, possibly by triggering similar events in all layers and areas of cortex and perhaps in even larger regions of the nervous system. In view of the relationship that may exist, as speculated above, between synaptogenesis and axon elimination, it is interesting that at least in the monkey cortex (data are not available for the cat) synaptogenesis is also synchronous in all layers and in several areas, possibly through the whole neocortex (Rakic, Bourgeois, Eckenhoff, Zecevic, and Goldman-Rakic 1986).

HOW?

A major difference between the elimination of transitory cortical and retinal projections is that the latter is due to neuronal death whereas the former occurs through axon elimination generally without the death of the parent neuron. Neuronal death seems to occur in the developing neocortex (Heumann, Leuba, and Rabinowicz 1978; Finlay and Slattery 1983; Price and Blakemore 1985a), although the criteria on which it is claimed have usually been, for difficulties intrinsic to this structure, less stringent than those applied elsewhere in the brain. Thus neuronal death may play a role in the refinement of cortical connections, but this role turns out to be difficult to document with certainty. On the contrary, cortical neurons labelled retrogradely with suitably long lasting tracers via a transitory projection remain visible long after this projection has been eliminated (Innocenti 1981a; O'Leary, Stanfield, and Cowan 1981; Ivy and Killackey 1982; Stanfield *et al.* 1982; Innocenti and Clarke 1984a; Tolbert and Panneton 1984). Those neurons must therefore have established a projection to another structure. Indeed, in the rat, at least some of the S1 neurons which give rise to transitory callosal projections can later be found to project to ipsilateral motor cortex (Ivy and Killackey 1982). Similarly, at least some of the visual cortex neurons which send transitory projections to the spinal cord later project to the pons or superior colliculus but not to the contralateral hemisphere (O'Leary and Stanfield 1985). In the kitten, cortical neurons projecting to the cerebellum were later found to project to the brain stem or spinal cord (Tolbert and Panneton 1984).

Figure 16.5. illustrates a series of experiments, the aims of which were to determine: (i) the final target of area-17 neurons, which transitorily project through the corpus callosum; (ii) whether a relationship exists between a neuron's initial and final choice of a target; and (iii) whether the transitory projections are collaterals of initially branched axons (i.e. whether the formation of the adult connections consists of selective elimination of collaterals) (Innocenti, Clarke, and Kraftsik 1986).

The results of these experiments indicate strong selectivity in the choice of the final target (Fig. 16.6). Area-17 neurons which form transitory callosal projections to contralateral areas 17/18 can be relabelled, when this projection has been eliminated, from ipsilateral area 18 but only exceptionally from other visual areas. These results might have suggested that neurons (at least the subclass which form callosal connections) are guided by selective affinity to an area, irrespective of which side of the brain it is in. This is not the case, however, since the neurons which form transitory callosal projections from area 17 to contralateral area PMLS (an 'association' visual area; Palmer, Rosenquist, and Tusa 1978) later project to ipsilateral area 18 but not to PMLS.

At the roots of the early and late target selection there seems to be a factor related to the position of neurons in the cortex. Indeed we found that each of the corticocortical projections from area 17 originates from a neuronal population with slightly different and characteristic radial distribution. The second choice of transitory callosal neurons seems to be the most appropriate one given their radial location, which is very similar to that of the neurons projecting to ipsilateral area 18 (Fig. 16.7). The transitory callosal neurons are but a small fraction of this projection. The fact that a neuron's position in the cortex reflects where it will establish connections may suggest that the cortex uses positional information in its development (for this concept, see Wolpert 1969). More probably, however, the projection of a neuron is largely determined by its birth-date, which, in the cortex, is reflected in radial position. Indeed, in the reeler mouse neurons projecting to the corpus callosum have abnormal radial locations but probably normal birth-dates (Caviness 1977).

As to the question illustrated in Fig. 16.5., some area-17 neurons can be double-labelled by two different tracers, one injected in contralateral areas 17 and 18 and one in ipsilateral area 18 at birth (Fig. 16.6). Some of these neurons can then be triple-labelled by another tracer injected in the ipsilateral area 18 after the transitory callosal axon was eliminated. Thus the evidence from these and other experiments (Ivy and Killackey 1982) tends to the hypothesis that neurons with transitory projections may have from the beginning an axon collateral to their permanent target, although other interpretations are also possible (for discussion, see Innocenti *et al.* 1986).

In view of the importance that transitory projections may have as a substrate for development a brain plasticity with adaptive or maladaptive consequences it is crucial to understand what signals some axons to be eliminated, and others to be stabilized.

The key events are likely to occur at the terminal site. Here, anterograde transport studies of callosal development (see references in Innocenti 1986) suggest the following sequence of events. Axons stop their growth, for some time once they have reached the border between white and grey matter. Then they grow into the cortex, but selectively at the restricted locations where they will also terminate in the adult. At birth, in kittens, callosal axons have already grown selectively into the 17/18 border. In addition, there is a more diffusely distributed axonal population which does not grow in the cortex to any great extent (Innocenti 1981a; Innocenti and Clarke 1984b; Fig. 16.8). At least some transitory association axons do grow into the cortex (Dehay *et al.* 1984; Clarke and Innocenti 1986) while others terminate with growth cones in the

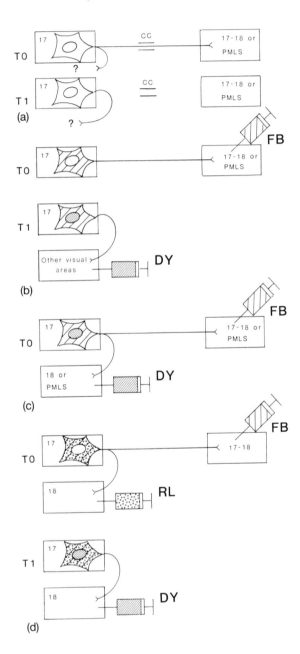

white matter (Clarke and Innocenti 1986). Most of the callosal axons which grow into the cortex are probably maintained, most of those which do not are eliminated (Innocenti and Clarke 1984*b*). Having access to the cortex, though, does not ensure maintenance, since virtually all the auditory-to-visual axons and probably some of the callosal axons which did enter the cortex (Innocenti *et al.* 1985) are eliminated.

The findings summarized above suggest that, unlike what would have been predicted from a literal interpretation of the chemo-affinity theory, the mechanisms responsible for the growth of an axon towards a target are different from those leading to its permanent colonization of the target. What could the latter factors be? The transitory projections do not seem to be eliminated because they are intrinsically 'wrong'. Several conditions are known which lead to stabilization of normally transitory projections (for references see Innocenti 1981*b*, 1986). In particular, transitory callosal connections from area 17 in the cat can be stabilized by genetic abnormalities as well as by manipulation of visual experience during a critical period. In rodents, abnormal stabilization of visual callosal connections results from early lesions to the visual pathways.

Another question concerns the mechanism of disappearence of transitory axons. To this date there is no compelling evidence that the axons to be eliminated undergo important ultrastructural modifications. Either these modifications are subtle, or the axons are eliminated very quickly. One possibility is that transitory axons are engulfed by transitory phagocytes (*gitter cells*) which appear in the developing white matter (Innocenti, Clarke, and Koppel 1984; Innocenti, Koppel, and Clarke 1984; Fig. 16.9).

Fig. 16.5. Questions, methods, and results of a study aimed at determining where area-17 neurons with transitory callosal projection establish their final projection. (a) At time T0 (first post-natal week) some area-17 neurons project temporarily to contralateral areas 17 and 18; other area-17 neurons project temporarily to contralateral PMLS. At time T1 (second post-natal month) these neurons have eliminated their callosal axon. Where do they project? And did they already have a collateral to their final target at T0? (b) fast blue (FB) was injected into areas 17–18 or PMLS at T0; this tracer provides long-lasting labelling of neuronal cytoplasm. At T1, diamidino yellow (DY) was injected in various visual areas contralateral to the FB injection; some neurons that previously projected through the corpus callosum are relabelled, but rather selectively from area 18. (c) FB is injected as in (b); DY is simultaneously injected at T0 in either area 18 or PMLS, double-labelling some transitorily callosal neurons; unlike in (b) and (d), the animal is killed after a few days' survival. (d) At T0, FB is injected as in (b) and (c), and rhodamine-labelled latex beads (RL) are injected in area 18. At T1, DY is re-injected in area 18. The results are consistent with the hypothesis that some of the transitory callosal neurons in area 17 have an axon collateral to ipsilateral area 18 and maintain it after eliminating their transitory callosal axon. [Reproduced from Innocenti *et al.* (1986) by kind permission of the Society for Neuroscience, Bethesda, MD.]

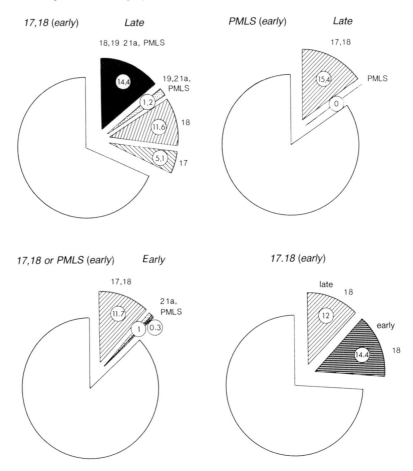

Fig. 16.6. Diagrams showing which proportions of area-17 neurons with transitory callosal axons (labelled by early FB injections in the contralateral hemisphere) could be relabelled by injections of a second tracer (DY or RL) in different areas of the same hemisphere. Which per cent of the FB-labelled population is also labelled by the second tracer is indicated by size of sectors as well as by the number on each sector. Top left: FB was injected in contralateral areas 17 and 18 during the first post-natal week; DY was injected in the different ipsilateral visual areas (in different animals) during the second post-natal month. Top right: FB was injected in contralateral PMLS during the first week; DY was injected in ipsilateral areas 17–18 or in PMLS (in different animals) during the second month. Bottom left: FB was injected in contralateral areas 17–18 or in PMLS, and DY in ipsilateral areas 17–18 or 21a-PMLS (in different animals) during the first week. Bottom right: FB was injected in contralateral areas 17–18 and RL in ipsilateral area 18 during the first week (sector marked 'early'). In the same animal, DY was re-injected in ipsilateral area 18 during the second month (sector marked 'late'). [Reproduced from Innocenti *et al.* 1986 by kind permission of the Society for Neuroscience, Bethesda, MD.]

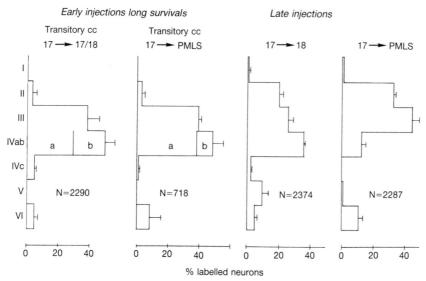

Fig. 16.7. Histograms showing radial distributions of four sets of efferent neurons in area 17, each defined as projecting to a different target. In each histogram, columns represent the fraction of the total population (number below each histogram); in two of the histograms, the fractions of neurons in the upper and lower half of layer IVab are represented separately. The histograms are derived from counts pooled from different animals; bars above each column are standard deviations. The two histograms on the left represent the distributions of area-17 neurons labelled by FB injected in contralateral areas 17–18 during the first post-natal week; the animals were killed during the second post-natal month. The two histograms on the right represent the distributions of area-17 neurons projecting to ipsilateral area 18 or PMLS. Notice that neurons projecting transitorily through the corpus callosum (transitory cc) are most common in layers IVab and III, the same as the neurons projecting to ipsilateral area 18. The neurons projecting to ipsilateral PMLS are located more superficially, with maxima in layers III and II. [Reproduced from Innocenti *et al.* (1986) by kind permission of the Society for Neuroscience, Bethesda, MD.]

WHY?

This question can be asked in connection with all the instances in which, during development, transitory structures are generated which do not assume obvious functional roles. The question has disturbing teleological undertones. It is obviously possible to interpret exuberance as errors and regressive phenomena as error-eliminating devices (for an application of this concept to neuronal death in other structures, see Clarke 1981; Cowan, Fawcett, O'Leary, and Stanfield 1984). This view was already supported by Cajal (1929), but in the case of neocortical development it is unsatisfactory, for at least two reasons. First, it fails to explain why such enormous errors are made

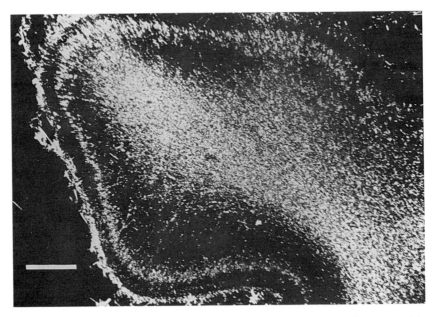

Fig. 16.8. Polarized light photomicrograph showing the distribution of anterogradely labelled callosal axons in the lateral gyrus of a kitten injected with WGA-HRP in the homotopic contralateral region on day 1 and sacrificed on day 2. Callosal axons have a widespread distribution in the white matter but they enter the cortex selectively at the 17/18 border (top left) and in a small part of area 19 (top right). The continuous band of neuronal labelling corresponds to layer 3. Scale bar: 500 μm. [Reproduced from Innocenti (1986) by kind permission of Plenum Press, New York.]

in the development of neo-cortex requiring elimination of more than 50 per cent of the axons involved in a projection. Second, an error is usually defined with respect to a goal and a strategy to reach this goal. Both are difficult to define rigorously. For example, what we call 'errors' varies if we assume that the goal of the axonal growth preceding axon elimination is the formation of the adult network or, else, of a juvenile network (see Innocenti and Clarke, 1984*b*). The latter may be as different from the former as an adult holometabolous insect from its larva. An interpretation devoid of value judgment is that cortical exuberance is the outcome of developmental processes crucial for the formation of connections but operating at a time when the information necessary to specify the detailed organization of connections is not yet available or useable in the system concerned. This notion is compatible with a hierarchical model of development (genes at the top, phenotype at the bottom; for example, see Alberch 1982), in which part of the information relevant for the establishment of a pattern comes from the environment and/or from interactions between the phenotypic expression of different sets of genes, late in ontogenesis.

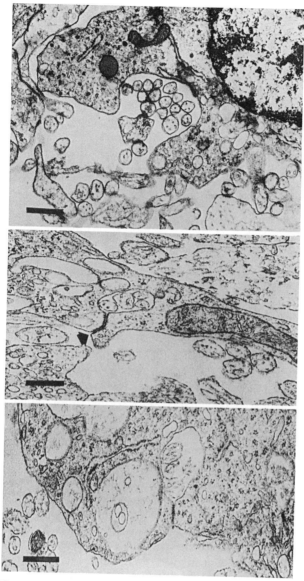

Fig. 16.9. Ultrastructural evidence suggesting involvement of 'gitter cells' in the phagocytosis of axons. Kitten perfused on day 12.5. Top: 'gitter cell' cytoplasm partially surrounds a group of axons. Distribution of chromatin, dumb-bell-shaped mitochondria, and vacuoles are characteristic of the 'gitter cell'. Middle: at what may be a later stage, a 'gitter cell' process has completely surrounded a group of axons, and the apposing surface membranes (arrow-head) may be fusing prior to detachment of the vacuole. Bottom: the large vacuole contains an element which could be an axon and floccular material; on the right of this vacuole there is another nearly completely formed vacuole at a stage resembling that described above. Scale bars: 0·5 μm. [Reproduced from Innocenti *et al.* (1984*b*) by kind permission of Alan R. Liss, Inc., New York.]

The development by exuberance provides an enormous flexibility for matching the phenotypic expressions of the various sets of genes at the level at which they come to interact. For example, in the case of neo-cortex, the genes responsible for the order in the afferent pathways through the thalamus are probably at least partially different from those dictating the cell composition of neo-cortex, and the development of corticocortical connections may depend on still other sets of genes. These various sets may be independently and differentially regulated by extrinsic and intrinsic factors, although their expression is probably co-ordinated to some extent. In the adult, corticocortical connections connect neurons with appropriate functional properties which, however, are largely determined by the pattern of thalamocortical connections. For example, neurons with the same orientation specificity and similar receptive field location are connected through the corpus callosum (Berlucchi and Rizzolatti 1968); presumably the matching of neurons with such functional properties is made possible or facilitated by developmental exuberance. The probable role of neuronal death in matching pre- and post-synaptic neuronal populations of different size was already discussed by Cowan (1973), Katz and Lasek (1978), and Rager (1978). Changeux and Danchin (1976) have emphasized how exuberance and selective, activity-dependent stabilization afford economy of early genetic information.

The above interpretations, though, sound like a *post hoc* justification of exuberance. Could the matching of pre- and post-synaptic elements not have been achieved with less waste? Are there systems where exuberance plays no role in development? Unfortunately, at least one of the systems which was previously considered a clear example of a precise and selective axon–target encounter by selective growth has now been shown to develop (and/or regenerate) largely, through exuberance [e.g. see this volume: Wetts, O'Rourke, and Fraser (Chapter 3); Stuermer (Chapter 11); Schmidt (Chapter 19)].

The issue may be further clarified by a phylogenetic perspective. Developmental strategies may not have remained invariant in evolution (for discussion, see Sander 1983). Rather, they may have undergone changes and selection. While this notion should caution against imprudent generalization of developmental mechanisms across systems and species, it also allows guesses on why development by exuberance should have become such a general phenomenon. What could have been the criteria for the selection of a developmental strategy? Presumably certain strategies gave rise to individuals that were better adapted for survival and reproduction. It is appealing to think that the cause for the success of developmental exuberance in phylogenesis may be the flexibility it allows in the late stages of neural development. Of the two types of developmental exuberance acting at the level of pathway formation, neuronal death and axon elimination, the latter is more economical, and provides even more flexibility than neuronal death. Indeed, neurons, rather than being eliminated when they do not reach an adequate target, are given either multiple choices or the possibility of modifying their choice late.

Interestingly, axonal elimination plays an important role in the development of what might be hierarchically the highest structure in the mammalian brain; a well-wired neocortex is probably useful for competitive survival and reproduction.

Although it may have been selected for its ontogenetic efficacy, a developmental strategy can have evolutionary consequences, since it may allow only certain genetic mutations to become phenotypically expressed (for example, see Alberch 1982; Maderson 1982; Kauffman 1983). From this perspective it appears that developmental exuberance may have favoured phylogenetic changes and indeed is compatible with the evolutionary invasion of new territories by a projection, as well as with segregation of projections into separate territories (Katz, Lasek, and Silver 1983; Ebbesson 1984). In the development of neo-cortex, an example of the first may have been the invasion of the lumbar and spinal cord levels and of the motorneurons by corticospinal projections (for references, see Kuypers 1981). An example of the second may be the stabilization of commissural connections from area 17 in marsupials (Moreland, Granger, Masterton, and Glendenning 1985) and rodents but not in cats or monkeys, or of projections from auditory cortex to visual areas in rodents (Miller and Vogdt 1984). If this view is correct the developmental mechanisms described above may have played a major role in the enormous variation of neo-cortical evolution across the various mammalian radiations.

ACKNOWLEDGEMENTS

I wish to thank my colleagues P. Clarke and S. Catsicas for their comments on this paper, and C. Vaclavik for typing the manuscript. The work was supported by the Swiss National Science Foundation, grant no. 3.359–0.86.

REFERENCES

Alberch, P. (1982). Developmental constraints in evolutionary processes. In *Evolution and development* (ed. J. T. Bonner), *Dahlem Konferenzen*, pp. 313–32. Springer-Verlag, Berlin.

Berlucchi, G. and Rizzolatti, G. (1968). Binocularly driven neurons in visual cortex of split-chiasm cats. *Science* **159**, pp. 308–10.

Bunt, S. M. and Lund, R. D. (1981). Development of a transient retinoretinal pathway in hooded and albino rats. *Brain Res.* **211**, pp. 399–404.

Cajal, S. R. y (1929). *Etudes sur la neurogenèse de quelques vertébrés*. Tipografía Artística, Madrid.

Caviness, V. S. (1977). *Reeler* mutant mouse: a genetic experiment in developing mammalian cortex. In *Approaches to the cell biology of neurons* (eds. W. M. Cowan and J. A. Ferrendelli), pp. 27–46. Society for Neuroscience, Bethesda, MD.

Changeux, J. -P. and Danchin, A. (1976). Selective stabilisation of developing synapses as a mechanism for the specification of neuronal networks. *Nature* **264**, pp. 705–12.

Chow, K. L., Baumbach, H. D., and Lawson, R. (1981). Callosal projections of the striate cortex in the neonatal rabbit. *Exp. Brain Res.* **42**, pp. 122–6.

Clarke, P. G. H. (1981). Chance, repetition, and error in the development of normal nervous systems. *Perspect. Biol. Med.* **25**, pp. 2–19.

Clarke, P. G. H. (1985). Neuronal death in the development of the vertebrate nervous system. *Trends Neurosci.* **8**, pp. 345–9.

Clarke, S. and Innocenti, G. M. (1986). Organization of immature intrahemispheric connections. *J. Comp. Neurol.* **251**, pp. 1–22.

Cowan, W. M. (1973). Neuronal death as a regulative mechanism in the control of cell number in the nervous system. In *Development and aging in the nervous system* (ed. M. Rockstein), pp. 19–41. Academic Press, New York.

Cowan, W. M., Fawcett, J. W., O'Leary, D. D. M. and Stanfield, B. B. (1984). Regressive events in neurogenesis. *Science* **225**, pp1258–65.

Crandall, J. E., Whitcomb, J. M., and Caviness, V. S., Jr. (1985). Development of the spinal-medullary projection from the mouse barrel field. *J. Comp. Neurol.* **239**, pp. 205–15.

D'Amato, C. J. and Hicks, S. P. (1978). Normal development and post-traumatic plasticity of corticospinal neurons in rats. *Exp. Neurol.* **60**, pp. 557–69.

Dehay, C., Bullier, J., and Kennedy, H. (1984). Transient projections from the fronto-parietal and temporal cortex to areas 17, 18 and 19 in the kitten. *Exp. Brain Res.* **57**, pp. 208–12.

Distel, H. and Holländer, H. (1980). Autoradiographic tracing of developing subcortical projections of the occipital region in fetal rabbits. *J. Comp. Neurol.* **192**, pp. 505–18.

Ebbesson, S. O. (1984). Evolution and ontogeny of neural circuits. *Behav. Brain Sci.* **7**, pp. 321–66.

Feng, J. Z. and Brugge, J. F. (1983). Postnatal development of auditory callosal connections in the kitten. *J. Comp. Neurol.* **214**, pp. 416–26.

Finlay, B. L. and Slattery, M. (1983). Local differences in the amount of early cell death in neocortex predict adult local specializations. *Science* **219**, pp. 1349–51.

Frost, D. O. (1984). Axonal growth and target selection during development: regional projections to the ventrobasal complex and other 'nonvisual' structures in neonatal syrian hamsters. *J. Comp. Neurol.* **230**, pp. 576–92.

Frost, D. O., So, K. -F., and Schneider, G. E. (1979). Postnatal development of retinal projections in syrian hamsters: a study using autoradiographic and anterograde degeneration techniques. *Neuroscience* **4**, pp. 1649–77.

Heumann, D., Leuba, G., and Rabinowicz, T. (1978). Postnatal development of the mouse cerebral neocortex. IV. Evolution of the total cortical volume, of the population of neurons and glial cells. *J. Hirnforsch.* **19**, pp. 385–93.

Hubel, D. H., Wiesel, T. N., and LeVay, S. (1977). Plasticity of ocular dominance columns in monkey striate cortex. *Phil. Trans. R. Soc. Lond. B.* **278**, pp. 377–409.

Innocenti, G. M. (1981*a*). Growth and reshaping of axons in the establishment of visual callosal connections. *Science* **212**, pp. 824–7.

Innocenti, G. M. (1981*b*). Transitory structures as substrate for developmental plasticity of the brain. In *Developments in neuroscience, vol. 13* (eds. M. W. Van Hof and G. Mohn), pp. 305–33. Elsevier/North-Holland Biomedical Press, Amsterdam.

Innocenti, G. M. (1986). General organization of callosal connections in the cerebral cortex. In *Cerebral cortex, vol. 5* (eds. E. G. Jones and A. Peters), pp. 291–353 Plenum Press, New York.

Innocenti, G. M. and Caminiti, R. (1980). Postnatal shaping of callosal connections from sensory areas. *Exp. Brain Res.* **38**, pp. 381–94.

Innocenti, G. M. and Clarke, S. (1984*a*). Bilateral transitory projection to visual areas from auditory cortex in kittens. *Dev. Brain Res.* **14**, pp. 143–8.

Innocenti, G. M. and Clarke, S. (1984*b*). The organization of immature callosal connections. *J. Comp. Neurol.* **230**, pp. 287–309.

Innocenti, G. M., Clarke, S., and Koppel, H. (1984). Transitory macrophages in the white matter of the developing visual cortex. II. Development, relations with axonal pathways. *Dev. Brain Res.* **11**, pp. 55–66.

Innocenti, G. M., Clarke, S., and Kraftsik, R. (1986). Interchange of callosal and association projections in the developing visual cortex. *J. Neurosci.* **6**, pp. 1384–409.

Innocenti, G. M., Fiore, L., and Caminiti, R. (1977). Exuberant projection into the corpus callosum from the visual cortex of newborn cats. *Neurosci. Lett.* **4**, pp. 237–42.

Innocenti, G. M., Frost, D. O., and Illes, J. (1985). Maturation of visual callosal connections in visually deprived kittens: a challenging critical period. *J. Neurosci.* **5**, pp. 255–67.

Innocenti, G. M., Koppel, H., and Clarke, S. (1984). Transitory macrophages in the white matter of the developing visual cortex. I. Light and electron microscopic characteristics and distribution. *Dev. Brain Res.* **11**, pp. 39–53.

Insausti, R., Blakemore, C., and Cowan, W. M. (1985). Postnatal development of the ipsilateral retinocollicular projection and the effects of unilateral enucleation in the golden hamster. *J. Comp. Neurol.* **234**, pp. 393–409.

Ivy, G. O. and Killackey, H. P. (1981). The ontogeny of the distribution of callosal projection neurons in the rat parietal cortex. *J. Comp. Neurol.* **195**, pp. 367–89.

Ivy, G. O. and Killackey, H. P. (1982). Ontogenetic changes in the projections of neocortical neurons. *J. Neurosci.* **2**, pp. 735–43.

Kato, N., Kawaguchi, S., and Miyata, H. (1984). Geniculocortical projection to layer I of area 17 in kittens: orthograde and retrograde HRP studies. *J. Comp. Neurol.* **225**, pp. 441–7.

Katz, M. J. and Lasek, R. J. (1978). Evolution of the nervous system: role of ontogenetic mechanisms in the evolution of matching populations. *Proc. Natl. Acad. Sci. USA* **75**, pp. 1349–52.

Katz, M. J., Lasek, R. J., and Silver, J. (1983). Ontophyletics of the nervous system: development of the corpus callosum and evolution of axon tracts. *Proc. Natl. Acad. Sci. USA* **80**, pp. 5936–40.

Kauffman, S. A. (1983). Developmental constraints: internal factors in evolution. In *Development and evolution* (eds. B. C. Goodwin, N. Holder, and C. C. Wylie), pp. 196–225. Cambridge University Press, Cambridge.

Killackey, H. P. and Chalupa, L. M. (1986). Ontogenetic change in the distribution of callosal projection neurons in the postcentral gyrus of the fetal rhesus monkey. *J. Comp. Neurol.* **244**, pp. 331–48.

Koppel, H. and Innocenti, G. M. (1983). Is there a genuine exuberancy of callosal projections in development? A quantitative electron microscopic study in the cat. *Neurosci. Lett.* **41**, pp. 33–40.

Kuypers, H. G. J. M. (1981). Anatomy of the descending pathways. In *Handbook of physiology—the nervous system II* (eds. J. Brookhart and V. Mountcastle), pp. 597–666. American Physiological Society, Bethesda, MD.

La Mantia, A. -S. and Rakic, P. (1984). The number, size, myelination, and regional variation of axons in the corpus callosum and anterior commissure of the developing rhesus monkey. *Neurosci. Abstr.* **10**, p. 1081.

La Mantia, A. -S. and Rakic, P. (1985). Organization and development of the hippocampal commissure in primates: overproduction and elimination of commissural axons in infant rhesus monkeys. *Soc. Neurosi. Abstr.* **11**, p. 494.

Land, P. W. and Lund, R. D. (1979). Development of the rat's uncrossed retinotectal pathway and its relation to plasticity studies. *Science* **205**, pp. 698–700.

LeVay, S. and Stryker, M. P. (1979). The development of ocular dominance columns in the cat. In *Aspects of developmental neurobiology, vol. VI* (ed. J. A. Ferendelli), pp. 83–98. Society for Neuroscience, Bethesda, MD.

LeVay, S., Stryker, M. P., and Shatz, C. J. (1978). Ocular dominance columns and their development in layer IV of the cat's visual cortex: a quantitative study. *J. Comp. Neurol.* **179**, pp. 223–44.

Maderson, P. F. A. (1982). The role of development in macroevolutionary change. Group report. In *Evolution and development* (ed. J. T. Bonner), pp. 279–312. Springer-Verlag, Berlin.

Marler, P. and Peters, S. (1982). Developmental overproduction and selective attrition: new processes in the epigenesis of birdsong. *Dev. Psychobiol.* **15**, pp. 369–78.

McLoon, S. C. and Lund, R. D. (1982). Transient retinofugal pathways in the developing chick. *Exp. Brain Res.* **45**, pp. 277–84.

Mihailoff, G. A. and Bourell, K. W. (1986). Synapse formation and other ultrastructural features of postnatal development in the basilar pontine nuclei of the rat. *Dev. Brain Res.* **28**, pp. 195–212.

Mihailoff, G. A., Adams, C. E., and Woodward, D. J. (1984). An autoradiographic study of the postnatal development of sensorimotor and visual components of the corticopontine system. *J. Comp. Neurol.* **222**, pp. 116–27.

Miller, M. W. and Vogt, B. A. (1984). Direct connections of rat visual cortex with sensory, motor, and association cortices. *J. Comp. Neurol.* **226**, pp. 184–202.

Moreland Granger, E., Masterton, R. B., and Glendenning, K. K. (1985). Origin of interhemispheric fibers in acallosal opossum (with a comparison to callosal origins in rat). *J. Comp. Neurol.* **241**, pp. 82–98.

O'Leary, D. D. M. and Stanfield, B. B. (1985). Occipital cortical neurons with transient pyramidal tract axons extend and maintain collaterals to subcortical but not intracortical targets. *Brain Res.* **336**, pp. 326–33.

O'Leary, D. D. M. and Stanfield, B. B. (1986). A transient pyramidal tract projection from the visual cortex in the hamster and its removal by selective collateral elimination. *Dev. Brain Res.* **27**, pp. 87–99.

O'Leary, D. D. M., Stanfield, B. B., and Cowan, W. M. (1981). Evidence that the early postnatal restriction of the cells of origin of the callosal projection is due to the elimination of axonal collaterals rather than to the death of neurons. *Dev. Brain Res.* **1**, pp. 607–17.

Palmer, L. A., Rosenquist, A. C., and Tusa, R. J. (1978). The retinotopic organization of lateral suprasylvian visual areas in the cat. *J. Comp. Neurol.* **177**, pp. 237–56.

Price, D. J. and Blakemore, C. (1985*a*). Regressive events in the postnatal development of association projections in the visual cortex. *Nature* **316,** pp. 721–4.

Price, D. J. and Blakemore, C. (1985*b*). The postnatal development of the association projection from visual cortical area 17 to area 18 in the cat. *J. Neurosci.* **5,** pp. 2443–52.

Rager, G. (1978). Systems-matching by degeneration. II. Interpretation of the generation and degeneration of retinal ganglion cells in the chicken by a mathematical model. *Exp. Brain Res.* **33,** pp. 79–90.

Rakic, P. (1976). Prenatal genesis of connections subserving ocular dominance in the rhesus monkey. *Nature* **261,** pp. 467–71.

Rakic, P. (1977). Prenatal development of the visual system in rhesus monkey. *Phil. Trans. R. Soc. Lond. B.* **278,** pp. 245–60.

Rakic, P., Bourgeois, J. -P., Eckenhoff, M. F., Zecevic, N., and Goldman-Rakic, P. S. (1986). Concurrent overproduction of synapses in diverse regions of the primate cerebral cortex. *Science* **232,** pp. 232–5.

Reh, T. and Kalil, K. (1982). Development of the pyramidal tract in the hamster. II. An electron microscopic study. *J. Comp. Neurol.* **205,** pp. 77–88.

Sander, K. (1983). The evolution of patterning mechanisms: gleanings from insect embryogenesis and spermatogenesis. In *Development and evolution* (eds. B. C. Goodwin, N. Holder, and C. C. Wylie), pp. 138–59. Cambridge University Press, Cambridge.

Schmidt, J. T. (1987). Activity-dependent sharpening of the retinotopic projection of the tectum of goldfish in regeneration and development. In *The making of the nervous system* (eds. J. G. Parnavelas, C. D. Stern, and R. V. Stirling), pp. 380–94 Oxford University Press, Oxford.

Sperry, R. W. (1963). Chemoaffinity in the orderly growth of nerve fiber patterns and connections. *Proc. Nat. Acad. Sci. USA* **50,** pp. 703–10.

Sretavan, D. and Shatz, C. J. (1984). Prenatal development of individual retinogeniculate axons during the period of segregation. *Nature* **308,** pp. 845–8.

Stanfield, B. B., O'Leary, D. D. M., and Fricks, C. (1982). Selective collateral elimination in early postnatal development restricts cortical distribution of rat pyramidal tract neurones. *Nature* **298,** pp. 371–3.

Stein, B. E., McHaffie, J. G., Harting, J. K., Huerta, M. F., and Hashikawa, T. (1985). Transient tectogeniculate projections in neonatal kittens: an autoradiographic study. *J. Comp. Neurol.* **239,** pp. 402–12.

Stuermer, C. A. O. (1987). Navigation of normal and regeneration axons in the goldfish. In *The making of the nervous system* (eds. J. G. Parnavelas, C. D. Stern, and R. V. Stirling), pp. 204–27 Oxford University Press, Oxford.

Tolbert, D. L. and Panneton, W. M. (1983). Transient cerebrocerebellar projections in kittens: postnatal development and topography. *J. Comp. Neurol.* **221,** pp. 216–28.

Tolbert, D. L. and Panneton, W. M. (1984). The transience of cerebrocerebellar projections is due to selective elimination of axon collaterals and not neuronal death. *Dev. Brain Res.* **16,** pp. 301–6.

Wetts, R., O'Rourke, N. A., and Fraser, S. E. (1987). Vital-dye analyses of neuronal development and connectivity. In *The making of the nervous system* (eds. J. G. Parnavelas, C. D. Stern, and R. V. Stirling), pp. 52–69 Oxford University Press, Oxford.

Wolpert, L. (1969). Positional information and the spatial pattern of cellular differentiation. *J. Theoret. Biol.* **25,** pp. 1–47.

17

Dynamic aspects of synaptic connections at the vertebrate neuromuscular junction

JEFF W. LICHTMAN

Although the nervous system begins to function very early on in development, usually well before birth or hatching, the neural circuitry is far from complete. Neural connections continue to be elaborated, eliminated, and, in certain cases, remodelled, not only during post-natal development but throughout life. This ongoing neural change might reasonably be split into two broad categories, ontogenetic and epigenetic.

Ontogenetic changes in the nervous system continue to occur for a sizeable fraction of an animal's lifetime because of the protracted nature of many developmental events. The most obvious ontogenetic reasons for post-natal changes in neural connections are growth (i.e. change in size), ageing (i.e. change in maturity), and the reaching of late developmental milestones such as puberty. Each of these developmental phenomena lead quite directly to alterations in neural connections.

Epigenetic (extrinsic) influences also modify synaptic connections throughout life. There are several sources of these influences. Ordinary wear and tear on tissues requires renewal of cellular and chemical constituents. In most organ systems, this give rise to normal turnover of cells. The nervous system is a special case because most populations of neurons are post-mitotic. However, even though neurons are not replaced, the constituents of each cell are turning over. Another epigenetic factor that brings about changes in neural connections is the response of the nervous system to injury. Neurons and glia possess a number of compensatory mechanisms that permit functional recovery from damage. The best studied compensatory reaction is the sprouting of undamaged axons and their subsequent formation of new synaptic connections in response to partial denervation of a target. Perhaps the most interesting extrinsic causes for neural change are the adaptive modifications brought about by environmental stimuli. Such changes range from rather simple modification of synapses that stem from changes in levels of neural activity to the still largely unknown synaptic correlates of learning and memory.

TECHNICAL PROBLEMS IN STUDYING NEURAL CHANGE

Despite the variety of reasons for ongoing changes in synaptic connections, very little is known about the underlying mechanisms. Indeed it is conceivable that only a small number of cellular processes could account for the various alterations seen. Even more problematic is that evidence for change itself is hard to come by and most of the evidence that has been obtained is indirect.

Ignorance about long-term change stems from two problems. First, synaptic connections are difficult to study. They are essentially subcellular organelles and, although each neuron may establish hundreds or thousands of them, their behaviour is, to some degree, individualized; that is, not all the synapses established by a neuron are doing the same things. This autonomy is based on the fact that the local environment of each synapse determines its behaviour. Thus, which post-synaptic cell a synapse is in contact with, the presence of other synapses in its vicinity, the activity pattern of the post-synaptic cell, and so on, will all effect the long-term stability of that synapse. The uniqueness of the local millieu for any one synapse prevents simple conclusions being drawn about how synapses generally change over time.

A further problem is that dynamic phenomena such as synaptic change are not easily studied with techniques that give static information. Anatomical evidence for neural change is usually inferential: a series of still images of different elements from different time-points are used to argue what the progression of changes would be like for a single element if it could be viewed over time. Large numbers of samples must be obtained for each time-point before one can have much confidence in the results. But if the sample is not homogeneous to begin with, as may often be the case, the aggregate behaviour may not represent the way any individual element behaves. Furthermore, the outcome is very much dependent upon picking relevant time intervals. Some dynamic events may cause change gradually over years, others over minutes. Another difficulty stems from the necessity to draw inferences about dynamic events from the still pictures themselves. Thus a thin, small axonal branch emanating from an established synapse must be interpreted either as a new sprout growing out or as an old process in the midst of being resorbed. These difficulties in data acquisition and interpretation probably deter a good deal of effort in studying long-term change in the nervous system and call into question the interpretations of work already done.

THE NEUROMUSCULAR JUNCTION AS A PARADIGM

One part of the nervous system where information about dynamic aspects of synaptic connections has been obtained is the vertebrate neuromuscular junction. From almost any standpoint, this synapse is the best understood neural connection. Because of its accessibility and simplicity, the resolution of the questions that can be asked and the answers obtained is unparalleled. A major drawback of the neuromuscular junction, however, is that it remains unclear whether this synapse is 'typical'. In two important respects it is certainly exceptional. First, in contrast to most synapses, the post-synaptic cells are not neurons, but muscle fibres. Second, this synapse is not located in the central nervous system (CNS) but in the periphery. Thus how likely is it that the neural changes underlying CNS phenomena such as learning will be clarified by studies of the neuromuscular junction? Although the answer to that question is not known, it is important to realize that many dynamic phenomena that were first described at the neuromuscular junction were subsequently shown to occur at more 'typical' synapses (e.g. sprouting, synapse elimination, facilitation, etc.). Given the dearth of information on long-term change elsewhere in the nervous system, however, the ability to generalize from the neuromuscular junction remains moot. Until a great deal more is known about dynamic events at more typical synapses, the information gleaned from the neuromuscular junction will have to serve as a paradigm for questions about the dynamic aspects of synaptic connections.

It is my aim to review briefly some of the evidence for the various categories of long-term change in synaptic connections as discerned from studies of the neuromuscular junction. Two points that emerge are: (1) there is much indirect evidence to suggest that neuromuscular junctions are highly dynamic, and (2) new experimental strategies are needed to transform many of these suggestions into facts.

GROWTH-RELATED CHANGES AT THE NEUROMUSCULAR JUNCTION

The vertebrate neuromuscular junction is functional long before it obtains its mature form. Indeed, the first synaptic potentials occur well before any specialized pre- or post-synaptic elements can be discerned (Kelly and Zacks 1969; Atsumi 1971, 1977; Sisto Daneo and Filogamo 1973; Kullberg, Lentz, and Cohen 1977). Over the remaining embryonic period, neuromuscular junctions become increasingly specialized; synaptic terminals become laden with vesicles, basal lamina forms between the nerve and muscle, and the localization of acetylcholine receptors in the muscle fibre membrane under the nerve terminal becomes more obvious. But even with these prenatal changes, the neuromuscular synapse is quite rudimentary at birth. In newborn kittens and rodents the motor terminals, junctional cholinesterase staining, and the underlying acetylcholine receptors are found within small round discs (Nyström 1968a, 1968b; Steinbach 1981; Slater 1982). It is difficult to get good staining of nerve terminals at early stages; thus the 'disc-shaped' nerve terminal is not necessarily a contiguous structure as some have suggested (Nyström 1968b). In mammalian muscle at birth, it is likely that the neuromuscular junction is made up of a number of fine processes that reside in a dense network that is round in shape (Rosenthal and Taraskevich 1977; Slater 1982). Similarly, in the chick at the time of hatching, the end-plate appears round with a ring-shaped network of branches (Atsumi 1971; Jacob and Lentz 1979). Although the neuromuscular junction is simple in shape perinatally, the number of innervating axons at each end-plate site is at a maximum (Bennett and Pettigrew 1974; Dennis, Ziskind-Conhaim, and Harris 1981). Over a several week perinatal period polyneuronal innervation is eliminated from twitch fibres, leaving most end-plates with a single axon (for a review, see Brown, Holland, and Hopkins 1981). The mechanism underlying this dynamic reorganization of synaptic connections is still unclear. It is uncertain whether the axonal branches to be eliminated degenerate (Rosenthal and Taraskevich 1977; Ko 1985) or retract (Kornelliusen and Jansen 1976; Riley 1981). Silver staining at the light microscopical level suggests that perhaps both degeneration and retraction are occurring concurrently (Riley 1977). A detailed electron microscopical examination of several hundred sections through end-plates fixed at the peak time of synapse elimination has revealed, however, no signs of degeneration (Bixby 1981). At the light microscopical level, very fine axons have swollen ends that have been described as 'retraction bulbs' (O'Brien, Ostberg, and Vrbova 1978; Riley 1981; also see Morrison-Graham 1983). These swollen processes have also been described ultrastructurally (Riley 1981). Unfortunately, the techniques used have not permitted unambiguous differentiation of growing and retracting processes. Thus even the 'retraction bulbs' may not be what they seem.

At around the stage that synapse elimination is coming to completion and most of the neuromuscular junctions are becoming singly innervated, a further series of changes in the structure of the neuromuscular junction become manifest. These changes have been referred to as 'perforation' or a breaking up of the round plaque-like terminal (Nyström 1968*b*). What may be happening is that the remaining axon's terminal branches increase in size, permitting better staining, and, as a result, gaps become evident in the end-plate region not occupied by the axon. Each of the expanded branches is interconnected by very thin processes. During this period of reorganization the post-synaptic acetylcholine receptors go through a similar transformation (Steinbach 1981; Slater 1982; also see Courtney and Steinbach 1981). During early postnatal life the receptors form a contiguous plaque under the nerve terminal. In parallel with the nerve terminal itself, the uniform distribution of receptors gradually breaks up, resulting in areas within the confines of the original plaque of high and low receptor density. The exact temporal relation between the elimination of multiple axons and the breaking up of the end-plate remains unclear. Thus, do the areas of low nerve and receptor density occur because axons are being eliminated (Steinbach 1981) or do they occur only once all but one axon remains (Slater 1982)?

Once the end-plate is singly innervated and has completed the process of breaking up, the shape of the nerve terminal for the first time resembles its fully mature form. Even so, end-plate structure continues to change as animals grow. A recent study carefully followed the number and length of axon branches at neuromuscular junctions in three different mouse muscles from twelve days to three years of age with silver stains (Hopkins, Brown, and Keynes 1985). The results of this work show that during the post-natal period after synapse elimination is complete there is a very large amount of nerve terminal growth. This growth gives rise to up to a two-fold increase in nerve terminal length, an increase in the number of branches within an end-plate, and an increase in the number of myelinated branches that enter the end-plate. The end-plate enlargement is largely complete between the ages of 2–3 months in mice. The phase of rapid growth correlates with an increase in fibre diameter which also peaks between the ages of 2–3 months in mice. But it is difficult to decide which is cause and which is effect. Animal weight in mice peaks at a somewhat later stage (4–5 months), perhaps indicating that the relation between somatic and nerve terminal growth may not be direct.

What happens following this growth phase seems to be very variable, depending on which muscle, which animal, and even which strain is being used. Thus the number of branches continues to incresae in the slow soleus muscle of mice (Wernig, Carmody, Anzil, Hansert, Marciniak, and Zucker 1984), but remains constant or even decreases slightly in a fast muscle (Hopkins *et al.* 1985). In another study, branching of nerve terminals at end-plates increased in the fast diaphragm but decreased in two hindlimb muscles (one fast the other slow) (Rosenheimer and Smith 1985). Furthermore, in this latter study in which many time-points were taken, the fluctuations in the measures of end-plate size in any one muscle at three-month intervals were often greater than the average differences between these measures at different muscles. At this point, generalizations are difficult (see the discussion in Rosenheimer and Smith 1985, and see below).

CHANGES IN THE NEUROMUSCULAR JUNCTION OF AGED ANIMALS

There is, of course, no clear deliniation of when development stops and ageing begins. Indeed, many animals (e.g. frogs, rats, carp) continue to grow throughout their lives, thus growing and growing old at the same time. There are, however, a number of studies that make the case for senile changes in neuromuscular junctions, but it is often impossible to rule out that these changes are not simply continuations of the ongoing growth-related changes already mentioned (for a discussion of this problem, see Robbins and Fahim 1985). Furthermore, the conclusions here, as with the growth-related changes occurring earlier in life, are complicated by the fact that not all of the changes seem to happen at all the junctions in all of the muscles. Thus, for example, increased tortuosity, which has often been implicated as a feature of senile neuromuscular junctions (Fahim and Robbins 1982; Fahim, Holley, and Robbins 1983), plateaus in the young adult for the soleus muscle, whereas it progressively increases with age in the extensor digitorum longus (Robbins and Fahim 1985).

Other age-related changes may be more consistent. In senescent animals end-plates generally appear to become less contiguous with increased numbers of discrete regions or islands (Robbins and Fahim, 1985). This 'regionalization' is thought to come about through the abandonment of some post-synaptic areas rather than through axonal sprouting into nearby new regions, because this change is seen in muscles in which the total linear dimensions of the end-plate do not change. Furthermore, electron microscopical studies suggest the presence of vacated post-synaptic folds in aged neuromuscular junctions (Fahim and Robbins 1982; Cardasis 1983; Wernig *et al.* 1984).

Another change seen in senile animals suggests frank motoneuronal loss and compensatory collateral sprouting. Many junctions that are ordinarily singly innervated become innervated by more than one axon (as judged anatomically) and many terminals show evidence of terminal sprouts (Fagg, Scheff, and Cotman 1981; Hopkins *et al.* 1985). At the ultrastructural level as well, signs of multiple innervation (several axons in one gutter) have also been documented (Cardasis 1983). These changes may be secondary to a loss of motor neurons which results in denervated muscle fibres which attract other axons to occupy the vacated end-plate site. Whether this multiple innervation is a stable feature of aged junctions is not known.

TURNOVER AT THE NEUROMUSCULAR JUNCTION

Barker and Ip (1966) were probably the first to suggest that a motor axon's terminals might be in a state of dynamic equilibrium in which continual sprouting and degeneration kept the motor unit in a state of constant renewal. They suggested a 'replacement hypothesis' in which 'sprouting effects the replacement of old endplates which degenerate after a limited life-span'.

At the frog neuromuscular junction the case of continual remodelling is especially strong. Several groups have presented evidence consistent with the idea that neuromuscular synapses are continually undergoing sprouting and regression (Wernig, Pecot-Dechavassine, and Stöver 1980a, 1980b; Wernig, Anzil, and Bieser 1981; Haiman, Mallart, Ferré, and Zilber-Gachelin 1981; see also Fig. 15 in Letinsky, Fischbeck, and McMahan 1976). Thus by using silver staining for nerve terminals and cholinesterase staining to delineate the post-syanptic specializations, Wernig *et al.* (1980a) found that emanating distally from the long terminal branches which are underlain by cholinesterase are small-diameter nerve branches which have only patchy islands of cholinesterase under them. These are thought to be sprouts at recently formed synaptic sites. At the ultrastructural level such small processes were not above well-differentiated synaptic gutters, also suggesting they are newly formed synapses. In other regions, the opposite picture was seen: cholinesterase bands located over synaptic gutters but no nerve or Schwann cell elements were present. These sites are interpreted to be areas of axonal regression. These features, indicative of remodelling (partially occupied gutters, empty gutters, nerve sprouts), are found at 7 per cent of the synaptic sites of normal frogs. 'Winter' frogs (caught during the seasonal nadir of frog activity) and frogs treated with curare showed the identical remodelling features but with a much higher incidence (24 per cent and about 50 per cent of the end-plates, respectively showed signs of remodelling).

There is also evidence for similar reorganizations taking place at mammalian end-plates (Barker and Ip 1966; Tuffery 1971; Kemplay and Stolkin 1980; Cardasis and Padykula 1981; Wernig *et al.* 1984). In the most recent of these studies (Wernig *et al.* 1984) anatomical evidence showed that end-plates in soleus muscle of adult mice become more complex with age, as has been described for a number of different muscles (see previous sections). The number of branch points and end-plate length seemed to increase continually between ages 3–11. Serial electron micrographs of potential sprouts (light microscopically appearing as thin axon branches arising from an end-plate) showed that they were in fact synaptic regions overlying fully differentiated post-synaptic regions (i.e. with secondary infoldings). Thus these images do not provide unequivocal support for newly forming junctions. On the other hand, synaptic gutters devoid of axons were seen and usually located distal to the terminations of axons. The finding of a net increase in the size of end-plates coupled with unoccupied gutters invites the speculation that, as in frog, synaptic sprouting and regression are continually taking place. Indeed, from the average values Wernig *et al.* (1984) obtained at each time-point they calculate that at each end-plate at least one additional branch is produced every 10–11 days between ages 3–6 months. Furthermore, they suggest that this number is the bare minimum because it does not take into account ongoing retraction. Thus they suggest a remarkable degree of remodelling at the mouse neuromuscular junction (see, however, Lichtman *et al.* 1987 and below).

CHANGES AT THE NEUROMUSCULAR JUNCTION IN RESPONSE TO INJURY

Motor axons are generally able to grow and form synaptic connections after injury. In mammals such regrowth does not necessarily result in motor axons finding their original muscle fibres or even the same muscle (Weiss and Hoag 1946; Brushart, Tarlov, and Mesulam 1983). Despite this lack of specificity it has long been known that motor axons will often reinnervate muscle fibres in the vicinity of their old end-plate sites (Tello 1907; Miledi 1960; Saito and Zacks 1969; Bennett, McLachlan, and Taylor 1973). The most detailed study of the site of reinnervation suggests that, in frogs at least, axons return precisely to the same post-synaptic sites that were originally innervated. This reinnervation thus results in neuromuscular junctions that with only a very few minor changes are identical in shape to the original end-plate sites (Letinsky *et al.* 1976). This conclusion was possible because the original end-plate sites remain largely intact following denervation. Letinsky *et al.* found that the cholinesterase staining does not diminish very much, if at all, at the synaptic basal lamina, so that the location and size of the original end-plate site could be monitored during the period of reinnervation. Thus, in an important respect, this study differs from most studies of end-plate change in that each muscle fibre contains information from two different time-points, making interpretation of the results much less complicated. Within two weeks of crushing the nerve to the cutaneous pectoris muscle, about 98 per cent of the original synaptic sites were reoccupied by nerve terminals. This remained constant for as long as they looked (three months). This conclusion is based on the absence of any change in the total length of cholinesterase-positive regions on the muscle fibres throughout the three-month period following nerve crush. The constant amount of cholinesterase argues that no new synaptic ending formed (control experiments ruled out the presence of new synapses without cholinesterase). Only if a new axon induced new cholinesterase and post-synaptic specializations, and caused the old cholinesterase and synaptic gutters to disappear at exactly equal rates, would their interpretation be wrong.

There were a few changes in the reinnervated frog end-plates. About half had small regions unoccupied by the returning axons. The incidence of unoccupied gutters was at least twice the normal degree of unoccupied post-synaptic regions (see above). Another feature found only rarely in normal muscle was 'escaped' branches; that is, sprouts going from one neuromuscular junction to either other junctions or sometimes just ending blindly in the connective tissue space between the fibres. A related change was an increased incidence of multiple axons innervating the same end-plate—often co-occupying the same post-synaptic gutters (see also Rotshenker and McMahan 1976, and below).

In mammals, the precision of reoccupation of the old end-plate site is less clear. Most workers in this field seem to agree that old post-synaptic sites are reoccupied to some extent by regrowing axons (Shulka and Aitken 1963; Iwayama 1969; Lüllman-Rauch 1971; Bennett *et al.* 1973). There is, however, also evidence for nerve endings near the old end-plate site but not directly over the old junctional folds (Iwayama 1969; Bennett *et al.* 1973). That new sites are being innervated is suggested by the absence of post-synaptic gutters at the sites of nerve termination and the discontinuous appearance of cholinesterase staining which differs from the continuous staining at the old junctional regions. It has also been suggested that another change at the reinnervated mammalian neuromuscular junction is the presence of post-synaptic junctional folds often extending beyond the point of contact with the reinnervating axon (Bennett *et al.* 1973). However, other workers have seen examples of vacated gutters at normal and aged adult end-plates (Cardasis and Padykula 1981; Fujisawa 1976; Cardasis 1983).

Another significant difference at the reinnervated junction is the presence of multiple innervation. Physiological evidence suggests that during reinnervation multiple axons innervate end-plates that would ordinarily be singly innervated (Tate and Westerman 1973; Jansen and Van Essen 1975; McArdle 1975; Gorio, Carminoto, Finesso, Polato, and Nunzi 1983). Anatomical evidence for multiple axons within the same gutter (Lüllman-Rauch 1971; Rotshenker and McMahan 1976; Letinsky *et al.* 1976) and for terminal sprouts crossing from one end-plate to another (Gutmann and Young 1944; Letinsky *et al.* 1976; Gorio *et al.* 1983) support this conclusion.

Multiple innervation at reinnervated mammalian end-plates is apparently unstable since both physiologically and anatomically the signs of multiple innervation decrease to low values two months after reinnervation (McArdle 1975; Gorio *et al.* 1983). According to Gorio *et al.* (1983) the end-plates continue to change, even after eliminating the multiple innervation, by very gradually reoccupying all the old synaptic gutters. In contrast to the mammal, reinnervated frog neuromuscular junctions remain multiply innervated for at least seven months without any signs of regression (Rotshenker and McMahan 1976). This difference may have less to do with species differences than with animal age and the muscle used. A recent study in mammals suggests that the elimination of multiple axons during reinnervation is age dependent and is more likely to occur in a slow than in a fast muscle (Hopkins, Liang, and Barrett 1986).

There is evidence to suggest that changes in synaptic connections also occur in end-plates contralateral to the site of the damage (for a review see Grinnell and Herrera 1981). These changes are difficult to generalize as many seem to be species specific and even muscle specific.

ACTIVITY-DEPENDENT CHANGES OF NEUROMUSCULAR SYNAPSES

One of the most natural and simple ways to reduce neuromuscular activity is by immobilization (e.g. a cast on a limb) (Booth 1982). In distinction to pharmacological blockade of neuromuscular transmission in which only muscle fibre activity is eliminated, or the use of tetrodotoxin which inhibits action potentials in the nerve but also blocks sodium channels in muscle fibres, immobilization reduces normal muscle activity without preventing it. Several workers have studied neuromuscular connections following limb immobilization (Cole 1960; Malathi and Batmanabane 1983; Pachter and Eberstein 1984). The most recent of these studies compared ultrastructural end-plate appearance in muscles that were immobilized in a shortened position within a plaster cast for three weeks. Fibres in the immobilized muscles were quite atrophic (30–40 per cent of the normal cross-sectional area) and some of the end-plates showed abnormalities suggesting both degeneration and compensatory regeneration of nerve terminals (Pachter and Eberstein 1984). The signs of disruption at end-plates included exposed junctional folds, myelin-like debris in the Schwann cells, nerve terminals overlying post-synaptic areas without junctional folds, and increased numbers of small nerve terminals often residing together in the same primary synaptic cleft. Light microscopical studies of end-plates in immobilized muscles also suggest increased sprouting (Eldridge *et al.* 1981; Malathi and Batmanabane 1983; however, see Cole 1960). A number of workers have made the point that junctions in aged animals resemble junctions in inactive muscles, suggesting that decreased activity may be an important factor in senile changes at the neuromuscular junction (Smith and Rosenheimer 1982; Fahim and Robbins 1983; Cardasis 1983). However, a recent study suggests that in some old animals activity levels and patterns are not significantly changed even though the junctions are already showing senile changes (Robbins and Fahim 1985).

Exercise-related changes in neuromuscular junctions also occur (Roy, Gillian, Taylor, and Heusner 1983; Stebbins, Schultz, Smith, and Smith 1985; Rosenheimer 1985). As with so many of the other phenomena discussed here, species, strain, and muscle type all seem to influence the result. Furthermore, stress, which frequently accompanies increased activity, may have an antagonistic influence to that of increased levels of activity (Rosenheimer 1985). What seems clearly *not* to be the case in that increased activity, as occurs in chronic exercise, has the opposite effect to decreased activity because, in aged animals at least, sprouting is observed in some chronically exercised muscles (Stebbins *et al.* 1985).

FUTURE DIRECTIONS

Even a cursory review of the literature indicates that fundamental difficulties exist in the field of dynamic aspects of synaptic connections at the neuromuscular junction. It is just not possible to come to firm conclusions about many of the phenomena. Rosenheimer and Smith (1985) recently studied a large number of morphometric parameters of end-plates in three rat muscles studied between ages 10–31 months. Their study is carefully controlled and large numbers of end-plate (60) were measured in each muscle at each of eight time-points at intervals of three months. The results indicate a surprising degree of statistically significant fluctuation. For example, at 22 months of age the soleus end-plates are 860 μm^2 in area, at 25 months are 1050 μm^2, at 28 months they are 850 μm^2, and at 31 months they are 1100 μm^2. The authors rightly conclude that, if these fluctuations are true, data in which only two time-points are used (e.g. 22 months and 31 months) would yield conclusions exactly opposite than if two other time-points were used (e.g. 25 and 28 months), If, on the other hand, we imagine that some unforeseen artefact caused these fluctuations (for a discussion of the possibilities, see Robbins and Fahim 1985), how much confidence can we have in comparing the results of different laboratories using different techniques, different animals, different strains, and different muscles?

The solution to this problem is probably not more carefully controlled studies but new experimental strategies. Over the past several years, neurobiologists have begun to look at dynamic aspects of the nervous system with techniques that permit the viewing of the same elements at multiple times (Purves and Hadley 1985; Purves, Hadley, and Voyvodic 1986; Eisen, Myers, and Westerfield 1986; Lichtman *et al.* 1987). The advantage of this sort of approach is that it is far more direct and interpretation is reserved for questions concerning what the data *means* rather than what the data *is*. The recent development of strains that vitally mark the neuromuscular junction (Yoshikami and Okun 1984; Lichtman, Wilkinson, and Rich 1985; Magrassi, Purves, and Lichtman 1987; Kelly, Avis, and Robbins 1985) permit the viewing of the same neuromuscular junction at more than one time-point. Our own work in this field suggests that it is possible to view the same mammalian junctions at intervals as short as one day or so long that they represent a significant portion of an animal's lifetime (six months or more in mice) (Lichtman *et al.* 1987; Rich and Lichtman 1986 and in preparation). It is our hope that such techniques may allow more direct approaches to the intriguing questions of neuromuscular plasticity.

REFERENCES

Albani, M. and Vrbova, G. (1985). Physiological properties and pattern of innervation of regenerated muscles in the rat. *Neuroscience.* **15,** pp. 489–98.

Atsumi, S. (1971). The histogenesis of motor neurons with special reference to the correlation of their endplate formation. *Acta Anat.* **80,** pp. 161–82.

Atsumi, S. (1977). Development of neuromuscular junctions of fast and slow muscles in the chick embryo: a light and electron microscopic study. *J. Neurocytol.* **6,** pp. 691–709.

Banker, B. Q., Kelly, S. S., and Robbins, N. (1983). Neuromuscular transmission and correlative morphology in young and old mice. *J. Physiol. (Lond.)* **339,** pp. 355–77.

Barker, D. and Ip, M. C. (1966). Sprouting and degeneration of mammalian motor axons in normal and de-afferentated skeletal muscle. *Proc. R. Soc. Lond.* B **163,** pp. 538–54.

Bennett, M. R. and Pettigrew, A. G. (1974). The formation of synapses in striated muscle during development. *J. Physiol. (Lond.)* **241,** pp. 515–45.

Bennett, M. R., McLachlan, E. M., and Taylor, R. S. (1973). The formation of synapses in reinnervated mammalian striated muscle. *J. Physiol. (Lond.)* **233,** pp. 481–500.

Bevan, S. and Steinbach, J. H. (1977). The distribution of α-bungarotoxin binding sites on mammalian skeletal muscle developing in vivo. *J. Physiol. (Lond.)* **267**, pp. 195–213.

Bixby, J. L. (1981). Ultrastructural observations on synapse elimination in neonatal rabbit skeletal muscle. *J. Neurocytol.* **10**, pp. 81–100.

Booth, F. W. (1982). Effect of limb immobilization on skeletal muscle. *J. Appl. Physiol.* **52**, pp. 1113–8.

Brown, M. C., Holland, R. L., and Hopkins, W. G. (1981). Excess neuronal inputs during development. In *Development of the nervous system* (eds. D. R. Garrod and J. D. Feldman) pp. 245–62. Cambridge University Press, Cambridge.

Brown, M. C., Jansen, J. K. S., and Van Essen, D. (1976). Polyneuronal innervation of skeletal muscle in new-born rats and its elimination during maturation. *J. Physiol.* **261**, pp. 387–422.

Brushart, T. M., Tarlov, E. C., and Mesulam, M. -M. (1983). Specificity of muscle reinnervation after epineurial and individual fascicular suture of the rat sciatic nerve. *J. Hand. Surg.* **8**, pp. 248–53.

Cardasis, C. A. (1983). Ultrastructural evidence of continued reorganization at the aging (11–26 months) rat soleus neuromuscular junction. *Anat. Rec.* **207**, pp. 399–415.

Cardasis, C. A. and Padykula, H. A. (1981). Ultrastructural evidence indicating reorganization at the neuromuscular junction in the normal rat soleus muscle. *Anat. Rec.* **200**, pp. 41–59.

Cole, W. V. (1960). The effect of immobilization on striated muscle and the myoneuronal junction. *J. Comp. Neurol.* **115**, pp. 9–13.

Courtney, J. and Steinbach, J. H. (1981). Age changes in neuromuscular junction morphology and acetylcholine receptor distribution on rat skeletal muscle fibres. *J. Physiol. (Lond.)* **320**, pp. 435–47.

Dennis, M. J. and Miledi, R. (1974). Non-transmitting neuromuscular junctions during an early stage of and-plate reinnervation. *J. Physiol.* **239**, 553–70

Dennis, M. J., Ziskind-Conhaim, L., and Harris, A. J. (1981). Development of neuromuscular junctions in rat embryos. *Dev. Biol.* **81**, pp. 266–79.

Eisen, J. S., Myers, P. Z., and Westerfield, M. (1986). Pathway selection by growth cones of identified motoneurones in live zebra fish embryos. *Nature* **320**, pp. 269–71.

Eldridge, L., Liebhold, M., and Steinbach, J. H. (1981). Alterations in cat skeletal neuromuscular junctions following prolonged inactivity. *J. Physiol. (Lond.)* **313**, pp. 529–45.

Fagg, G. E., Scheff, S. W., and Cotman, C. W. (1981). Axonal sprouting at the neuromuscular junction of adult and aged rats. *Exp. Neurol.* **74**, pp. 847–59.

Fahim, M. A. and Robbins, N. (1982). Ultrastructural studies of young and old mouse neuromuscular junctions. *J. Neurocytol.* **11**, pp. 641–56.

Fahim, M. A., Holley, J. A., and Robbins, N. (1983). Scanning and light microscopic study of age changes at a neuromuscular junction in the mouse. *J. Neurocytol.* **12**, pp. 13–25.

Fahim, M. A., Holley, J. A., and Robbins, N. (1984). Topographic comparison of neuromuscular junctions in mouse slow and fast twitch muscles. *Neuroscience.* **13**, 227–35.

Frolkis, V. V., Martynenko, O. A., and Zamostyan, V. P. (1976). Aging of the neuromuscular apparatus. *Gerontol.* **22**, pp. 244–79.

Fujisawa, K. (1974). Some observations on the skeletal musculature of aged rats. I. Histological aspects. *J. Neurol. Sci.* **22**, pp. 353–66.

Fujisawa, K. (1976). Some observation on the skeletal musculature of aged rats. III. Abnormalities of terminal axons found in motor end-plates. *Exp. Gerontol.* **11,** pp. 43–7.

Gorio, A., Carmignoto, G., Finesso, M., Polato, P., and Nunzi, M. G. (1983). Muscle reinnervation. II. Sprouting, synapse formation and repression. *Neuroscience.* **8,** pp. 403–16.

Grinnell, A. D. and Herrera, A. A. (1981). Specificity and plasticity of neuromuscular connections: long-term regulation of motoneuron function. *Prog. Neurobiol.* **17,** pp. 203–82.

Guth, L. (1969). Effect of immobilization on sole-plate and background cholinesterase of rat skeletal muscle. *Exp. Neurol.* **24,** pp. 508–13.

Gutmann, E. and Hanzlikova, V. (1965). Age changes of motor endplates in muscle fibres of the rat. *Gerontologia,* **11,** pp. 12–24.

Gutmann, E. and Young, J. Z. (1944). The re-innervation of muscle after various periods of atrophy. *J. Anat.* **78,** pp. 15–43.

Gutmann, E., Hanzlíková, V., and Jakoubek, B. (1968). Changes in the neuromuscular system during old age. *Exp. Gerontol.* **3,** pp. 141–6.

Haimann, C., Mallart, A., Ferré, J. T. I., and Zilber-Gachelin, N. F. (1981). Patterns of motor innervation in the pectoral muscle of adult Xenopus laevis: evidence for possible synaptic remodelling. *J. Physiol. (Lond.)* **310,** pp. 241–56.

Hirano, H. (1967). Ultrastructural study on the morphogenesis of the neuromuscular junction in the skeletal muscle of the chick. *Z. Zellforsch* **79,** pp. 198–208.

Hopkins, W. G., Brown, M. C., and Keynes, R. J. (1985). Postnatal growth of motor nerve terminals in muscles of the mouse. *J. Neurocytol.* **14,** pp. 525–40.

Hopkins, W. G., Liang, J., and Barrett, E. J. (1986). Effect of age and muscle type on regeneration of neuromuscular synapses in mice. *Brain Res.* **372,** pp. 163–6.

Iwayama, T. (1969). Relation of regenerating nerve terminals to original endplates. *Nature* **224,** pp. 81–2.

Jacob, M. and Lentz, T. L. (1979). Localization of acetylcholine receptors by means of horseradish peroxidase-α-bungarotoxin during formation and development of the neuromuscular junction in the chick embryo. *J. Cell Biol.* **82,** pp. 195–211.

Jansen, J. K. S. and van Essen, D. C. (1975). Re-innervation of rat skeletal muscle in the presence of α-bungarotoxin. *J. Physiol. (Lond.)* **250,** pp. 651–67.

Kelly, S. S. (1978). The effect of age on neuromuscular transmission. *J. Physiol.* **274,** pp. 51–62.

Kelly, S. S. and Robbins, N. (1983). Progression of age changes in synaptic transmission at mouse neuromuscular junctions. *J. Physiol.* **343,** pp. 375–83.

Kelly, A. M. and Zacks, S. I. (1969). The fine structure of motor endplate morphogenesis. *J. Cell. Biol.* **42,** pp. 154–69.

Kelly, S. S., Anis, N., and Robbins, N. (1985). Fluorescent staining of living mouse neuromuscular junctions. *Pflugers Arch. Eur. J. Physiol.* **404,** pp. 97–9.

Kemplay, S. and Stolkin, C. (1980). Endplate classification and spontaneous sprouting in the sternocostalis muscle of the rat: a new whole mount preparation. *Cell Tissue Res.* **212,** pp. 333–9.

Ko, C. -P. (1985). Formation of the active zone in developing neuromuscular junctions in larval and adult bullfrogs. *J. Neurocytol.* **14,** pp. 487–512.

Korneliussen, H. and Jansen, J. K. S. (1976). Morphological aspects of the elimination of polyneuronal innervation of skeletal muscle fibres in newborn rats. *J. Neurocytol.* **5**, pp. 591–604.

Kullberg, R. W., Lentz, T. L., and Cohen, M. W. (1977). Development of the myotomal neuromuscular junction in Xenopus laevis: an electrophysiological and fine structural study. *Dev. Biol.* **60**, pp. 101–29.

Letinsky, M. S., Fischbeck, K. H., and McMahan, U. J. (1976). Precision of reinnervation of original postsynaptic sites in frog muscle after a nerve crush. *J. Neurocytol.* **5**, pp. 691–718.

Lichtman, J. W., Magrassi, L., and Purves, D. (1987). Visualization of neuromuscular junctions over periods of several months in living mice. *J. Neurosci.* **7**, pp. 1215–22.

Lichtman, J. W., Wilkinson, R. S., and Rich, M. M. (1985). Multiple innervation of tonic endplates revealed by activity-dependent uptake of fluorescent probes. *Nature* **314**, pp. 357–9.

Lüllmann-Rauch, R. (1971). The regeneration of neuromuscular junctions during spontaneous re-innervation of the rat diaphragm. *Z. Zellforsch. Mik. Anat.* **121**, pp. 593–603.

Magrassi, L., Purves, D., and Lichtman, J. W. (1987). Fluorescent probes that stain living nerve terminals. *J. Neurosci.* **7**, pp. 1207–14.

Malathi, S. and Batmanabane, M. (1983). Alterations in the morphology of the neuromuscular junctions following experimental immobilization in cats. *Experientia* **39**, pp. 547–9.

McArdle, J. J. (1975). Complex end-plate potentials at the regenerating neuromuscular junction of the rat. *Exp. Neurol.* **49**, pp. 629–38.

Miledi, R. (1960). Properties of regenerating neuromuscular synapses in the frog. *J. Physiol. (Lond.)* **154**, pp. 190–205.

Morrison-Graham, K. (1983). An anatomical and electrophysiological study of synapse elimination at the developing frog neuromuscular junction. Dev. Biol. **99**, pp. 298–311.

Nyström, B. (1968a). Histochemical studies of end-plate bound esterases in 'slow-red' and 'fast-white' cat muscles during postnatal development. *Acta. Neurol. Scand.* **44**, pp. 295–318.

Nyström, B. (1968b). Postnatal development of motor nerve terminals in 'slow-red' and 'fast-white' cat muscles. *Acta. Neurol. Scand.* **44**, pp. 363–83.

O'Brien, R. A. D., Östberg, A. J. C., and Vrbova, G. (1978). Observations on the elimination of polyneuronal innervation in developing mammalian skeletal muscle. *J. Physiol. (Lond.)* **282**, pp. 571–82.

Pachter, B. R. and Eberstein, A. (1984). Neuromuscular plasticity following limb immobilization. *J. Neurocytol.* **13**, pp. 1013–25.

Purves, D. and Hadley, R. D. (1985). Changes in the dendritic branching of adult mammalian neurones revealed by repeated imaging in situ. *Nature* **315**, pp. 404–6.

Purves, D., Hadley, R. D., and Voyvodic, J. T. (1986). Dynamic changes in the dendritic geometry of individual neurons visualized over periods of up to three months in the superior cervical ganglion of living mice. *J. Neurosci.* **6**, pp. 1051–60.

Rich, M. M. and Lichtman, J. W. (1986). Remodelling of endplate sites during muscle reinnervation in the living mouse. *Soc. Neurosci. Abstr.* **12**, p. 390.

Riley, D. A. (1977). Spontaneous elimination of nerve terminals from the endplates of developing skeletal myofibers. *Brain Res.* **134**, pp. 279–85.

Riley, D. A. (1981). Ultrastructural evidence for axon retraction during the spontaneous elimination of polyneuronal innervation of the rat soleus muscle. *J. Neurocytol.* **10,** pp. 425–40.

Robbins, N. and Fahim, M. A. (1985). Progression of age changes in mature mouse motor nerve terminals and its relation to locomotor activity. *J. Neurocytol.* **14,** pp. 1019–46.

Roberts, J., Baskin, S. I., and Goldberg, P. B. (1977). Age changes in the neuromuscular system of rats. *Exp. Aging Res.* **3,** pp. 75–84.

Rosenheimer, J. L. (1985). Effects of chronic stress and exercise on age-related changes in end-plate architecture. *J. Neurophysiol.* **53,** pp. 1582–9.

Rosenheimer, J. L. and Smith, D. O. (1985). Differential changes in the end-plate architecture of functionally diverse muscles during aging. *J. Neurophysiol.* **53,** pp. 1567–81.

Rosenthal, J. L. and Taraskevich, S. P. (1977). Reduction of multiaxonal innervation at the neuromuscular junction of the rat during development. *J. Physiol. (Lond.)* **270,** pp. 299–310.

Rotshenker, S. and McMahan, U. J. (1976). Altered patterns of innervation in frog muscle after denervation. *J. Neurocytol.* **5,** pp. 719–30.

Roy, R. R., Gilliam, T. B., Taylor, J. F., and Heusner, W. W. (1983). Activity-induced morphologic changes in rat soleus nerve. *Exp. Neurol.* **80,** pp. 622–32.

Saito, A. and Zacks, S. I. (1969). Fine structure observations of denervation and reinnervation of neuromuscular junction in mouse foot muscle. *J. Bone Joint Surg.* **51-A,** pp. 1163–78.

Shukla, P. L. and Aitken, J. T. (1963). Formation of motor end-plates in denervated voluntary muscles of the rat. *J. Anat.* **97,** p. 152.

Sisto Daneo, L. and Filogamo, G. (1973). Ultrastructure of early neuro-muscular contacts in the chick embryo. *J. Submicrosc. Cytol.* **5,** pp. 219–25.

Slater, C. R. (1982). Postnatal maturation of nerve-muscle junctions in hindlimb muscles of the mouse. *Dev. Biol.* **94,** pp. 11–22.

Smith, D. O. and Rosenheimer, J. L. (1982). Decreased sprouting and degeneration of nerve terminals of active muscles in aged rats. *J. Neurophysiol.* **48,** pp. 100–9.

Spector, S. A. (1985). Trophic effects. *J. Neurosci.* **5**(8), pp. 2189–96.

Stebbins, C. L., Schultz, E., Smith, R. T., and Smith, E. L. (1985). Effects of chronic exercise during aging on muscle and end-plate morphology in rats. *J. Appl. Physiol.* **58,** pp. 45–51.

Steinbach, J. H. (1981). Developmental changes in acetylcholine receptor aggregates at rat skeletal neuromuscular junctions. *Dev. Biol.* **84,** pp. 267–76.

Tate, K. and Westerman, R. A. (1973). Polyneuronal self-reinnervation of a slow-twitch muscle (soleus) in the cat. *Proc. Aust. Physiol. Pharm. Soc.* **4,** pp. 174–5.

Tello, F. (1907). Degeneration et regeneration des plaques matrices apres la section des nerfs. *Trav. Lab. Res. Biol. Madrid* **5,** pp. 117–49.

Terävainen, H. (1968). Development of the myoneural junction in the rat. *Z. Zellforsch.* **87,** pp. 249–65.

Tuffery, A. R. (1971). Growth and degeneration of motor end-plates in normal cat hind limb muscles. *J. Anat.* **110,** pp. 221–47.

Tweedle, C. D. and Stephens, K. E. (1981). Development of complexity in motor nerve endings at the rat neuromuscular junction. *Neuroscience.* **6,** pp. 1657–62.

Wallinga, De Jonge, W. *et al.* (1985). The different intracellular. *Electroencephal. Clin. Neurophysiol.* **60**(6) pp. 539–47.

Weiss, P. and Hoag, A. (1946). Competitive reinnervation of rat muscles by their own and foreign nerves. *J. Neurophysiol.* **9**, pp. 413–18.

Wernig, A., Anzil, A. P., and Bieser, A. (1981). Light and electron microscopic identification of a nerve sprout in muscle of normal adult frog. *Neurosci. Lett.* **21**, pp. 261–6.

Wernig, A., Pecot-Dechavassine, M., and Stöver, H. (1980a). Sprouting and regression of the nerve at the frog neuromuscular junction in normal conditions and after prolonged paralysis with curare. *J. Neurocytol.* **9**, pp. 277–303.

Wernig, A., Pecot-Dechavassine, M., and Stöver, H. (1980b). Signs of nerve regression and sprouting in the frog neuromuscular synapse. In *Ontogenesis and Functional Mechanisms of Peripheral Synapses* (ed. J. Taxi). pp. 255–38. In *INSERM Symp. No. 13*.

Wernig, A., Carmody, J. J., Anzil, A. P., Hansert, E., Marciniak, M., and Zucker, H. (1984). Persistence of nerve sprouting with features of synapse remodelling in soleus muscles of adult mice. *Neuroscience.* **11**, pp. 241–53.

Yoshikami, D. and Okun, L. M. (1984). Staining of living presynaptic nerve terminals with selective fluorescent dyes. *Nature* **310**, pp. 53–6.

18

Competition in the development
of the visual pathways

R. W. GUILLERY

Tweedledum and Tweedledee
Agreed to have a battle;
For Tweedledum said Tweedledee
Had spoiled his nice new rattle.

Just then flew down a monstrous crow,
As black as a tar-barrel;
Which frightened both the heroes so,
They quite forgot their quarrel.

(From *Through the looking-glass* by Lewis Carroll.)

'Competition', as an interpretative structure for events occurring in neural development, provides a mechanism that is easy to invoke but often difficult to demonstrate experimentally. It can produce control of population numbers or of synaptic territories, both crucial in the development of the nervous system. If one understood how neuronal numbers and the topographical distribution of synaptic connections between axonal and dendritic arbors are controlled, then some of the most puzzling aspects of neural development would become comprehensible.

In recent years, competitive interactions, acting in a variety of ways, have been postulated in many different developmental situations. In this brief essay I do not plan to review them all. Rather, I hope to show that in some situations the experimental evidence forces one to recognize a competitive interaction, whereas in others the facts that are currently available merely make competition appealing as a picturesque interpretation of events, without as yet giving competition any necessary function. I shall try to define different types of competitive interaction, and to look particularly at the nature of the experimental evidence that may or may not suffice to provide a convincing demonstration of competition having occurred. In the long run it will be important to define where in development competitive interactions do play a role. For this one will need an agreed view about what competition is, and how it can be demonstrated. The current literature is weak on critical experimental tests of the competition hypothesis and until the hypothesis can be widely challenged it is not likely to make a robust contribution to developmental neurobiology. I shall therefore be mainly concerned with the experimental evidence in favour of competition. Theoretical models that require competitive interactions (e.g. Prestige and Willshaw 1975; Whitelaw and Cowan 1981) will not be considered. For the experimentalist the difficult problem is the convincing demonstration of the interactions postulated by the theoretician.

Since much of the experimental evidence has come from the developing visual system, where two almost identical but easily distinguishable populations (labelled 'crossed' and 'uncrossed' rather than 'Dum' and 'Dee') are seen to be pitted against each other, most of my examples will be drawn from this system. However, it will become clear that the visual system can serve as a useful example of many other systems in vertebrates and in invertebrates. The issue is to define the extent to which competitive interactions play a demonstrable and crucial role in visual development, and to distinguish where the 'monstrous crow', which makes the occurrence or non-occurrence of the competition quite trivial, has to be recognized. Readers may choose to interpret the crow as representative of other, non-competitive mechanisms that can adequately explain the developmental events, or of our profound ignorance about the mechanism of competition itself. Commonly, when one looks at possible competitive interactions, the nature of the interaction, in terms of cellular or molecular processes, remains unknown and is generally not addressed (however, see Stent 1973; Changeux and Danchin 1976). Although eventually the mechanisms will prove to be the most interesting aspect of competitive interactions, at present it is still necessary to look carefully at the evidence defining where and when these interactions occur. As yet there is, unfortunately, little to be said about how they occur.

DEFINITIONS AND GENERAL CONSIDERATIONS

In general, competition is defined on the basis of experimental outcomes. It is commonly thought of as an interaction between nerve cells or neuronal processes that all require the same resource in a developmental situation where a limited supply of this resource is available. One postulates that not all of the neural elements can obtain enough of the resource for survival. The loss of neural elements during normal development, their increased loss when the resource is experimentally removed or decreased, and their reduced loss when more of the resource is made available are regarded as evidence that competition has occurred. The resource is often not defined, although it is commonly regarded as being a trophic material or the availability of synaptic space either pre- or post-synaptic to the elements being considered. However, 'competition' does not always have precisely the same empirical meaning when it is used by developmental neurobiologists. In a review of experimental situations in which the term can be useful one is led to the view that more than one type of competition can be defined. Each may be based on similar mechanisms (or each may even be represented by several different mechanisms), but since the demonstration of each calls for different experimental evidence, and these have different experimental outcomes, the distinction is useful.

Type-I competition

Type-I competition is the relatively simple interaction between members of a single population of neurons which are all dependent for survival upon a limited resource. In principle, any resource will satisfy the definition, provided that its manipulation can produce the appropriate changes in the neuronal population. Type-I competition can produce developmental changes in numbers but not in the topography of connections. This type of competition has been proposed as a mechanism for matching the size of neuronal populations within two interconnected neuron groups (Cowan, Fawcett, O'Leary, and Stanfield 1984) and is illustrated by the changes that can be produced in the number of ventral horn cells in the chick spinal cord by limb removal, which reduces the number of surviving cells, or by transplantation of supernumerary limbs, which increases the numbers that survive (Hamburger 1975; Hollyday and Hamburger 1976). There are several experiments providing comparable evidence for a competitive interaction in the control of neuron numbers (see Cowan *et al.* 1984) but only a few that raise serious questions about the role that competition might play. A recent intriguing example involves the transplantation of quail neural tissues into duck embryos (Sohal, Stoney, Arumugam, Yamashita, and Knox 1986). It was shown that the number of quail neurons formed were appropriate for the quail brain in spite of a muscle field that could have supported a larger number of duck neurons.

In type-I competition the cell population must be homogeneous from the experimenter's point of view. There may be hidden or unidentified subpopulations, but if the experiment only discriminates a single population, then (by definition) one is dealing with type-I competition, which can also be called 'internal competition' since it occurs within a single population, having the same identifiable perikaryal distribution and axonal termination.

One interesting problem about type-I competition arises when one asks why an organism might need such a control of population size. The extent to which closely related members of the same species resemble each other in terms of neuronal numbers must reflect the degree to which population size can be controlled by genetic mechanisms alone, with no competitive 'fine tuning' of neuron numbers based on interactions between synaptically connected neuron groups. Where small numbers are concerned, as in many invertebrate systems (e.g. Sulston and White 1980), we know that the genetic control can be quite accurate, so that little or no competitive interaction needs to be postulated. With larger numbers one can never be certain whether individual differences in a single species reflect genetic variability, experimenter's errors, or the degree to which population size may not be under genetic control. For example, the highly variable numbers obtained for cells sending fibres into the optic nerve of cats (Hughes 1975; Hughes and Wässle 1976; Stone 1978; Stone and Campion 1978; Williams, Bastiani, and Chalupa 1983) or for ipsilaterally projecting retinal ganglion cells in rodents (Dräger and Olson 1980; Jeffery, Cowey, and Kuypers 1981; Linden and Perry 1982; Dreher, Potts, Ni, and Bennett 1984; Godement 1984; Jeffery 1984) could be taken as an indication of weak genetic control if one knew more about the other variables (genetic variability, observer errors). The degree to which type-I competition is necessary in normal development for the control of population size is not defined, although it clearly plays a role in development that has been experimentally modified.

We know all too little about the normal development of population numbers. Information about the extent to which the stage of cell death in one population is related to the stage of cell production or loss in synaptically related populations will be useful in understanding the mechanisms by which the size of one population is matched to that of another. However, the analysis may well prove complex. For example, the evidence presented by Brown, Jansen, and Vantssen (1976), Harris (1981), and Oppenheim (1986) suggests that in the rat the production of new muscle continues long after the period of the relevant motor neuronal cell death. This does not rule out the view that the neuronal loss plays a part in the size matching, it simply adds a possible temporal delay to the proposed mechanism and makes its analysis more complex. Critical evidence about cell death, type-I competition, and size matching could be obtained if one recognized that size matching is, by definition, a developmental process establishing a definable ratio between the numbers of pre- and post-synaptic components in any single system, a ratio that depends upon an interaction between the two cell populations and that cannot be accurately produced by genetic controls acting independently upon each population. If this is the case, then the ratio of pre-synaptic to post-synaptic cell numbers, measured in single individuals and recorded for a significant population of individuals of any one species, should become less variable with increasing age wherever a size matching process is active. Further, the stage during which the variability decreased should provide clues about the period of the competitive interaction.

Type-II competition

Type-II competition involves an interaction between two (or more, but generally two) distinguishable neuron populations and can be regarded as 'external' competition for this reason. Two populations can be said to show a competitive interaction if both are interacting in normal development so that a weakening of one, generally by its destruction or deprivation, leads to an increased growth of the other. The second part of this definition can usually be dealt with quite simply because experimentally one can reduce the size or efficacy of one system and demonstrate a corresponding increase in the development of the other. When, however, one addresses the first half of the definition and asks whether the two systems interact in normal development, then it becomes difficult to define the type of evidence that might convince one that two systems undergo a competitive interaction during normal development, as distinct from showing an interaction that only occurs under the special conditions created by a particular experiment.

This distinction, between experimentally induced and naturally occurring competition, is best illustrated by examples and is considered in more detail in the next two sections. It will become clear that examples of experimentally induced competition that do not reflect a naturally occurring competition in the same system are readily identified, and the reasons for this will become evident. Once the existence of this type of competition is acknowledged, the demonstration of a naturally occurring type-II competition becomes extremely difficult. The simple interpretation, that an increase in one component produced by the removal of another is evidence for normally ocurring type-II competition (e.g. Rakic and Riley 1983; Williams *et al.* 1983; Murphey and Lemere 1984; Linden and Serfaty 1985), can no longer be accepted. However, in the final sections I hope to show that there are situations in which one can at least approach a reasonably convincing demonstration of naturally occurring competition.

An argument that is commonly produced at this point claims that all an experimenter can ever do is to define what happens in an experiment. One can never expect to demonstrate what happens normally. But this is too pessimistic and too simplistic. By reducing the *severity* of the experimental interference one can approach an appreciation of what normally happens, and by varying the *nature* of the experimental approach one can see where a particular postulated developmental process survives a multiplicity of experimental attacks. I have indicated above that critical evidence about the role of cell death in size matching may be obtained from counts with no pre-mortem experimental manipulations necessary, and it will be shown later that the evidence we have about binocular competition in the geniculocortical system is based on several distinct and related lines of evidence. Our views of cell migration and axonal growth have been refined by experimental approaches that are richer and more subtle than most of those that are today widely accepted as 'demonstrating' competition.

The relationships between type-I and type-II competitions are of interest. The mechanisms involved may well be the same; the outcomes differ. Type-I competition may underlie the production of type-II competition, or, stated another way, type-II competition can be regarded as a special case of type-I competition. If one focuses attention separately on one population, A, competing for a limited resource with another, B, then weakening B can be seen as simply a way of increasing the total resource available to A. However, in spite of this resemblance, the difference is crucial to an understanding of neural development. Whereas interaction within a single population can only produce control of population size, the interaction between two distinguishable populations can produce a sharing out of territories. Type-II competition, then, has important additional implications because it can produce topographical borders or gradients and provides a possible mechanism for subdividing the brain at any level from the synaptic to the architectonic.

THE FORMATION OF OCULAR DOMINANCE STRIPES IN THE OPTIC TECTUM OF NON-MAMMALIAN VERTEBRATES

When afferents from two eyes, or from two separate, non-continuous retinal segments, are forced to innervate a single tectal lobe in fish, amphibians, or birds, the terminals from the two inputs form alternating stripes (Levine and Jacobson 1975; Constantine-Paton 1978; Fawcett and Willshaw 1982; Meyer 1983; Boss and Schmidt 1984; Fawcett and Cowan 1985). These stripes can be demonstrated by labelling one set of fibres with an axonal marker while leaving the other set unlabelled, or by labelling each set with a different marker, [³H]-proline being used for one eye and horseradish peroxidase for the other (Law and Constantine-Paton 1980, 1981; Boss and Schmidt 1984). The formation of these tectal stripes appears to be dependent upon activity in the afferent fibres, since the stripe formation is prevented by tetrodotoxin (TTX; this blocks sodium channels and thus blocks axonal impulses) applied to both sets of afferents. If only one of the sets of afferents is subjected to the TTX block, then the patches survive but are less sharply defined than normal (Meyer 1982; Schmidt and Thieman 1985; Reh and Constantine-Paton 1985). If one set of afferents is crushed, the other changes from a striped to a continuous projection (Reh and Constantine-Paton 1985).

These tectal 'ocular dominance' stripes have been regarded as a good experimental model for the formation of the ocular dominance columns that are formed in normal development in the mammalian visual cortex (see Hubel and Wiesel 1977; LeVay, Wiesel, and Hubel 1980), where competitive interactions are thought to play a crucial role (see below). The parallels are close in many respects, so that one can reasonably expect studies of the tectal stripes to define some of the general mechanisms that produce this type of segregation.

The formation of the tectal stripes can be regarded as type-II competition produced by experimental manipulation. The effect of crushing one set of afferents (see above) satisfies the second part of the definition proposed earlier, that weakening one system should lead to the strengthening of the other, although in this instance the experiment is not really needed, it only recreates the normal situation of one eye innervating the whole tectum and forming an uninterrupted innervation. However, it is not yet clear whether this is merely a competition for territory or a competitive interaction involving neuronal numbers, numbers of axonal branches, or numbers of synapses made. Possibly one may eventually need to distinguish an interaction that produces a segregation of two distinct axon populations from an interaction producing a numerical increase of one population at the expense of the other. The possibility that these represent two distinct developmental processes merits study.

It is also clear that the pattern of competition seen in this experiment cannot represent interactions that occur in normal development, since the normal tectum has a monocular, unstriped innervation. It can be argued that the experiment reveals a capacity for competitive interactions that is latent in the retinotectal axons and possibly plays a role in the formation of monocular maps. However, it cannot be argued that the experimentally demonstrated binocular interaction ever plays a role in normal development, except perhaps to define the midline border between afferents from the left and the right eyes. The normal retinotectal system of teleosts is essentially monocular and the binocular interactions that occur in the frog's tectum do not involve interactions between primary afferents from the two eyes (e.g. Anders and Hibbard 1974; Grobstein, Comer, Hollyday, and Archer 1978; Gruberg and Udin 1978). The experiment may illustrate a tendency of individual retinotectal axons to form stripes of a particular width and orientation (this remains to be shown), but it clearly does not show the capacity of the fibres to form binocular interactions in normal development, since the stripes, which are so far the only sign of the interaction, do not form as a part of normal development. The point may seem all too obvious. It is worth stressing here because the same point applies to many other experimental situations where it is less obvious and generally not appreciated.

THE INCREASE OF ONE RETINOFUGAL SYSTEM PRODUCED BY THE REMOVAL OF THE OTHER IN MAMMALIAN DEVELOPMENT

The interaction between the two retinofugal pathways of mammals is of interest because in normal development the two pathways share terminal territories for a period before each establishes its own independent terminal zone (Rakic 1976, 1977; Linden, Guillery, and Cucchiaro 1981; Shatz 1983). The rules according to which the pathways segregate and share out the terminal territory vary according to the relay under consideration and upon the species. In many species the geniculate terminals segregate to form distinct layers, although the order of the layers varies greatly (see below). The tectal terminals can be arranged so that terminals from one eye (the ipsilateral eye) form patches among those from the other eye; or the tectal terminals may also show some segregation into different layers (Tigges and Tigges 1970; Graybiel 1975; Harting and Guillery 1976; Frost, So, and Schneider 1979; Huerta and Harting 1983). The degree to which these several patterns of normal segregation depend upon competition is not well defined, although it is clear that competitive interactions can be experimentally induced within the system.

The experimental production of an interaction that forms no directly comparable part of normal development is well demonstrated if one eye is removed in a young, 0–10-day-old kitten. One set of geniculate layers is denervated and fibres from the surviving eye in adjacent layers invade the denervated layers to a limited extent (Guillery 1972a; Hickey 1975), forming synaptic contacts in this foreign territory (Robson, Mason, and Guillery 1978). An important feature of this experiment is that retinogeniculate terminals are already completely segregated into separate layers before birth (Kalil 1973; Shatz 1983); that is, before the one set of layers was denervated. The postnatal trans-laminar growth shows that the surviving axons can be induced to do something that is not a part of their normal post-natal repertoire. This experiment, again, demonstrates experimentally induced type-II competition but itself provides no evidence that such competition plays any role in normal development.

One can argue that the growth of the trans-laminar sprouts represents a normal potential for competitive interactions which has survived for some time after it has completed its normal developmental role, but one can argue with equal conviction that the geniculate denervation served to produce abnormal conditions which themselves provided the stimulus for the trans-laminar sprouting. This latter argument, which claims that the experimental manipulation was too severe for a critical demonstration of normally occurring type-II competition (see above), is worth exploring in more detail. Suppose that in the developing retinogeniculate system there is initially type-I competition between all fibres coming from both eyes. The sharing out of territory betwen left- and right-eye afferents may well be a separate, non-competitive development (see below), occurring prenatally and dependent upon specific topographic cues that guide crossed and uncrossed fibres to different layers. Since growth of the axonal terminals in the layers continues during the first postnatal weeks (Mason 1982a, 1982b; Sur, Weller, and Sherman 1984; Friedlander, Martin, and Vahle-Hinz 1985) the type-I competition is likely to continue postnatally, and axons that have already settled in their appropriate laminae may be stimulated to behave abnormally if attracted into adjacent territories by the presence of (abnormal) denervated geniculate cells or, more specifically, by an abnormally high concentration of trophic substances. The important issue is to distinguish between a normal terminal topography that is produced by competitive interactions and one that is produced by site specific cues; the experiment under consideration does not address this issue.

Had the experimental eye removal been done at an earlier, prenatal stage the interpretation of the result would have been more difficult, because at the time of the experiment the two sets of terminals would have been overlapping. The removal of one set of afferents, followed during the subsequent development by the occupation of all surviving geniculate territory by the other, could then easily have been taken as evidence for type-II competition occurring in normal development (e.g. Rakic 1981, 1986). However, formally, the two experiments, the early and the late enucleation, are similar; we cannot tell in either case whether the severe nature of the denervation experiment has produced an abnormal situation which stimulated growth of the surviving axons on the basis of type-I competition, or whether the denervation revealed a normally occurring type-II competition.

There are many experiments in which an increase in terminal distribution, axon numbers, or perikaryal numbers of one retinofugal component can be produced by removal of the other component early in development (e.g. Lund, Cunningham, and Lund 1973; Land and Lund 1979; Godement, Saillour, and Imbert 1980; Rakic and Riley 1983; Williams *et al.* 1983; Chalupa, Williams, and Henderson 1984; Insausti, Blakemore, and Cowan 1984, 1985; Jeffery 1984; Campbell, So, and Lieberman 1985; Guillery, La Mantia, Robson, and Huang 1985). There are closely comparable experiments in other systems (e.g. Liestal, Maehlen, and Nja 1986), including interactions between identified single neurons in invertebrates (Murphey and Lemere 1984). The commonly held view that this increase, *in itself*, represents evidence for competition can only be accepted in the limited sense that it is type-I competition or experimentally induced type-II competition. The experiments provide no strong evidence about the role that competition may play during normal development in the topographical segregation of the two components.

A recent modification of this experimental design uses blockade with TTX of one retinofugal component instead of removal of one eye. Thus, in rats, Cowan *et al.* (1984) and Fawcett, O'Leary, and Cowan (1985) have described an increased cell survival in the normal, unblocked retinotectal pathway (however, see Holt and Thompson 1984). To the extent that TTX blockage produces a less severe, non-competitive change at the terminal site than does monocular enucleation, these experiments can be considered to provide stronger evidence in favour of a competitive interaction. However, the experiments need to be evaluated in terms of the severity of the non-competitive damage or retardation produced by the TTX alone. There is evidence that TTX modifies axonal transport (Edwards and Grafstein 1986) and that retinogeniculate terminals fail to develop normally when retinal ganglion cells are exposed to TTX. This evidence comes from a study (Kalil,

Dubin, and Scott 1986) showing that retinogeniculate terminals fail to mature normally when retinal ganglion cells are exposed to TTX in new-born kittens. This retardation is seen in one set of geniculate layers even though normal retinogeniculate terminals (in adjacent layers) coming from an untreated eye fail to invade the abnormal layers; that is, the developmental retardation cannot readily be ascribed to competition. TTX, like enucleation, must be regarded as having a significant, non-competitive action on the growth of retinofugal axons and therefore, may not represent a significant advance over enucleation as an experimental technique for evaluation competitive interactions between retinofugal axons.

CHANGES PRODUCED IN THE GENICULOCORTICAL PATHWAYS BY MONOCULAR VISUAL DEPRIVATION

When one eyelid is sutured early in the post-natal life of a cat or a monkey, a number of changes occur, and these can be seen as reflecting the disturbance of a normal competitive balance within the developing geniculocortical pathways. One important point that distinguishes monocular deprivation from deafferentation is the severity of the experimental manipulation. Another is that the effects produced by the deprivation itself can be distinguished from those produced by the changed competitive balance. The present discussion will be largely limited to cats and will focus on two quite distinct types of change. One reflects an interaction between the crossed and the uncrossed pathways in each hemisphere, and the other reflects an interaction between two of the functionally distinct pathways (X and Y) that arise from each eye.

Binocular interactions

In a cat, an early monocular deprivation produces changes in the visual cortex (area 17) and in the lateral geniculate nucleus (summarized in Hubel and Wiesel 1977; Sherman and Spear 1982). In the cortex the normal pattern of binocular input fails to develop. Cortical cells that can be activated mainly by stimuli delivered to the deprived eye are abnormally rare and, correspondingly, the ocular dominance columns demonstrable by electrophysiological or autoradiographic methods appear to be abnormally small for the deprived eye and large for the normal eye. In the lateral geniculate nucleus the layers that are innervated by the deprived eye develop cells that are abnormally small, while those innervated by the normal eye develop cells that are larger than normal. Further, while the cat responds normally to visual stimulation of the normal eye, visual performance with the deprived eye (after lid opening) is grossly abnormal. In terms of many details, especially as regards the early development of the changes, or their reversibility, the situation is more complex, but, for the purpose of considering possible competitive interactions, the changes outlined above are crucial.

It can be seen that the changes described are in accord with the definition suggested for type-II competition. They show the ocular segregation seen above in the dually innervated tectum, but, in addition, they show the clear reduction of one component at the expense of the other. One only needs to ask whether these cortical changes represent a naturally occurring type-II competition or one that has been induced experimentally. At this point a comparison with the geniculate changes produced by an early monocular enucleation is instructive. Whereas the enucleation itself produces major structural and functional changes that cannot be ascribed to competition (the loss and degeneration of retinogeniculate synapses), it can be shown that the monocular deprivation produces only relatively mild changes other than those due to the competition. In a monocularly deprived animal the effects of deprivation itself and of competition can, in fact, be directly compared. In the binocular segment of the geniculocortical pathway, which views the binocular segment of the visual field, and within which competition between the pathways innervated by the left and the right eye is possible, one sees the changes summarized above. In contrast, in the monocular segment, there are fewer changes: cortical cells can still be activated from the deprived eye, geniculate cells show only a mild loss of normal growth, and, if tested appropriately, a cat will respond to visual stimuli in the monocular segment of the visual field of the deprived eye even though it fails to respond in the binocular segment (Guillery and Stelzner 1970; Sherman 1973, 1974; Sherman, Guillery, Kaas, and Sanderson 1974).

Since the monocular segment of the retina is also peripheral it can be argued that this monocular 'sparing' does not relate specifically to the absence of competition, but reflects a difference between parts of the pathway representing peripheral and central parts of the retina. However, the production of an artificial monocular segment by a limited lesion in a more central binocular segment of the non-deprived eye shows that any monocular segment within the geniculocortical pathways, whether artificial or natural, shows the sparing described above in terms of geniculate cell growth, activation of cortical cells, and visual behaviour (Guillery 1972b; Sherman et al. 1974).

In so far as the changes that are seen when competition can play a role are not seen when competition must be absent, one is led to the reasonable, but not entirely unavoidable, conclusion that competition between geniculocortical axons for cortical synaptic space (or trophic factors) also occurs in normal development. The argument that the mild changes produced by the deprivation itself initiate a competitive interaction that does not occur normally is unappealing, but is also unanswerable in the absence of clear knowledge of the cellular and molecular mechanisms of the competition.

The normal pattern of development of the geniculo cortical axons, whose terminals are initially overlapping, at least as demonstrated by the trans-neuronal transport of labelled axonal markers (Rakic 1977; Le Vay, Stryker, and Shatz 1978), and which separate out during development, can also be taken to support the view that a competitive interaction occurs normally. If there were no demonstrable stage of overlap, competition would be ruled out as a reasonable hypothesis unless one were willing to entertain a novel form of competition at a distance. However, it should be stressed that the evidence for overlap is still only indirect (trans-neuronal transport or recording from cortical cells whose geniculate activation is not necessarily monosynaptic) and that an early transient overlap is not itself sufficient evidence for competition. Non-competitive interactions could produce the same developmental sequence, and in other systems such as the retinogeniculate they probably do. The point is considered further below.

Interactions between X- and Y-cell pathways

The discussion so far, together with most accounts of binocular interactions, has assumed a uniform population of retinofugal axons all with the same developmental sequence and the same competitive interactions. However, it is clear that in a cat's visual pathways different classes of retinal ganglion cell develop at different times (Walsh, Polley, Hickey, and Guillery 1983; Walsh and Polley 1985) and their axons react differently in response to monocular deprivation (Sur, Humphrey, and Sherman 1982) or enucleation (Garraghty, Sur, and Sherman 1986a, Garraghty, Sur, Weller, and Sherman 1986b). The X- and the Y-cell pathways have been studied in most detail (for the structural and functional distinctions of these pathways, see Lennie 1980, Sherman and Spear 1982, Rodieck and Brening 1983; Stone 1983; Sherman 1985a). It has been shown that X-cells are formed earlier in the retina (Walsh et al. 1983) and develop their terminal arbors in the lateral geniculate nucleus earlier (Sur et al. 1984). Further, wheras the geniculate cells that are innervated by X-cells show little change in response to visual deprivation, a significant loss of geniculate cells is produced in the Y pathway (Sherman, Hoffmann, and Stone 1972; Sherman and Spear 1982). Recent investigations (Friedlander, Stanford, and Sherman 1982; Sur et al. 1982, 1984), in which geniculate cells were first studied electrophysiologically so that their functional characterization in terms of X- or Y-like properties could be defined, and were then filled intracellularly with horse-radish peroxidase for subsequent morphological study, have shown not only that the X and the Y pathways behave differently in terms of possible binocular interactions, but also that the X and Y pathways may themselves be competing with each other.

In the normal cat the major geniculate layers (the A layers) are innervated by X and Y retinal ganglion cells. Any one geniculate cell generally receives its predominant input from either the X or the Y pathway, so that the geniculate cells in the normal A layers can be regarded as either X cells or Y cells (Friedlander, Lin, Stanford, and Sherman 1981). After monocular depriva-

nucleus (Linden *et al* 1981) and the crossed outnumber the uncrossed fibres in all parts of the nucleus, even in those destined to be occupied by uncrossed terminals only.

While an explanation on the basis of competition alone might account for the characteristic laminar sequence in carnivores, where crossed and uncrossed innervations alternate, it would be difficult to extend such an explanation to monkeys, in which two layers with uncrossed innervations lie adjacent to each other, to tree shrews, where one finds three adjacent layers all receiving a crossed innervation, or to *Galago* (bush baby), where three ipsilaterally innervated layers are adjacent (see Kaas, Guillery, and Allman 1972; Kaas, Huerta, Weber, and Harting 1978; Itoh, Conley, and Diamond 1982). It is simpler to suppose that the sequence of geniculate layers, with each having a characteristic monocular innervation and architecture, is determined by an intrinsic developmental programme not itself dependent upon competitive interactions.

This view of geniculate development is reinforced by studies of the geniculate structures that form in ferrets or mink under the influence of only a monocular input. In contrast to monkeys, where the difference between the crossed and the uncrossed components is small in normal animals, and where the asymmetry of the nuclei that develop in a monocular animal is minor (Rakic 1981), mustelids show a more marked asymmetry normally and after a monocular enucleation (Guillery *et al.* 1985). If one eye is removed very early in development, either before the retinal innervation of the nucleus or before the formation of distinguishable geniculate layers, then the nucleus that develops under the influence of only the crossed input differs significantly from the one that develops in relation to the uncrossed input. Comparable observations have recently been made in cats (Sretavan and Shatz 1986). The two nuclei differ in size, in the architectonic borders that separate the lateral geniculate cells from adjacent nuclei, and in the details of laminar structure. Only the side in receipt of a crossed input develops a magnocellular C layer; this corresponds to the situation in a normal animal where there is no ipsilaterally innervated counterpart to the magnocellular C layer. That is, each retinogeniculate component, the crossed and the uncrossed, is programmed to relate to a particular type of geniculate architectonic organization. This aspect of geniculate development is not influenced by any binocular competitive interactions. It must depend upon site specific markers. The claim that the retinogeniculate axons of a monocular animal have a laminar distribution apparently replicating the eye specific layers seen in a normal animal (Sretavan and Shatz 1986) also leads to the conclusion that geniculate markers must be playing a role in the laminar arrangement of retinal terminals. However, the distinction established between one set of retinogeniculate axons and another in a monocular animal that allows such a replica of the binocular arrangement to develop is obscure. I have shown that there is no compelling evidence for any competitive interactions in geniculate development since the effects of monocular enucleation can be interpreted in other ways. Once one recognizes the necessity for site specific markers, competitive interactions begin to look superfluous.

The differences between the developmental capacities of the X and the Y pathways summarized above also hint at an intrinsic, non-competitive programme for the formation of geniculate layers. The translaminar sprouting that was described earlier has recently been shown to involve Y cells but not X cells (Garraghty *et al.* 1986*a*, 1986*b*). The evidence available suggests that X cells do not sprout under any circumstances but are limited to their 'appropriate' lamina no matter what the potentially competing X cells from the other eye are doing. It is as though the earliest arriving retinogeniculate axons (the axons of retinal X cells) are firmly committed to a particular geniculate layer by an intrinsic label and only later arrivals have the freedom to demonstrate a competitive capacity by extending across laminar borders into denervated zones, should these become available.

The distribution of the geniculocortical pathways

In contrast to the development of geniculate layers, which depends largely upon topographically specified programmes, the development of ocular dominance columns in the cortex may depend to a major extent upon competitive interactions. Although the columns tend to lie perpendicular to the border between cortical areas 17 and 18, and to have a relatively constant width for any one species, (Hubel, Wiesel, and LeVay 1977; LeVay *et al.* 1980), these are features that can be taken as representing the ground rules for the competition. They do not require independent topographic clues that specify particular portions of a cortical area for one input or the other. It may be appropriate to think of the normal cortical columns as comparable to the tectal columns of three-eyed frogs, where the topography of the recipient tissue contributes little or nothing to the final distribution of the competing afferent components. It is the lack of a *known* constancy of topography of the ocular dominance columns (seen in terms of their position rather than their size or orientation) that helps to convince us that we are dealing with a normally occurring competitive interaction, although, as has been shown, the most convincing evidence comes from studies of monocular deprivation.

The origin of the retinofugal pathways

In a normal adult, non-primate mammal essentially all of the ganglion cells in the nasal retina send their axons to the contralateral hemisphere. In the temporal retina some cells send their axons to the ipsilateral hemisphere and others to the contralateral hemisphere. (In primates, essentially all temporal ganglion cells have uncrossed axons.) The evidence for the mechanisms producing this pattern of projection is limited, but it appears that at early stages there must be topographical clues related to retinal position that lead

Hickey, T. L. (1975). Translaminar growth of axons in the kitten dorsal lateral geniculate nucleus following removal of one eye. *J. Comp. Neurol.* **161,** pp. 359–82.

Hollyday, M. and Hamburger, V. (1976). Reduction of the naturally occurring motor neuron loss by the enlargement of the periphery. J. Comp. Neurol. **170,** pp. 311–20.

Holt, C. E. and Thompson, I. D. (1984). The effects of tetrodotoxin on the development of hamster retinal projections. *J. Physiol. (Lond.)* **357,** p. 24P.

Hubel, D. H. and Wiesel, T. N. (1977). Functional architecture of macaque monkey visual cortex. *Proc. R. Soc. Lond. B* **198,** pp. 1–59.

Hubel, D. H., Wiesel, T. N., and Le Vay, S. (1977). Plasticity of ocular dominance columns in monkey striate cortex. *Phil. Trans. R. Soc. Lond. B* **278,** pp. 377–409.

Huerta, M. F. and Harting, J. K. (1983). The mammalian superior colliculus: studies of its morphology and connections. In *The comparative neurology of the optic tectum* (ed. H Vanegas), pp. 687–773. Plenum Press, New York.

Hughes, A. (1975). A quantitative analysis of the cat retinal ganglion cell topography. *J. Comp Neurol.* **163,** pp. 107–28.

Hughes, A. and Wässle, H. (1976). The cat optic nerve: fibre total count and diameter spectrum. *J. Comp. Neurol.* **169,** pp. 171–84.

Insausti, R., Blakemore, C., and Cowan, W. M. (1984). Ganglion cell death during development of ipsilateral retino-collicular projection in golden hamster. *Nature* **308,** pp. 362–5.

Insausti, R., Blakemore, C., and Cowan, W. M. (1985). Postnatal development of the ipsilateral retino-collicular projection and the effects of unilateral enucleation in the golden hamster. *J. Comp. Neurol.* **234,** pp. 393–409.

Itoh, K., Conley, M., and Diamond, I. T. (1982). Retinal ganglion cell projection to individual layers of the lateral geniculate body in *Galago crassicaudatus. J. Comp. Neurol.* **205,** pp. 282–90.

Jeffery, G. (1984). Retinal ganglion cell death and terminal field retraction in the developing rodent. *Dev. Brain Res.* **13,** pp. 81–96.

Jeffery, G., Cowey, A., and Kuypers, H. G. J. M. (1981). Bifurcating retinal ganglion cell axons in the rat, demonstrated by retrograde double labelling. *Exp. Brain Res.* **44,** pp. 34–40.

Kaas, J. H., Guillery, R. W., and Allman, J. H. (1972). Some principles of organization in the dorsal lateral geniculate nucleus. *Brain Behav. Evol.* **6,** pp. 253–99.

Kaas, J. H., Huerta, K. F., Weber, J. T., and Harting, J. K. (1978). Patterns of retinal terminations and laminar organization of the lateral geniculate nucleus of primates. *J. Comp. Neurol.* **182,** pp. 517–54.

Kalil, R. E. (1973). Formation of new retinogeniculate connections in kittens: effect of age and visual experience. *Anat. Rec.* **175,** p. 353.

Kalil, R. E., Dubin, M. W., and Scott, G. (1986). Elimination of action potentials blocks the structural development of retinogeniculate synapses. *Nature* **323,** pp. 156–8.

Land, P. W. and Lund, R. D. (1979). Development of the rat's uncrossed pathway and its relationship to plasticity studies. *Science* **205,** pp. 698–700.

Law, M. and Constantine-Paton, M. (1980). Right and left eye bands in frogs with unilateral tectal ablations. *Proc. Natl. Acad. Sci. USA.* **77,** pp. 2314–18.

Law, M. and Constantine-Paton, M. (1981). Anatomy and physiology of experimentally produced striped tecta. *J. Neurosci.* **1,** pp. 741–59.

Lennie, P. (1980). Parallel visual pathways. *Vision Res.* **20,** pp. 561–94.

Le Vay, S. and McConnell, S. K. (1982). On and off layers in the lateral geniculate nucleus of the mink. *Nature* **300**, pp. 350–1.

Le Vay, S., Stryker, M. P., and Shatz, C. J. (1978). Ocular dominance columns and their development in layer IV of the cat's visual cortex: a quantitative study. *J. Comp. Neurol.* **179**, pp. 223–44.

Le Vay, S., Wiesel, T. N. and Hubel, D. H. (1980). The development of ocular dominance columns in normal and visually deprived monkeys. *J. Comp. Neurol.* **191**, pp. 1–51.

Levine, R. and Jacobson, M. (1975). Discontinuous mapping of retina into tectum innervated by both eyes. *Brain Res.* **98**, pp. 172–6.

Liestl, K., Maehlen, J., and Nja, A. (1986). Selective synaptic connections: significance of recognition and competition in mature sympathetic ganglia. *Trends Neurosci.* **9**, pp. 21–4.

Linden, D. C., Guillery, R. W., and Cucchiaro, J. (1981). The dorsal lateral geniculate nucleus of the normal ferret and its postnatal development. *J. Comp. Neurol.* **203**, pp. 189–211.

Linden, R. and Perry, V. H. (1982). Ganglion cell death within the developing retina: a regulatory role for retinal dendrites? *Neuroscience* **7**, pp. 2813–27.

Linden, R. and Serfaty, C. A. (1985). Evidence for differential effects of terminal and dendritic competition upon developmental neuronal death in the retina. *Neuroscience* **15**, pp. 853–68.

Lund, R. D., Cunningham, T. J., and Lund, J. S. (1973). Modified optic projections after unilateral eye removal in young rats. *Brain Behav. Evol.* **8**, pp. 51–72.

Lund, R. D., Land, P. W., and Boles, J. (1980). Normal and abnormal uncrossed retinotectal pathways in rats: an HRP study in adults. *J. Comp. Neurol.* **189**, pp. 711–20.

Mason, C. A. (1982*a*). Development of terminal arbors of retinogeniculate axons in the kitten. I. Light microscopical observations. *Neuroscience* **2**, pp. 541–60.

Mason, C. A. (1982*b*). Development of terminal arbors of retinogeniculate axons in the kitten. II. Electron microscopical observations. *Neuroscience* **7**, pp. 561–82.

Meyer, R. L. (1982). Tetrodotoxin blocks the formation of ocular dominance columns in goldfish. *Science* **218**, pp. 589–91.

Meyer, R. L. (1983). The growth and formation of ocular dominance columns by deflected optic fibres in goldfish. *Dev. Brain Res.* **6**, pp. 293–8.

Morgan, J. E. (1986). The organization of the retinogeniculate pathways in normal and neonatally enucleated pigmented and albino ferrets. *PhD thesis,* University of Oxford, Oxford, UK.

Murphey, R. K. and Lemere, C. A. (1984). Competition controls the growth of an identified axonal arborization. *Science* **224**, pp. 1352–5.

Oppenheim, R. W. (1986). The absence of significant postnatal motoneuron death in the branchial and lumbar spinal cord of the rat. *J. Comp. Neurol.* **246**, pp. 281–6.

Prestige, M. and Willshaw, D. (1975). On a role for competition in the formation of patterned neural connections. *Proc. R. Soc. Lond. B* **190**, pp. 77–98.

Rakic, P. (1976). Prenatal genesis of connections subserving ocular dominance in the rhesus monkey. *Nature* **261**, pp. 467–71.

Rakic, P. (1977). Prenatal development of the visual system in rhesus monkey. *Phil. Trans. R. Soc. Lond. B* **278**, pp. 245–60.

Rakic, P. (1981). Development of visual centers in the primate brain depends on binocular competition before birth. *Science* **214**, pp. 928–31.

Rakic, P. (1986). Mechanism of ocular dominance segregation in the lateral geniculate nucleus: competitive elimination hypothesis. *Trends Neurosci.* **9**, pp. 11–15.

Rakic, P. and Riley, K. P. (1983). Regulation of axon number in primate optic nerve by binocular competition. *Nature* **305**, pp. 135–7.

Reh, T. and Constantine-Paton, M. (1985). Eye-specific segregation requires neural activity in three-eyed *Rama pipiens*. *J. Neurosci.* **5**, pp. 1132–43.

Robson, J. A., Mason, C. A., and Guillery, R. W. (1978). Terminal arbors of axons that have formed abnormal connections. *Science* **201**, pp. 635–7.

Rodieck, R. W. and Brening, R. K. (1983). Retinal ganglion cells: properties, types, genera, pathways and trans-species comparisons. *Brain Behav. Evol.* **23**, pp. 121–64.

Schmidt, J. T. and Thieman, S. B. (1985). Eye-specific segregaton of optic afferents in mammals, fish, and frogs: the role of activity. *Cell. Mol. Neurobiol.* **5**, pp. 5–34.

Shatz, C. J. (1983). The prenatal development of the cat's retinogeniculate pathway. *J. Neurosci.* **3**, pp. 482–99.

Sherman, S. M. (1973). Visual field defects in monocularly and binocularly deprived cats. *Brain Res.* **49**, pp. 25–45.

Sherman, S. M. (1974). Permanence of visual field perimetry deficits in monocularly and binocularly deprived cats. *Brain Res.* **73**, pp. 491–501.

Sherman, S. M. (1985a). Functional organization of the W-, X-, and Y-cell pathways: a review and hypothesis. In *Progress in psychobiology and physiological psychology, Vol. II* (eds J. M. Sprague and A. N. Epstein), pp. 233–314. Academic Press, New York.

Sherman, S. M. (1985b). Development of retinal projections to the cat's lateral geniculate nucleus. *Trends Neurosci.* **8**, pp. 350–5.

Sherman, S. M. and Spear, P. D. (1982). Organization of the visual pathways in normal and visually deprived cats. *Physiol. Rev.* **62**, pp. 738–855.

Sherman, S. M., Hoffmann, K. -P., and Stone, J. (1972). Loss of a specific cell type from dorsal lateral geniculate nucleus in visually deprived cats. *J. Neurophysiol.* **35**, pp. 532–41.

Sherman, S. M., Guillery, R. W., Kaas, J. H., and Sanderson, K. J. (1974). Behavioral, electrophysiological and morphological studies of binocular competition in the development of the geniculocortical pathways of cats. *J. Comp. Neurol.* **158**, 1–18.

Sohal, G. S., Stoney, S. D., Arumugam, T., Yamashita, Y., and Knox, T. S. (1986). Influence of reduced neuron pool on the magnitude of naturally occurring motor neuron death. *J. Comp. Neurol.* **247**, pp. 516–28.

Sretavan, D. W. and Shatz, C. J. (1986). Prenatal development of cat retinogeniculate axon arbors in the absence of binocular interactions. *J. Neurosci.* **6**, pp. 990–1003.

Stent, G. S. (1973). A physiological mechanism for Hebb's postulate of learning. *Proc. Natl. Acad. Sci. USA* **70**, pp. 997–1001.

Stone, J. (1978). The number and distribution of ganglion cells in the cat's retina. *J. Comp. Neurol.* **124**, pp. 337–52.

Stone, J. (1983). *Parallel processing in the visual system*. Plenum Press, New York.

Stone, J. and Campion, J. E. (1978). Estimate of the number of myelinated axons in the cat's optic nerve. *J. Comp. Neurol.* **180**, pp. 799–806.

Stryker, M. P. and Zahs, K. R. (1983). On and off sublaminae in the lateral geniculate nucleus of the ferret. *J. Neurosci.* **3**, 1943–51.

Sulston, J. and White, J. G. (1980). Regulation and cell autonomy during postembryonic development of *Caenorhabditis elegans*. *Dev. Biol.* **78**, 577–97.

Sur, M., Humphrey, A. L., and Sherman, S. M. (1982). Monocular deprivation affects X- and Y- cell retino geniculate terminations in cats. *Nature* **300,** pp. 183–5.

Sur, M., Weller, R. E, and Sherman, S. M. (1984). Development of X- and Y-cell retinogeniculate terminations in kittens. *Nature* **310,** pp. 246–9.

Tigges, M. and Tigges, J. (1970). The retinofugal fibers and their terminal nuclei in *Galago crassicaudatus* (primates). *J. Comp. Neurol.* **138,** pp. 87–102.

Walsh, C. and Polley, E. H. (1985). The topography of ganglion cell production in the cat's retina. *J. Neurosci.* **5,** pp. 741–50.

Walsh, C., Polley, E. H., Hickey, T. L., and Guillery, R. W. (1983). Generation of cat retinal ganglion cells in relation to central pathways. *Nature* **302,** pp. 611–4.

Whitelaw, V. A. and Cowan, J. D. (1981). Specificity and plasticity of retinotectal connections: a computational model. *J. Neurosci.* **1,** pp. 1369–87.

Williams, R. W., Bastiani, M. J., and Chalupa, L. M. (1983). Loss of axons in the cat optic nerve following fetal unilateral enucleation: an electron microscopical analysis. *J. Neurosci.* **3,** pp. 133–44.

19

Activity-dependent sharpening of the retinotopic projection on the tectum of goldfish in regeneration and development

JOHN T. SCHMIDT

Because much of the brain contains maps of body surfaces and of visual and auditory space, the developmental mechanisms responsible for the formation of such maps have been topics of great interest. The most intensively studied map, the direct retinal projection to the optic tectum of fish and frogs, can be studied both during development in the embryo and during regeneration of the optic nerve in the adult. The central question is: How does each ingrowing retinal fibre select its correct termination site in the tectum?

Hypothesized mechanisms for retinotopic ordering can be grouped into three classes: (1) differential chemospecific adhesion between retinal fibres and tectal cells (Sperry 1943, 1963; Bonhoeffer and Huf 1982); (2) fibre self-ordering and pathway interactions *en route* to the tectum (Horder and Martin 1977; Schmidt 1982; Stuermer and Easter 1984; Bonhoeffer and Huf 1985); (3) activity-dependent stabilization of a retinotopic pattern after a diffuse early innervation (Willshaw and von der Malsburg 1976; Meyer 1983; Schmidt and Edwards 1983). In this chapter, I will briefly review the evidence that the first two mechanisms are capable of forming only a crude map; then I will review in more detail the evidence that the third mechanism serves to sharpen the retinotectal map and probably also many other topographic maps.

CHEMO-AFFINITY MECHANISMS HAVE LIMITED RESOLUTION

The earliest suggested mechanism is a selective chemo-affinity of each retinal fibre for appropriate tectal cells, based upon the position of the ganglion cell in the retina and the tectal cell in the tectum. Sperry (1943) initially postulated general biochemical gradients across the tectum, but later made his interpretation much more rigid by postulating unique surface markers for each cell (Sperry 1963). Unique markers appeared to be supported by the anatomical experiments of Attardi and Sperry (1963), who used a modified silver stain to study the pathways and termination sites of optic fibres that regenerated from a half-retina. They reported that the optic fibres grew back selectively to their original sites, even if they had to bypass open sites *en route*. More modern methods have not upheld this finding (see next section). Further evidence against the notion of unique markers came in experiments demonstrating dramatic plastic rearrangements made by the projection either following surgical intervention (reviewed by Schmidt 1982) or during normal development (reviewed by Easter 1983).

Surgically induced reorganizations include the compression of the full projection onto a half tectum, and the expansion of a half-retinal projection over the full tectum. In both cases, retinotopic order is maintained even though each retinal fibre terminates at a different tectal site than it normally does. These movements of arbors can be made consistent with relative preferences if one postulates a competition between retinal fibres for tectal sites so that optic fibres could be made to occupy lesser preferred sites (Schmidt 1982). Recently, we have been staining optic arbors following compression onto a half tectum and find evidence both for the movement of arbors and for heightened competition (Fig. 19.1). The arbors were found to be generally smaller than normal with fewer branch endings and terminal swellings. This was predicted during compression because synaptic counts per unit area in an electron micrographic study were found to remain constant so that, with the double density of pre-synaptic arbors, each arbor could have only half its normal number (Murray and Edwards 1982). In addition, the trajectories of the axons, which normally proceed from rostral to caudal, very frequently looped back on themselves, furnishing evidence that the arbors had moved from caudal to more rostral sites during compression (Fig. 19.1).

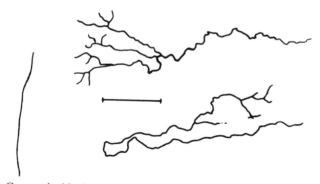

Fig. 19.1. Camera lucida drawings of a normal optic arbor (top, small class) and of a corresponding arbor (bottom) from a compressed half-tectal projection. Caudal is to the left. Note how the normal arbor grows caudally giving off branches, while the arbor from the compressed projection (18 months post-surgery) doubles back on its parent axon. This reflects the movement of the arbor rostrally to accommodate caudal arbors near the edge of the lesion (line at far left). Scale bar: 100 μm.

During development in fish and frogs, similar movements of optic arbors occur, but always in a rostral to caudal direction, because of the disparate geometric growth patterns of the retina and tectum (Easter 1983; Stuermer this volume, Chapter 11). The movements of the optic arbors imply a continual changing of post-synaptic partners. These movements, as well as the surgically induced rearrangements, are consistent with general chemo-affinity gradients (which may in fact be necessary to orientate the projection), but they are not consistent with unique positional markers on the tectum.

Clearly, factors other than chemospecific fibre-target interactions must contribute to the precision of these retinotopic maps. A second mechanism is selective fibre-fibre chemo-affinity, which could maintain the relative ordering of retinal fibres in the pre-synaptic array (Horder and Martin 1977; Schmidt 1982; Bonhoeffer and Huf 1985). Stuermer and Easter (1984) studied the degree of order in both normal and regenerated optic pathways in goldfish using horseradish-peroxidase (HRP) staining. The normal pathway is highly ordered, and undergoes several reorganizations along the way to the tectum. Normally, where the optic tract bifurcates, the fibres from dorsal retina all go ventrally and those from ventral retina all go dorsally. After regeneration, however, approximately one fibre in five enters through the wrong branch. This ratio of correct to incorrect pathways shows that pathway interactions may play some role in organizing the projection, but many mistakes are left to be corrected after entry into the tectum.

EARLY DIFFUSE PROJECTIONS IN REGENERATION

Anatomical studies

Many experiments demonstrate mistakes in the zone of tectal innervation. Meyer (1980) used autoradiography instead of silver staining to trace the projection from a partial retina, and determined that at least half of the retina would have to be removed to create any denervated zone in the tectum. Thus the regenerated projection was much more diffuse than normal. Both Stuermer and Easter (1984) and Rankin and Cook (1986) showed this same diffuseness by making punctate injections of HRP both in normal tecta and in tecta after regeneration. Normally the ganglion cells that are retrogradely labelled through their terminals are confined to a small retinal area. Early in regeneration, however, labelled cells were scattered over the entire retina with only a slight preponderance in the correct half. After two months or more, the labelled ganglion cells were once again compactly clustered, much as in the normal tecta (Rankin and Cook 1986).

These diffuse projections could result either from greatly enlarged individual optic arbors or from errors in targeting of individual regenerated arbors of normal size, or from a mixture of the two. In the newt, Fujisawa,

Tani, Watanabe, and Ibata (1982) were the first to stain regenerated optic arbors with HRP and to view them in tectal whole-mounts. The regenerated fibres often took aberrant paths into and through the tectum, and also made many branches in inappropriate tectal areas. We have used similar techniques in goldfish (Schmidt, Buzzard, and Turcotte 1984). Normal optic arbors range in size from 100 to 400 μm across (average of 217 μm), but early in regeneration many optic arbors make greatly enlarged arbors that are often more than two millimetres across (average of 1200 μm) but sparsely branched (Fig. 19.2). As time progresses, the arbors shrink back to their normal size, but the paths of the regenerated fibres often remain abnormal (see also Stuermer 1987, this volume).

In parallel studies of development, there is some evidence that early projections also tend to be diffuse in *Xenopus* (Sakuguchi and Murphey 1985), chick (McLoon 1982), rat (Fawcett and O'Leary 1985), and hamster (Schneider, Rava, Sachs, and Jhaveri 1981).

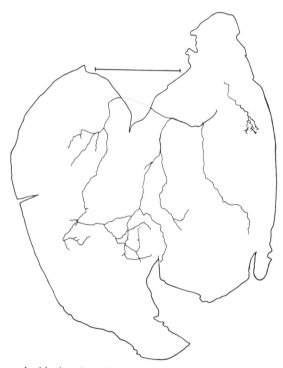

Fig. 19.2. Camera lucida drawing of a regenerated optic arbor, stained with HRP at 21 days after nerve crush, showing the widespread branching. The heavy lines at the outside mark the boundaries of the tectum, which was split both rostrally and caudally to allow it to lie flat. A normal optic arbor is shown for comparison. Scale bar: 1 mm. [Reproduced from Schmidt (1985) by kind permission of Plenum Press, New York.]

Electrophysiological studies

In the case of the goldfish, electrophysiological recordings during this early diffuse phase are difficult because the responses fatigue extremely rapidly. The earliest recordings at 34 days post-crush show maps that are already normal in organization. In the frog, however, the sharpening of the map can be followed with the electrophysiological mapping technique (Humphrey and Beazley 1982; Adamson, Burke, and Grobstein 1984). At 4–6 weeks, recording at each tectal point yielded many units responding to stimulation of a wide area of the visual field. This area is called a multiunit receptive field, and its large size indicates that only a very crude level of retinotopic organization was present on the tectum. Over the next 20–30 days, these large responsive areas shrunk to the normal size. In addition to the direct retinotectal projection, frogs also have an intertectal relay through the Nucleus Isthmi that is easily recorded. This relay allowed Adamson *et al.* (1984) to assess the post-synaptic effects of the crudely organized retinotopic projection. Early in regeneration, the receptive fields of single relay fibres in the normal tectum were greatly enlarged, reflecting the crude map on the opposite tectum. Thus the misdirected arbors or branches of arbors within the crude map appeared to have established effective synaptic connections. We will see below in the studies of goldfish regeneration that effective synaptic transmission appears to be necessary for the sharpening to occur.

DIFFUSE MAP SHARPENED BY ACTIVITY DURING REGENERATION

Effects of blocking activity with tetrotodoxin

In adult goldfish, both anatomical (Meyer 1983) and electrophysiological (Schmidt and Edwards 1983) studies have demonstrated that the sharpening of the initially diffuse regenerated projection is dependent upon activity by blocking all activity with intraocular injections of tetrodotoxin (TTX). Meyer (1983) used auto-radiographic tracing and lesions to show that the regenerated projection remains diffuse when activity is blocked. Although blocking from 32–80 days post-crush prevented the return to a normal topography, the map could still sharpen if allowed a further 24 days of activity after the TTX was discontinued. Thus, in small goldfish, activity could still sharpen the map several months after the fibres reached the tectum.

Schmidt and Edwards (1983) used electrophysiological recording to assess the sharpening of retinotectal maps in large goldfish. In control fish, maps recorded at 35 days post-crush were already normal both in organization and in the size of the multiunit receptive fields, which averaged 11°. In projections blocked for the first 28 days, however, the multiunit receptive fields were greatly enlarged, averaging around 30° (Fig. 19.3). The centres of these enlarged fields were in the retinotopically appropriate region of the visual field, indicating that the gross organization of the map was correct. The enlarged multiunit receptive fields reflect the convergence onto each tectal point of arbors from retinal ganglion cells distributed over a wide area of retina. The tectal recordings yielded many units at each site, which, when isolated by amplitude, were found to have receptive fields of normal size and characteristics for individual ganglion cells (Fig. 19.3). Additional recording of single ganglion cells made in the retinae of these same fish supported this conclusion. Thus the enlarged multiunit receptive fields reflect errors in the targeting of regenerated arbors that are usually corrected with activity. This interpretation is consistent with the finding of many enlarged arbors early in regeneration, and the presence of enlarged multiunit receptive fields in the frog as a normal phase in regeneration. Preliminary results from HRP-stained optic fibres in our fish suggest that TTX may prevent the arbors from concentrating their branches, which remain scattered over a somewhat wider area than normal.

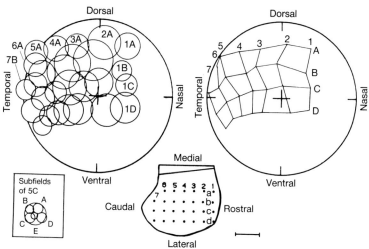

Fig. 19.3. Retinotectal map recorded 63 days after optic nerve crush in fish blocked intraocularly with TTX from 0–27 days. The two large circles are representations of the visual field that contain the outlines of the receptive fields and the positions of their centres. Below, electrode penetrations are marked on the drawing of the tectal surface. The receptive fields recorded at these points fall into an orderly array in the visual field similar to the array on the tectal surface and are numbered accordingly. The inset at the lower left diagrams the relationship between a multiunit receptive field and several of its single unit components, mapped separately with a spike height discriminator. Normally, the multiunit receptive fields are the size of single unit fields. Scale bar: 1 mm. [Reproduced from Schmidt and Edwards (1983) by kind permission of Elsevier, Amsterdam.]

A MODEL BASED ON CORRELATED ACTIVITY

The model

A proposed model for sharpening the map is based upon the correlated firing of neighbouring ganglion cells and the resultant summation of their excitatory post-synaptic potentials (EPSPs) in the post-synaptic tectal cells (Willshaw and von der Malsburg 1976; Schmidt and Edwards 1983). Neighbouring ganglion cells, which view the same part of the visual world, are likely to fire with a high degree of correlation if they are of the same type (e.g. ON or OFF; Ginsberg, Johnsen, and Levine 1984). Both Arnett (1978) and Ginsberg *et al.* (1984) have in fact demonstrated such correlations even in absolute darkness when only spontaneous activity is present. The model (Fig. 19.4) also assumes that the arbors in the initial diffuse projection are large, and have a high degree of overlap. For neighbouring ganglion cells having some overlap of their arbors and firing with a high degree of correlation, there would be a summation of the post-synaptic EPSPs. Finally, if the most effective synapses are differentially stabilized and retained (Hebb 1949; Changeux and Danchin 1976), then the correlated activity, resulting in larger EPSPs, would stabilize

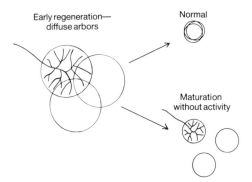

Fig. 19.4. Schematic diagram of the model for activity-dependent sharpening of the retinotectal map. On the left is the situation early in regeneration in which three neighbouring retinal ganglion cells have diffuse and inaccurately targeted arbors. Within the area of overlap, the three cells' synchronous firing would tend to stabilize their synapses more so than without. This would lead to a retraction of the other branches and a concentration of the arbors within the smaller area (see 'Normal' on right). The final arbor is depicted as smaller than that initially regenerated. Without activity, a similar retraction might take place, but the arbors would merely retract randomly towards their centres, leading to a loss of overlap and therefore a diminished capability for activity-dependent convergence later on. [Reproduced from Schmidt and Edwards (1983) by kind permission of Elsevier, Amsterdam.]

them in the region of overlap. Of course, arbors from distant ganglion cells would also overlap, but without correlated firing there would be no summation and no stabilization of those synaptic connections. Such a cue for convergence, therefore, would be specific to the arbors of neighbouring ganglion cells, because they would have correlated activity.

Without activity, the parent axon, because of a limited supply of axonally transported materials might be forced to retract branches randomly, and thereby fail to cluster its branches normally. Some retraction would explain why the sharpening that takes place after TTX wears off goes much slower, taking months to complete in the larger fish (Schmidt and Edwards 1983). It is not yet clear whether this difference with Meyer's (1983) report is due to the smaller size of his fish (which would imply a faster growing projection with more sliding of connections) or is merely due to differences in the methods of assessment.

Testing the model: strobe rearing

Recent experiments (Schmidt and Eisele 1985) have upheld the major features of this model. First, the model proposes that the sharpening would still be disrupted even if the ganglion cells were allowed activity as long as the strictly local correlation in firing of neighbouring ganglion cells is disrupted. Two methods were used: stroboscopic illumination and dark rearing. Stroboscopic illumination caused correlated firing in all ganglion cells, since single unit recordings from the retinae during regeneration showed that both 'OFF' cells and 'ON' cells fired one or two spikes at a constant latency after each flash. When all cells, not just near neighbours, fire in synchrony, correlated firing can no longer be a cue for finding neighbours from the retina. Projections regenerated under stroboscopic illumination, like those regenerated without activity, had enlarged multiunit receptive fields that averaged 33·2° in diameter (Fig. 19.5).

A recent anatomical study verified the finding that stroboscopic illumination prevents the sharpening of the retinotopic map. Cook and Rankin (1986) employed retrograde transport of HRP from a focal tectal injection to show that the labelled retinal ganglion cells remain scattered over a large area of retina at 70 days post-crush in fish exposed to stroboscopic illumination. In addition, our preliminary anatomical studies involving anterograde labelling of optic arbors suggest that strobe rearing may prevent the arbors from concentrating their branches into one area, as they do normally by this time.

Regeneration in total darkness also produced enlarged multi-unit receptive fields, averaging 28·7° in diameter. This is somewhat smaller than the average of 33·2° under strobe-light illumination or the 40° with the equivalent TTX block, and may reflect a slight degree of sharpening due to the correlation in the spontaneous activity of neighbouring ganglion cells (Arnett 1978). The

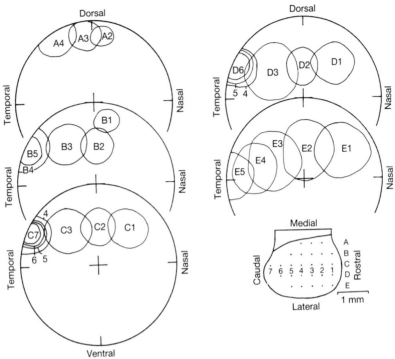

Fig. 19.5. Map of a retinotectal projection regenerated under stroboscopic illumination and recorded 55 days after nerve crush. At the lower right is a drawing of the tectal
surface viewed from above. Each point in the tectal array is an electrode penetration.
The receptive fields recorded at these points, although enlarged, fall into an orderly
array in the visual field similar to the array seen on the tectal surface and are numbered
accordingly. For clarity, five separate representations of the hemispherical visual field,
one for each row of points A through E on the tectum, are presented. Circles within the
visual field define the boundaries of the multiunit receptive fields. For convenience, the
drawing of the tectum has been inverted about one axis so that the arrays are oriented
in the same direction. [Reproduced from Schmidt and Eisele (1985) by kind permission
of Pergamon Press, Oxford.]

levels of spontaneous activity are very low in goldfish, but are relatively high in
rabbit and cat (Arnett 1978).

   The strobe and dark rearing experiments make unlikely the possibility that
the TTX effect upon sharpening was caused by the deficit in axonal transport
in regenerating optic fibres that was demonstrated by Edwards and Grafstein
(1983). The high and low levels of activity in the strobe and dark reared fish are
unlikely to be associated with similar decrements in axonal transport. The
experiments also show that sharpening depends upon the pattern of activity,
presumably the correlation in firing between neighbours in the retina.

Probable involvement of synaptic transmission

A second prediction from the model is that, in order for the synapses to be stabilized, the correlated activity must be transmitted to the post-synaptic tectal cell to allow summation of the EPSPs. To test this prediction, α-bungarotoxin (α-BTX) was used to decrease synaptic transmission during the period of early synaptogenesis (Schmidt 1985). An osmotic minipump was attached to the head of the fish to deliver a continuous infusion of α-BTX, previously shown to decrement retinotectal synaptic transmission (Freeman, Schmidt, and Oswald 1980). The resulting maps had enlarged multiunit receptive fields similar to those seen in the TTX-blocked, strobe reared and dark reared fish, averaging 28·5° in diameter. This experiment suggested that fibres with correlated activity may not interact directly, but rather through the transmission of their signals to the post-synaptic tectal cells, probably through the summation of EPSPs. At the present time, we cannot determine exactly what form of activity in the post-synaptic cell (whether EPSPs or spike activity) may be important in the stabilization of synaptic contacts, nor do we know the nature of the feedback to stabilize the pre-synaptic contact. This feedback might be direct or through feedback circuits either within the tectum or through the Nucleus Isthmi. Recent studies suggest that the Nucleus Isthmi may furnish cholinergic innervation that modulates retinotectal transmission (Ricciuti and Gruberg 1985) through nicotinic acetylcholine receptors located on pre-synaptic terminals of optic axons (Henley, Lindstrom, and Oswald 1986).

The sensitive period and synaptogenesis

The period of sensitivity corresponds to the period of synaptogenesis. The first synapses, as assessed by recording field potentials, were detectable on day 20 post-crush (Schmidt, Edwards, and Steurmer 1983). Neither blocking activity nor strobe illumination before this time (0–14 days) prevented the sharpening. Both treatments from 14–34 days, however, were extremely effective, producing enlarged fields averaging approximately 40°. Synaptogenesis probably continues at a declining rate until approximately 100 days post-crush, because counts of total synaptic density continue to increase until that time (Murray and Edwards 1982). Eisele and Schmidt (1985) have now assessed the effects of blocking activity and strobe illumination for two-week periods starting at later times (35, 50, 65, 80, 95, or 110 days post-crush). Results for the two treatments are virtually identical. Treatments imposed at 35 days cause the receptive fields, which had already sharpened, to become enlarged again. The size of this effect, however, becomes progressively smaller at later times, and no effect is seen in the mature projection, where synaptogenesis should be minimal. The results suggest a parallel between the rate at which synapses are added and the degree of disorder produced by disrupting normal patterns of activity.

Neither strobe illumination nor TTX appear to cause a decreased rate of synaptogenesis as judged by the field potentials elicited by optic nerve shock. A similar lack of effect of TTX was noted concerning neuromuscular synapse formation *in vitro* (Obata 1977). In the fish tectum, the amplitude of the field potentials from eyes blocked during regeneration was not decreased when they were recorded just after the block wore off (Schmidt *et al.* 1983). Similar results have now been obtained for strobe illumination. For the small field potentials in early regeneration, amplitude is likely to be a reasonably sensitive measure of the number of synapses formed. This result suggests that the manipulation of activity may not affect the number of synapses made, but instead may interfere with the deployment of the synapses in the retinotopically correct order.

Role of activity in development

To test the role of sharpening in development as well as in regeneration we recently reared newly hatched larval goldfish for more than a year under alternate 12-hour periods of darkness and stroboscopic illumination. The multiunit receptive fields of these one-year-old fish were enlarged to approximately the same degree as in the regenerates, demonstrating the relevance of this mechanism in the development of the retinotectal projection. Recently, Keating, Grant, Dawes, and Nancharal (1986) reported no effect of dark rearing on the development of the retinotectal projection in *Xenopus*. However, they examined only the multiunit receptive fields of event units (class III) which are normally large (21°), and not those of the smaller convexity or 'bug' detectors (class II). If the class-II multiunit receptive fields are shown to sharpen in the dark, then such sharpening might still be mediated by ongoing spontaneous activity, since spontaneous activity occurs at a much higher rate than in the goldfish. Otherwise, such a result, if found, could reflect real differences in the mechanisms employed by goldfish and *Xenopus*.

Activity and other projections

Several other central-nervous-system (CNS) maps are known to be sharpened, organized, or otherwise altered by activity-dependent mechanisms. In *Xenopus*, Keating (1975) has shown that the indirect retinotectal pathway, which relays information from the ipsilateral eye, can adjust itself, following rotation of one eye, to bring the maps from the two eyes into register. Dubin, Starke, and Archer (1986) have shown that the retinotopic map in the lateral geniculate nucleus of the cat is also sharpened by activity. In addition, they found that the segregation of receptive field types is also disrupted by intraocular TTX. The segregation of visual afferents into eye specific patches or stripes is activity dependent (Meyer 1982; Boss and Schmidt 1984; Reh and Constantine-Paton 1985; Stryker and Harris 1986), probably driven by the correlated activity of neighbouring ganglion cells within each eye but not between eyes. Also in the visual cortex, selection of neurons participating in the callosal connections may depend upon patterned visual activity, as a different subset remain connected when the animal is reared in the dark (Innocenti 1981, this volume, Chapter 16). Finally, in the auditory system of the owl, a tectal map of auditory space apparently aligns itself to the visual map already in place on the tectum via activity cues (Knudsen 1983).

The production and subsequent elimination of excess synaptic connections is also a familiar pattern outside the CNS, occurring in the autonomic ganglia (Purves and Lichtman 1980) and at the neuromuscular junction, where the elimination of polyneuronal innervation requires that pre-synaptic activity be transmitted to the post-synaptic muscle fibre (Thompson 1985).

CONCLUDING REMARKS

Activity-dependent mechanisms for the selective stabilization or elimination of the initially diffuse synaptic connections may represent a widespread phenomenon, occurring at all levels from the neuromuscular junction to the callosal connections between the cortices. Such mechanisms do not act alone, but in concert with the differential cell adhesion mechanisms commonly known as chemo-affinity. Activity-dependent stabilization of totally random synapses would not be able to generate the reproducibly oriented maps found in the nervous system. Instead, a random mix of retinal fibres would result either in randomly orientated maps or in 'mosaic' maps with occasional discontinuities (Willshaw and von der Malsburg 1976). Rather, the reproducible polarity must stem from the ability of differential affinity mechanisms to bring a greater number of temporal versus nasal retinal fibres to rostral tectum, and nasal fibres to caudal tectum, etc. On the other hand, a completely rigid developmental process (rigid chemo-affinity alone) might not be sufficiently flexible to succeed. Factors such as the variable geometry of the head, the separation between the eyes, between the ears, etc. might demand flexibility in the process of aligning the visual maps from the two eyes or aligning the auditory map with the visual maps. This can be accomplished economically through the initial elaboration of wider than normal arbors coupled with the stabilization of appropriate branches and the elimination of the others. A slightly less economical method is the death of those cells which grow arbors into inappropriate areas (again under control of activity), which apparently occurs sometimes in mammals (Fawcett and O'Leary 1985; Fawcett this volume, Chapter 20). These corrective mechanisms appear to play a prominent role in bringing the developing nervous system to the high level of order found in the adult.

REFERENCES

Adamson, J. R., Burke, J., and Grobstein, P. (1984). Re-establishment of the ipsilateral oculotectal projection after optic nerve crush in the frog: evidence for synaptic remodelling during regeneration. *J. Neurosci.* **4**, pp. 2635–49.

Arnett, D. W. (1978). Statistical dependence between neighbouring retinal ganglion cells in goldfish. *Exp. Brain Res.* **32**, pp. 49–53.

Attardi, D. G. and Sperry, R. W. (1963). Preferential selection of central pathways by regenerating optic fibers. *Exp. Neurol.* **7**, pp. 46–64.

Bonhoeffer, F. and Huf, J. (1982). *In vitro* experiments on axon guidance demonstrating an anterior-posterior gradient on the tectum. *EMBO J.* **1**, pp. 427–31.

Bonhoeffer, F. and Huf, J. (1985). Position-dependent properties of retinal axons and their growth cones. *Nature* **315**, pp. 409–10.

Boss, V. and Schmidt, J. T. (1984). Activity and the formation of ocular dominance patches in dually innervated tectum of goldfish. *J. Neurosci.* **4**, pp. 2891–905.

Changeux, J. P. and Danchin, A. (1976). Selective stabilization of developing synapses as a mechanism for the specification of neuronal networks. *Nature* **264**, pp. 705–12.

Cook, J. E. and Rankin, E. C. C. (1986). Impaired refinement of the regenerated retinotectal projection of the goldfish in stroboscopic light: a quantitative HRP study. *Exp. Brain Res.* **63**, pp. 421–30.

Dubin, M. W., Starke, L. A. and Archer, S. M. (1986). A role for action potential activity in the development of neuronal connections in the kitten retinogeniculate pathway. *J. Neurosci.* **6**, pp. 1021–36.

Easter, S. S. (1983). Postnatal neurogenesis and changing neuronal connections. *Trends Neurosci.* **6**, pp. 53–6.

Edwards, D. L. and Grafstein, B. (1983). Intraocular tetrodotoxin in goldfish hinders optic nerve regeneration. *Brain Res.* **269**, pp. 1–14.

Eisele, L. E. and Schmidt, J. T. (1985). Activity sharpens the regenerated retinotectal projection: sensitive period for strobe and TTX. *Neurosci. Abstr.* **11**, p. 101.

Fawcett, J. W. (1987). Retinotopic maps, cell death, and electrical activity in the retinotectal and retinocollicular projections. In *The making of the nervous system* (eds. J. G. Parnavelas, C. D. Stern, and R. V. Stirling), pp. 395–416 .Oxford University Press, Oxford.

Fawcett, J. W. and O'Leary, D. D. M. (1985). The role of electrical activity in the formation of topographic maps in the nervous system. *Trends Neurosci.* **8**, pp. 201–6.

Freeman, J. A., Schmidt, J. T., and Oswald, R. E. (1980). Effect of α-Bungarotoxin on retinotectal synaptic transmission in the goldfish and the toad. *Neuroscience* **5**, pp. 929–42.

Fujisawa, H., Tani, N., Watanabe, K., and Ibata, Y. (1982). Branching of regenerating retinal axons and preferential selection of appropriate branches for specific neuronal connection in the newt. *Dev. Biol.* **90**, pp. 43–57.

Ginsberg, K. S., Johnsen, J. A., and Levine, M. W. (1984). Common noise in the firing of neighbouring ganglion cells in goldfish retina. *J. Physiol. (Lond.)* **351**, pp. 433–44.

Hebb, D. O. (1949). *The organization of behavior.* John Wiley, New York.

Henley, J. M., Lindstrom, J. M., and Oswald, R. E. (1986). Acetylcholine receptor synthesis in retina and transport to optic tectum in goldfish. *Science* **232**, pp. 1627–9.

Horder, T. J. and Martin, K. A. C. (1977). Morphogenetics as an alternative to chemospecificity in the formation of nerve connections. In *Cell-cell recognition, 32 Symp. Soc. Exp. Biol.* (ed. A. S. G. Curtis), pp. 275–358. Cambridge University Press, Cambridge.

Humphrey, M. F. and Beazley, L. D. (1982). An electrophysiological study of early retinotectal projection patterns during optic nerve regeneration in *Hyla moorei. Brain Res.* **239,** pp. 595–602.

Innocenti, G. M. (1981). Growth and reshaping of axons in the establishment of visual callosal connections. *Science* **212,** pp. 824–6.

Innocenti, G. M. (1987). Loss of axonal projections in the development of the mammalian brain. In *The making of the nervous system* (eds. J. G. Parnavelas, C. D. Stern, and R. V. Stirling), pp. 319–40. Oxford University Press, Oxford.

Keating, M. J. (1975). The time course of experience dependent synaptic switching of visual connections in *Xenopus laevis. Proc. R. Soc. Lond. B* **189,** pp. 603–10.

Keating, M. J., Grant, S., Dawes, E. A., and Nanchanal, K. (1986). Visual deprivation of the retinotectal projection in *Xenopus laevis. J. Embryol. exp. Morphol.* **91,** pp. 101–15.

Knudsen, E. I. (1983). Early auditory experience aligns the auditory map of space in the optic tectum of the barn owl. *Science* **222,** pp. 939–41.

McLoon, S. (1982). Alterations in precision of the crossed retinotectal projection during chick development. *Science* **218,** pp. 1418–20.

Meyer, R. L. (1980). Mapping the normal and regenerating retinotectal project of goldfish with autoradiographic methods. *J. Comp. Neurol.* **189,** pp. 273–89.

Meyer, R. L. (1982). Tetrodotoxin blocks the formation of ocular dominance columns in goldfish. *Science* **218,** pp. 589–91.

Meyer, R. L. (1983). Tetrodotoxin inhibits the formation of refined retinotopography in goldfish. *Dev. Brain Res.* **6,** pp. 293–8.

Murray, M. and Edwards, M. A. (1982). A quantitative study of the reinnervation of the goldish optic tectum following optic nerve crush. *J. Comp. Neurol.* **209,** pp. 363–73.

Obata, K. (1977). Development of neuromuscular transmission in culture with a variety of neurons and in the presence of cholinergic substances and tetrodotoxin. *Brain Res.* **119,** pp. 141–50.

Purves, D., Lichtman, J. W. (1980). Elimination of synapses in the developing nervous system. *Science* **210,** pp. 153–7.

Rankin, E. C. C. and Cook, J. (1986). Topographic refinement of the regenerating retinotectal projection of the goldfish in standard laboratory conditions: a quantitative WGA–HRP study. *Exp. Brain Res.* **63,** pp. 432–46.

Reh, T. and Constantine-Paton, M. (1985). Eye specific segregation is dependent on neural activity in three eyed *Rana pipiens. J. Neurosci.* **5,** pp. 1132–43.

Ricciuti, A. and Gruberg, E. R. (1985). Nucleus isthmi provides most tectal choline acetyltransferase in the frog *Rana pipiens. Brain Res.* **341,** pp. 399–402.

Sakaguchi, D. S. and Murphey, R. K. (1985). Initial development of the retinotectal projection in *Xenopus*: an examination of ganglion cell terminal arborizations. *J. Neurosci.* **5,** pp. 3228–45.

Schmidt, J. T. (1982). The formation of retinotectal projections. *Trends Neurosci.* **5,** pp. 111–6.

Schmidt, J. T. (1985). Formation of retinotopic connections: selective stabilization by an activity dependent mechanism. *Cell. Mol. Neurobiol.* **5,** pp. 65–84.

Schmidt, J. T. and Edwards, D. L. (1983). Activity sharpens the map during regeneration of the retinotectal projection in goldfish. *Brain Res.* **269,** pp. 29–39.

Schmidt, J. T. and Eisele, L. E. (1985). Stroboscopic illumination and dark rearing block the sharpening of the regenerated retinotectal map in goldfish. *Neuroscience* **14,** pp. 535–46.

Schmidt, J. T., Buzzard, M., and Turcotte, J. (1984). Morphology of regenerated optic arbors in goldfish tectum. *Neurosci. Abstr.* **10,** p. 667.

Schmidt, J. T., Edwards, D. L., and Stuermer, C. (1983). The re-establishment of synaptic transmission by regenerating optic axons in goldfish: time course and effects of blocking activity by intraocular injection of tetrodotoxin. *Brain Res.* **269,** pp. 15–27.

Schneider, G., Rava, L., Sachs, G. M., and Jhaveri, S. (1981). Widespread branching of retinotectal axons: transient in normal development and anomalous in adults with neonatal lesions. *Neurosci. Abstr.* **7,** p. 732.

Sperry, R. W. (1943). Effect of 180 degree rotation of the retinal field on visumotor coordination. *J. Exp. Zool.* **92,** pp. 263–79.

Sperry, R. W. (1963). Chemoaffinity in the orderly growth of nerve fiber patterns and connections. *Proc. Natl. Acad. Sci. USA.* **50,** pp. 703–9.

Stryker, M. P. and Harris, W. A. (1986). Binocular impulse blockade prevents the formation of ocular dominance columns in cat visual cortex. *J. Neurosci.* **6,** pp. 2117–33.

Stuermer, C. A. O. (1987). Navigation of normal and regenerating axons in the goldfish. In *The making of the nervous system* (eds. J. G. Parnavelas, C. D. Stern, and R. V. Stirling), pp. 204–27. Oxford University Press, Oxford.

Stuermer, C. A. O. and Easter, S. S. (1984). A comparison of the normal regenerated retinotectal pathways of goldfish. *J. Comp. Neurol.* **223,** pp. 57–76.

Thompson, W. J. (1985). Activity and synapse elimination at the neuromuscular junction. *Cell. Mol. Neurobiol.* **5,** pp. 167–82.

Willshaw, D. J. and von der Malsburg, C. (1976). How patterned neural connections can be set up by self-organization. *Proc. R. Soc. Lond. B* **194,** pp. 431–45.

20

Retinotopic maps, cell death, and electrical activity in the retinotectal and retinocollicular projections

J. W. FAWCETT

A basic feature of brain architecture is the organization of neuronal projections into topographic maps. For example, the visual centres of the brain have their inputs retinotopically ordered, the motor and sensory cortex are ordered in body coordinates, and the auditory centres are tonotopically ordered. Unravelling the mechanisms responsible for the setting up of these ordered maps has been a major thrust in neurobiology. Much of the work has concentrated on the visual system, and in this chapter I will describe some of our work, and work from other laboratories, which relates to this subject.

THE FISH AND AMPHIBIAN VISUAL SYSTEMS

Elsewhere in this volume, Schmidt (1987) has described how fish and frogs are able to re-order a disordered retinotectal projection, using a mechanism which is driven by the patterns of electrical activity in the axons of the retinal ganglion cells. Why do fish and frogs need this mechanism? The answer probably lies in the phenomenon of 'shifting connections'. The anamniotes are very small when they first begin to live independently, and their nervous system relatively undeveloped, yet they have to be able to feed themselves and escape from predators from the beginning; in many species this means that they have to be able to see, and this in turn means that they have to have an ordered retinotopic map on their optic tectum. As the animals grow so do their retinae and tecta, but the pattern of growth of these two structures is quite different; cells are added to the retina all around its periphery, whereas cells are added to the optic tectum mainly at its caudal margin. Therefore, to maintain a retinotopic map on the optic tectum during growth, the earliest retinal fibres to arrive at the tectum have progressively to shift their termination sites on the tectum (Gaze, Keating, Ostberg, and Chung 1979; Fraser, 1983; Easter and Stuermer, 1984; Reh and Constantine-Paton 1985). If this shifting were simply driven by the terminal arbors competing for space on the tectum, and so filling up the newly created areas of tectum on its caudal margin, then the retinotectal map would gradually become disordered, and the animal's visual performance would be degraded. There must, therefore, be a mechanism that is capable of maintaining order in the projection as it grows, and it is this role that the electrically driven mechanism fulfills. In experimental animals, this mechanism can be assayed for, either by deliberately disordering the retinotectal map (as described by Schmidt this volume, Chapter 19), or by forcing two equivalent pieces of retina to compete for the same area of tectum, in which case the two projections separate out to form ocular dominance stripes (see Fig. 20.1) (Levine and Jacobson 1975; Constantine-Paton and Law 1978; Fawcett and Willshaw 1982; Meyer 1982).

THE AMNIOTE VISUAL SYSTEM

The amniotes have a very different pattern of development to frogs and fishes; by the time they are born, their nervous system is essentially fully developed, and there is usually no further neuronal cell division either in the retina or the optic tectum. However, there is a period during which around half the neurons in both the retina and tectum (or colliculus) die, which occurs shortly before hatching in the chick (Rager and Rager 1978) and around and after birth in the rat (for a review, see Cowan, Fawcett, O'Leary, and Stanfield 1984); there is no evidence at present for a similar period in frog or fish retinotectal development. Axonal growth from the amniote retina occurs over a relatively short period, which may decrease the need for any organized shifting of connections. Moreover, amniote development occurs in a protected environment, in which there is no need for a functional visual system. One can argue, therefore, that amniotes have no real need for a mechanism to re-order their retinofugal connections during development (but see later). We decided to see whether this is in fact the case, and we chose as our experimental model the chick. The chick develops to hatching in 21 days, by which time the nervous system has virtually reached its adult form; the retinotectal projection has formed, neuronal cell division in the tectum and retina has ceased, and the period of neuronal cell death is passed (Cowan, Adamson, and Powell 1961). Moreover, there is evidence that there is little plasticity in the chick retinotectal projection even during its development; if a proportion of the retina is removed before optic axons leave the eye, the remaining retina will still only connect to the same region of the tectum it would have innervated had the eye not been lesioned. The projection from the remaining small area of retina will not expand to occupy the whole tectum (Crossland, Cowan, Rogers, and Kelly 1974; McLoon 1982), as would be the case in a fish, for instance (Schmidt, Cicerone, and Easter 1978; Udin and Gaze 1983).

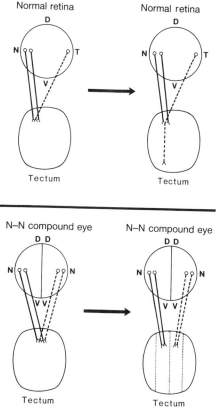

Fig. 20.1. The mechanism for shifting of connections in the frog or fish tectum. The upper pair of diagrams represents the sequence of events which occurs when an axon reaches an inappropriate region of the tectum. Two axons from nasal retina have made correct connections with caudal tectum, but one axon (dotted line) has reached the wrong area. This incorrectly targeted axon will gradually shift its terminal until it is correctly situated. The driving force for this process is probably the relative synchrony of electrical activity in neighbouring ganglion cells. Errors of this magnitude would generally only occur in regeneration. In the lower diagrams, the frog has been given a double nasal compound eye, by removing the temporal half-retina from a larva and replacing it with the nasal half-eye from a donor animal. The axons from both 'nasal' poles of the eye initially all terminate together in caudal tectum because they all share the same retinal positional label. When the fibres form functional synapses, the electrically driven mechanism will detect that the axons from the two half-eyes do not come from neighbouring ganglion cells, and the two sets of terminals will separate out into stripes. Within each stripe the terminals come from neighbouring areas of retina. D, dorsal; N, nasal; T, temporal; V, ventral.

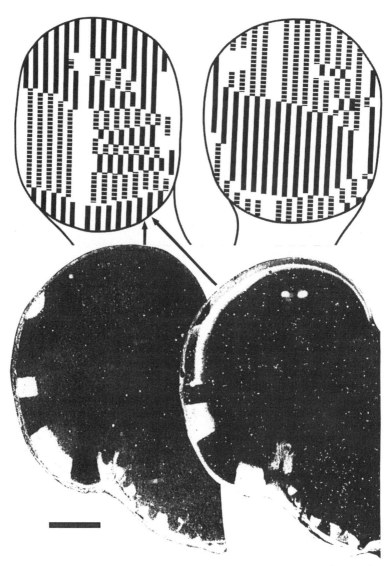

Fig. 20.3. The pattern of stripes in an E18 chick, whose chiasma was disrupted on E4. The two lower sections are neighbouring sections, the left-hand one processed for [³H] proline autoradiography and the right-hand one for HRP. The stripes in one section fit exactly into the gaps in the other. The diagrams above are reconstructions of the stripe pattern in the tecta. Scale bar: 1 mm. [Reproduced from Fawcett and Cowan (1985) by kind permission of Elsevier, Amsterdam.]

normally each tectum receives innervation from only one eye. In anamniotes the mechanism is there to ensure that axons from neighbouring ganglion cells project to neighbouring sites on the tectum, and it is therefore essentially a mechanism for correcting mapping errors in the retinotectal projection. Could it, therefore, exist in chicks to remove axons which have grown to inappropriate regions of the tectum subserving the process of systems matching by degeneration, as originally proposed by Rager and Rager (1978). There is evidence that such mapping errors do occur in chick development (McLoon 1982; McLoon 1985), and there is also evidence that errors artificially induced by surgical disruption of the optic tract are subsequently removed (Fujisawa, Thanos, and Schwarz 1984), so it seemed to us likely that the mechanism is present in the chick to correct topographic mapping errors. We decided to look into this possibility further, using, for technical reasons, the retinocollicular projection of the new-born rat as our experimental model.

One can define three categories of targeting error that retinocollicular axons could potentially make: in the *first category* axons grow to the wrong part of the brain entirely; in the *second* they reach the superior colliculus, but grow to the ipsilateral rather than the contralateral side; and in the *third category* they reach the correct superior colliculus but grow to the wrong part of it. All three types of targeting error have been observed (Frost 1984; and see later).

THE RAT IPSILATERAL RETINOCOLLICULAR PROJECTION

In the rat, there are fibres present at birth which project to the wrong (ipsilateral) colliculus, but during the first 10 days or so of life they nearly all disappear (Land and Lund 1979; Frost and Schneider 1979); those that remain mostly project from the binocular region in the temporal retinal margin to rostral superior colliculus. The ipsilaterally projecting fibres are not branches of axons which project to the contralateral colliculus, and are removed by the death of their ganglion cells during the period of naturally occurring ganglion cell death which happens in the rat during the first 10 days of life (Sengelaub and Finlay 1982; Jeffery and Perry 1982; Martin, Sefton, and Dreher 1983; O'Leary, Fawcett, and Cowan 1983; Jeffery 1984; Insausti, Blakemore, and Cowan 1984). Most of the ipsilaterally projecting axons and their ganglion cells can be rescued by removing the other eye at birth. This implies that some form of competition between the fibres from the two eyes normally plays a role in the death of the ipsilaterally projecting cells.

We investigated the mechanism responsible for the death of the ipsilaterally projecting ganglion cells. We reasoned that these cells had made a particular type of erroneous projection, leading to them being removed, together with their axons by a competitive mechanism, and that the mechanism by which this was achieved might be electrically driven. To test this hypothesis we looked at the elimination of the rat's ipsilaterally projecting ganglion cells and their axons over the first two weeks of life in normal animals, and in animals in which electrical conduction in the eyes was blocked by intraocular injection of the sodium channel blocker tetrodotoxin (TTX) (Fawcett, O'Leary, and Cowan 1984). We assayed the ipsilaterally projecting ganglion cells by intraocular injections of wheat-germ-agglutinin-conjugated HRP (WGA–HRP), which labels the axons, and with fast blue (FB), which labels retinal ganglion cells when injected into the colliculus. FB has the added advantage that it remains detectable in labelled cells for months, but disappears if the cell dies (Bentivoglio, Kuypers, and Catsman-Berrevoets 1980; Innocenti 1981; O'Leary, Stanfield, and Cowan 1981; Sawcenko and Swanson 1981).

Our findings in normal animals were essentially confirmatory of previous reports (see Fig. 20.4); in new-born Sprague-Dawley rats there are around 800 ganglion cells that project to the ipsilateral superior colliculus, not counting those in the binocular area of the retina, the temporal crescent. By postnatal day 12 (P12) all but about 120 of these cells have died. Our anterograde WGA–HRP fills showed that ipsilaterally projecting axons were plentiful at birth, and innervated the whole surface of the superior colliculus, but by P12 the projection was sparse, and restricted to the rostral and medial edges of the colliculus. However, if one eye was removed at birth, by P12 there were still around 800 ipsilaterally projecting ganglion cells outside the temporal crescent in the remaining eye, and their axons innervated the whole extent of the colliculus.

To see whether abolishing electrical activity in retinocollicular fibres reduces their competitive potential, we injected one eye of a group of animals with TTX over the first 12 days of life, injected the colliculus with FB, and counted the ipsilaterally projecting ganglion cells in the non-TTX treated eye. We found that we had rescued some but not all of the ipsilaterally projecting cells by this maneouvre; the average number of cells surviving to P12 was 273,

---

Fig. 20.4. Experiments on the rat ipsilateral retinocollicular projection. (a) At birth there is a projection from the eye to the entire ipsilateral superior colliculus, but by P12 this has largely disappeared. Removing one eye at birth allows ipsilaterally projecting fibres from the other eye to survive and innervate the entire colliculus. (b) Shows the same thing as (a), but by retrograde labelling of the ganglion cells with FB. At birth there are 820 ipsilaterally projecting ganglion cells outside the temporal crescent, but by P12 there are only 120. Removing one eye at birth rescues all the ipsilaterally projecting cells in the other eye. (c) The effects of TTX treatment: when one eye is treated with TTX, an extensive ipsilateral projection from the other eye survives to P12, but the ipsilateral projection from a TTX treated eye is even smaller than normal by P12. TTX treatment of one eye allows 270 ipsilaterally projecting cells in the other eye to survive, more than twice as many as normal. [Reproduced from Cowan *et al.* (1984) by kind permission of the American Association for the Advancement of Science, Washington, D.C.]

which is more than twice the number in normal P12 animals, but nevertheless considerably less than the 800 or so found in new-borns. There was a corresponding sparse fibre projection covering most of the ipsilateral superior colliculus. Blocking the competing fibres with TTX, therefore, rescues a proportion of the ipsilaterally projecting ganglion cells in rats. Holt and

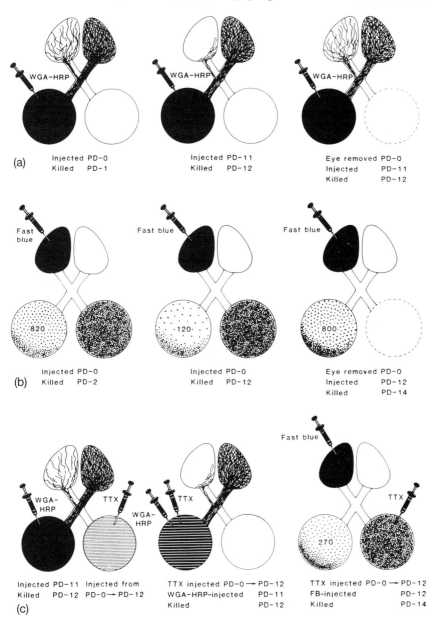

(a)

Injected PD-0
Killed   PD-1

Injected PD-11
Killed   PD-12

Eye removed PD-0
Injected   PD-11
Killed   PD-12

(b)

Fast blue

820

Injected PD-0
Killed   PD-2

Fast blue

·120·

Injected PD-0
Killed   PD-12

Fast blue

800·

Eye removed PD-0
Injected   PD-12
Killed   PD-14

(c)

WGA-HRP   TTX   WGA-HRP

Injected PD-11   Injected from
Killed   PD-12   PD-0 → PD-12

TTX   WGA-HRP

TTX injected PD-0 → PD-12
WGA-HRP-injected   PD-11
Killed   PD-12

Fast blue

TTX

270

TTX injected PD-0 → PD-12
FB-injected   PD-12
Killed   PD-14

Thompson (1984) have done essentially the same experiment in hamsters, and report the rescue of a small number of cells, all of which were in temporal retina. We conclude that electrical activity is involved to some degree in the competition for survival between ipsilaterally and contralaterally projecting ganglion cells, although, as one would expect, TTX blockade does not have the same effect as removing the contralaterally projecting axons altogether; the blocked axons are still present, and still presumably competing with the ipsilateral fibres, although less effectively than normal. Holt and Thompson (1984) were also able to demonstrate a phenomenon very similar to ocular dominance stripes in the hamster colliculus: in normal hamsters, the ipsilateral retinocollicular projection tends to be divided up into small clumps and they were able to prevent these clumps forming by treating both eyes with TTX.

ERRORS IN THE RETINOCOLLICULAR PROJECTION

The electrically controlled mechanism in the fish and frog retinotectal projection is essentially an error correction mechanism, designed to correct the third category of errors defined above; that is, axons which have reached the right target but the wrong region of it. We decided to look directly for evidence of targeting errors within the rat contralateral retinocollicular projection, for evidence of their removal, and for an involvement of electrical activity in the process (Fawcett and O'Leary 1985; O'Leary, Fawcett, and Cowan 1986). To see whether significant numbers of retinocollicular axons make targeting errors we made very localized injections of FB into the caudal superior colliculus of newborn rats, and then examined the contralateral retina to see the location of the labelled ganglion cells which had projected to this area. As expected, many ganglion cells in the nasal pole of the retina were labelled with FB (nasal retina projects to caudal colliculus), but there were also many labelled cells scattered over the surface of the rest of the retina (see Fig. 20.5). Thus, in the newborn rat, many ganglion cells, which, from their position on the retina one would expect to project elsewhere, project inappropriately to the caudal margin of the colliculus. To make a numerical estimate of the number of erroneously projecting cells we counted the number of labelled cells in the temporal retina (erroneously projecting) for every 100 correctly projecting cells in an equivalent area of nasal retina, and we called this figure the percentage error; this was 14 per cent in new-born animals. However, if the FB injection was given on the day of birth, but the animal was allowed to survive until P12, the labelling pattern was quite different; almost all the labelled cells were correctly situated in temporal retina, and the incorrectly projecting ganglion cells in the rest of the retina, which were labelled at the time of the FB injection, had died. The percentage error in these

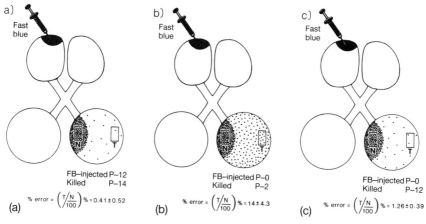

Fig. 20.5. Error correction in the rat contralateral retinocollicular projection. (a) A localized injection of FB into the caudal colliculus on P12 labels many cells in nasal retina, but few elsewhere. (b) If the injection is made at birth, many cells are labelled in nasal retina, but erroneously projectiong FB-labelled cells are 14 per cent as dense in temporal retina as in nasal retina. (c) If the FB injection is done at birth, so as to label both correctly and erroneously projecting ganglion cells, but the animal is not killed until P12, most of the erroneously projecting cells have died; the ratio of density of correctly projecting versus incorrectly projecting cells is only 1 per cent. T, temporal; N, nasal. [Reproduced from O'Leary *et al.* (1986) by kind permission of the Society for Neuroscience, Bethesda, MD.]

cases was only 1·26 per cent, roughly the same figure we obtained when the FB injection was done on P12 and the animal killed on P14.

This means that a substantial proportion of retinal ganglion cells project to inappropriate regions of the colliculus at birth, and nearly all these cells die during the period of naturally occurring cell death. According to our hypothesis, the mechanism which detects axons which have made erroneous connections and eliminates them should use electrical activity as its driving force; blocking electrical activity in the retina should therefore prevent the developing brain from being able to distinguish a correct from an incorrect connection. To see whether this is true, we made localized FB injections into the caudal colliculus of a group of new-born rats, so as to label both correctly and erroneously projecting ganglion cells. We then treated these animals with intraocular TTX for the first 12 days of life, killed them, and examined the retinal labelling pattern. The percentage error in these animals was the same as at birth, 13·8 per cent (see Fig. 20.6). TTX treatment had therefore prevented the preferential elimination of the ganglion cells which had made these gross targeting errors. However, TTX did not prevent ganglion cell death *per se*; over the first two weeks of life, the same number of ganglion cells die in TTX blocked as in untreated animals (Fawcett *et al.* 1984; Crespo, O'Leary, Fawcett, and Cowan 1985). In TTX treated eyes, ganglion cell death becomes

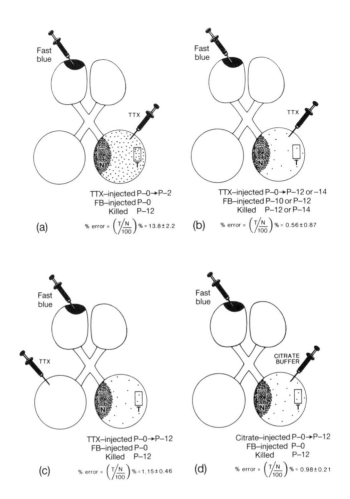

Fig. 20.6. The effects of TTX treatment on error elimination in the rat retinocollicular projection. (a) FB is injected into the colliculus at birth, so as to label both correctly and erroneously projecting ganglion cells, and TTX is injected over the first 12 days of life. When the animal is killed on P12, the percentage error is the same as at birth, indicating that there has been no preferential elimination of the erroneously projecting cells. (b) The animal is treated with TTX over the first 12 days of life, but the FB injection is not made until two days before the animal is killed. The percentage error is only 0.56 per cent, which indicates that the erroneously projecting cells, although still alive, are no longer connected to caudal colliculus. (c) and (d) are controls, to show that TTX injected into one eye has no effect on topographic error elimination in the other, and that the citrate buffer in which the TTX was dissolved has no effect. [Reproduced from O'Leary *et al.* (1986) by kind permission of the Society for Neuroscience, Bethesda, MD.]

a random event, rather than one which preferentially removes the erroneously projecting cells; TTX blocks the process which selects which cells are to die, but not cell death itself. Finally, to see whether the erroneous connections were maintained under TTX treatment, we injected TTX into rat eyes over the first 12 days of life, then made a localized FB injection on either P10 or P12, and killed the animals two days later. The labelling pattern in these retinae was normal for rats of this age: there were few cells outside nasal retina which were erroneously connected to caudal superior colliculus (SO), and we could not detect an abnormal number of gross targeting errors despite TTX treatment. This result indicates that the extensive terminal arbors which ganglion cells possess in the newborn rat (Schneider, Rava, Sachs, and Jhaveri 1981; Sachs, Jacobson, and Caviness 1986) will contract in size over the first two weeks of life, regardless of TTX [as do goldfish terminal arbors (Schmidt, pers. com., although often around an incorrect locus (Schmidt and Edwards (1983))]. Thus the gross targeting errors which we were seeing at birth were no longer detectable at two weeks; presumably the more far-flung branches of the terminal arbors had been withdrawn. Of course, this does not mean that the terminals of the erroneously projecting cells were now concentrated in the correct area of the tectum; our results simply show that they were no longer connected to the caudal part of the SC.

There appears, then, to be an electrically driven mechanism which is general to the retinotectal or retinocollicular projections, and which acts to sharpen the retinotopic map. In the anamniotes these refinements are achieved by a combination of terminal arbor pruning and shifting of connections. In the amniotes terminal arbor pruning has been observed in the rodent colliculus during the first days of life (Schneider *et al.* 1981; Sachs *et al.* 1986), and our experiments provide evidence that some of the map sharpening is achieved by the death of cells whose axons have made gross targeting errors. The sharpening of the map is thus probably achieved by a combination of these two separate processes; small positional errors are corrected by pruning away the part of the arbor which is misplaced, whereas major errors are eliminated by removing the whole axon and its ganglion cell. There is also evidence in the chick that erroneous connections may be removed in the absence of competition, presumably by a positional label-dependent process (McLoon 1982). Ganglion cell death therefore achieves two ends, the matching of the number of cells to the size of their target, and the refinement of topography; at present we have no way of estimating the amount of cell death attributable to the two roles.

MECHANISMS

How might this be accomplished? Almost all models have been based on Hebb's (1949) original hypothesis, subsequently developed by Stent (1973), of how modifiable synapses might function as a substrate for learning. The basic idea is that those synapses which fire synchronously with the post-synaptic cell will be strengthened, whereas those which fire asynchronously will become weaker. To make this sort of mechanism work as a tool for sharpening topographic maps, one has to propose that neighbouring cells in the input structure (the retina) must fire relatively synchronously, whereas non-neighbouring cells fire asynchronously. Since neighbouring input cells normally send their axons to neighbouring sites on the target, as they fire together they will strongly depolarize the post-synaptic cell, and their synapses will be strengthened. Conversely, an axon which has reached the wrong area of the target will fire out of synchrony with the majority of axons in this area, and will therefore be at a competitive disadvantage relative to the axons which belong there. This, of course, assumes that the initial retinal projection is ordered. There is good evidence in chicks, fish, and frogs that this non-randomness is provided by a combination of axonal guidance to the correct region of the target, and by the presence of positional addresses on it (Straznicky, Gaze, and Horder 1979; Harris 1980; McLoon 1982; Bonhoeffer and Huf 1982, Fawcett and Gaze 1982; O'Leary and Cowan 1983; Holt and Harris 1983; Stuermer and Easter 1984; Holt 1984; Rusoff 1984). There is direct evidence that neighbouring retinal ganglion cells do fire synchronously (Arnett 1978; Mastronarde 1983; Ginsberg, Johnsen, and Levine 1984), and also that firing all ganglion cells synchronously disables the mechanism responsible for the refinement of fish retinotectal topography (Schmidt and Eisele 1985). In higher vertebrates this electrical activity must represent spontaneous firing of the ganglion cells, since map sharpening in rats happens at a stage of development when the eyes are closed, and connections in the retina still forming, whereas stripe formation in chicks occurs while the animal is in darkness inside the egg, and the retina is similarly poorly developed; spontaneous activity is quite common in the developing nervous system.

If axons are competing, what factor are they competing for, and how is this factor given specifically to the appropriate terminals? Do they compete directly for synaptic space, or for a trophic factor, or for one of these via the other? There is no experimental evidence which addresses these questions at present. However, it is certainly reasonable to extrapolate a plausible mechanism from the example of NGF (nerve growth factor), which is released in limited amounts by the targets of sensory and sympathetic neurons and acts as a trophic and tropic factor to them. Among its many actions, NGF has been found to be able to maintain responsive neurons *in vitro* and also to strengthen individual neuronal processes when applied selectively (Levi-Montalcini 1982; Campenot 1982; Thoenen and Edgar 1985). It is possible that the weakening or strengthening of synapses in the brain could be mediated in this way via a trophic factor similar to NGF; target neurons may release more trophic factor when strongly depolarized by several synchronously firing synapses, and this factor could be selectively released to the active terminals, or selectively taken up by synapses which have recently fired, and which are therefore recycling vesicle material. This could control the synaptic strengths, and also the survival of branches of terminal arbors.

Disconnecting central nervous system (CNS) neurons from their targets during the 'critical period' of naturally occurring neuronal cell death usually leads to their death (for a review, see Cowan *et al.* 1984), and CNS neurons usually die *in vitro* unless cultured with some brain tissue, usually from their target region. Both these observations suggest that there are trophic factors in the CNS. In the amniote visual system, cutting the optic nerve leads to massive ganglion cell death, so there is probably a ganglion cell trophic factor produced by the central visual structures. It is possible, as with NGF, that the same trophic factor regulates synaptic strength, terminal arbor size and shape, and also ganglion cell survival. Thus a ganglion cell whose axon has connected to the correct area of its target would fire in synchrony with the other axons in the region, depolarize the post-synaptic cell, and therefore pick up large amounts of trophic factor, which, in turn, would stabilize the terminal arbor, be transported back to the retina, and prevent the ganglion cell dying during the period of cell death. Conversely, a cell whose axon has reached the wrong region of the target will fire at times when few other synapses are active, and therefore receive little factor, leading to its death (see Fig. 20.7).

There is a problem with this simple model; it makes the prediction that if all electrical activity is blocked in the retina, the post-synaptic cells in the colliculus will not be stimulated, will not release any trophic factor, and therefore all the ganglion cells will die. This does not happen; there is a normal amount of cell death in TTX treated retinae (Fawcett *et al.* 1984; Crespo *et al.* 1985). To account for this observation the model must be modified. One possibility is that unstimulated neurons will leak trophic factor at a roughly normal overall rate, but randomly to all synapses. Alternatively, there may be two different factors involved, one which is only released in response to electrical stimulation of the post-synaptic cells and which governs synaptic stability and terminal arbor shape, and a second factor which functions solely as a ganglion cell survival factor, and which is released equally to all synapses. At present there are no experimental data which point to any particular mechanism, although putative ganglion cell trophic factors have been identified (McCaffrey, Bennet, and Dreher 1982; Turner 1985).

SIMILAR EVENTS ELSEWHERE IN THE NERVOUS SYSTEM

It is likely that similar mechanisms will be found throughout the nervous system. For example, modification of transmission at the neuromuscular junction affects both cell death and terminal arbor shape (Oppenheim and

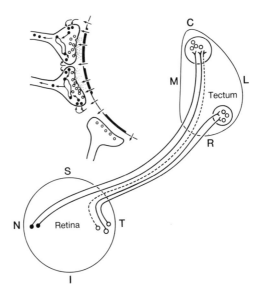

Fig. 20.7. A possible mechanism for the correction of topographic mapping errors. Two ganglion cells in nasal retina send their axons correctly to caudal tectum, but one cell from temporal retina projects there erroneously as well. The sequence of events is shown in the top left part of the diagram. The two top synapses are from the two nasal cells. They fire synchronously, releasing transmitter from their vesicles (fine dots), and depolarize the post-synaptic cell strongly. This leads the post-synaptic cell to release trophic factor (arrows). The factor is taken up preferentially by the terminals which have just fired, because they are actively taking up vesicle material (black circles). The trophic factor is now transported back to the ganglion cell body, enhancing its chance of survival. The lower synapse, from the cell in temporal retina, does not fire in synchrony with the majority of synapses on the cell, and therefore is not taking in vesicle material at times when trophic factor is being released. As a result, the synapse weakens and the ganglion cell dies. M, medial; L, lateral; R, rostral; S, superior; I, inferior; N, nasal; T, temporal. [Reproduced from Cowan *et al.* (1984) by kind permission of the American Association for the Advancement of Science, Washington, D.C.]

Chu-Wang, 1983; Bennet 1984; Lamb 1984), and there are several examples of changes in development after modifications of the sensory periphery (for instance, Sanes and Constantine-Paton 1985). Mechanisms similar to the one described above seem to be active elsewhere in the visual system. Two of the best studied examples are the intertectal connections of frogs and the geniculo cortical connections of higher mammals.

Frogs have completely crossed primary visual projections; all the axons from the eyes project to the contralateral optic tectum. However, frogs do have a degree of stereoscopic vision, which uses an intertectal connection via the nucleus isthmi. Each nucleus isthmi receives a topographically arranged input from the tectum on the same side, and sends outputs straight back to the same area of the ipsilateral tectum, and to the contralateral tectum. The connections from the nucleus isthmi to the contralateral tectum are so arranged as to ensure that an image seen in both eyes will stimulate the same area of tectum both directly and via the intertectal relay (Gruberg and Lettvin 1980; Grobstein and Comer 1983; Caine and Gruberg 1985). However, if one eye is rotated in its orbit this reciprocal mapping is suddenly disarranged. The frog brain responds to this perturbation by slowly rearranging the projection from the nucleus isthmi to the contralateral tectum so as to restore correct binocularity. This involves terminal arbors shifting their termination sites by distances of a millimetre or so (Udin and Keating 1983; Udin 1983). A similar process occurs during normal development in some frogs as the eyes shift their relative positions as the animal grows (Grant and Keating 1986). This shifting of connections must be driven by visual experience, since the direct retinotectal projection from the rotated eye does not change at all in response to eye rotation and the change in the isthmo–tectal projection seems to require normal visual experience. It seems reasonable to suppose that the driving force behind the superimposition of inputs to the tectum is a matching of patterns of electrical activity between the direct retinotectal and the indirect intertectal projection, although as yet there is no direct proof of this.

The geniculo-cortical projection of higher mammals has been intensively studied over the years. One of the striking features of cortical neurons in area 18 is that they are generally sensitive to input from either one eye or the other, and neighbouring cells have the same eye dominance, so that there are areas about 400 μm wide in which all the cells are primarily responsive to the same eye, called ocular dominance columns. These columns are modifiable by manipulating the visual experience of young animals, or by injecting the eyes with TTX (LeVay, Stryker, and Shatz 1978; Blakemore 1978; LeVay, Wiesel, and Hubel 1981; Stryker 1981; Swindale 1981). Stryker and Strickland (1984) have shown that asynchronous electrical activity in the optic nerves is critical to the formation of these ocular dominance columns. When spontaneous electrical activity in the eyes was blocked with TTX, and the optic nerves stimulated synchronously, no ocular dominance columns were formed, whereas if the optic nerves were stimulated asynchronously columns appeared normally. Although this experiment is complicated by the presence of a synapse between the retina and the cortex, it seems that the pattern of retinal activity is sufficiently well transmitted to the cortex to influence ocular dominance column formation. The overall mechanism of ocular dominance column formation is probably just the same as that which sharpens the retinotectal and retinocollicular maps and generates eye dominance stripes in the retinotectal projections. However, there is no evidence for any link between ocular dominance column formation in the cortex and neuronal cell death.

This similarity of basic mechanism between higher and lower vertebrates tempts one to speculate on the evolution of cortical ocular dominance columns. In lower vertebrates, whose retinal projections are completely crossed, ocular dominance stripes form whenever the projections from the two eyes are made experimentally to innervate the same structure; this appears to be a side effect of a mechanism whose actual function is to sharpen the retinotopicity of the retinotectal map during development. Perhaps when retinofugal projections evolved to innervate both sides of the brain, ocular dominance columns were an inevitable consequence.

ACKNOWLEDGEMENTS

I wish to thank Max Cowan and Dennis O'Leary for their collaboration in these experiments and for their suggestions on this manuscript. This work was supported by grant EY-03653 from the National Eye Institute, and by the Clayton Foundation for Research, California Division.

REFERENCES

Arnett, D. W. (1978). Statistical dependence between neighbouring retinal ganglion cells in the goldfish. *Exp. Brain Res.* **32,** pp. 49–53.

Bennet, M. R. (1983). Development of neuromuscular synapses. *Physiol. Rev.* **63,** pp. 915–1048.

Bentivoglio, M., Kuypers, H. G. J. M., Catsman-Berrevoets, C. E., and Dann, O. (1979). Fluorescent retrograde neuronal labelling in rat by means of substances binding specifically to adenine-thymine rich DNA. *Neurosci. Lett.* **12,** pp. 235–40.

Blakemore, C. (1978). In *Handbook of sensory physiology, vol. VIII.* perception (eds. R. Held, H. W. Leibowitz, and H. L. Teuber), pp. 377–436. Springer-Verlag, Berlin.

Bonhoeffer, F. and Huf, J. (1982). In vitro experiments on axon guidance demonstrating anterior–posterior gradient on the tectum. *EMBO J.* **1,** pp. 427–31.

Boss, V. C. and Schmidt, J. T. (1984). Activity and the formation of ocular dominance patches in dually innervated tectum of goldfish. *J. Neurosci.* **4,** pp. 2891–905.

Caine, H. S. and Gruberg, E. R. (1985). Ablation of nucleus isthmi leads to loss of specific visually elicited behaviours in the frog Rana pipiens. *Neurosci. Lett.* **54,** pp. 307–12.

Campenot, R. B. (1982). Development of sympathetic neurons in compartmentalized cultures II. Local control of neurite survival by nerve growth factor. *Dev. Biol.* **93,** pp. 13–21.

Constantine-Paton, M. and Law, M. T. (1978). Eye specific termination bands in tecta of three eyed frogs. *Science* **202,** pp. 639–41.

Cowan, W. M., Adamson, L., and Powell, T. P. S. (1961). An experimental study of the avian visual system. *J. Anat.* **95,** pp. 545–63.

Cowan, W. M., Fawcett, J. W., O'Leary, D. D. M., and Stanfield, B. B. (1984). Regressive events in Neurogenesis. *Science* **225,** pp. 1258–65.

Crespo, D., O'Leary, D. D. M., Fawcett, J. W., and Cowan, W. M. (1985). Minimal effect of intraocular Tetrodotoxin on the postnatal reduction in the number of optic nerve axons in the albino rat. *Soc. Neurosci. Abstr.* **11**, p. 259.

Crossland, W. J., Cowan, W. M., Rogers, L. A., and Kelly, J. P. (1974). The specification of the retinotectal projection in the chick. *J. Comp. Neurol.* **155**, pp. 127–64.

Easter, S. S., Jr. and Stuermer, C. A. O. (1984). An evaluation of the hypothesis of shifting terminals in the goldfish optic tectum. *J. Neurosci.* **4**, pp. 1052–63.

Fawcett, J. W. and Cowan, W. M. (1985). On the formation of eye dominance stripes and patches in the doubly innervated optic tectum of the chick. *Dev. Brain Res.* **17**, pp. 149–63.

Fawcett, J. W. and Gaze, R. M. (1982). The retinotectal fibre pathways from normal and compound eyes in Xenopus. *J. Embryol. exp. Morphol.* **72**, pp. 19–37.

Fawcett, J. W. and O'Leary, D. D. M. (1985). The role of electrical activity in the formation of topographic maps in the nervous system. *Trends Neurosci.* **8**, pp. 201–6.

Fawcett, J. W. and Willshaw, D. J. (1982). Compound eyes project stripes on the optic tectum in Xenopus. *Nature* **296**, pp. 350–2.

Fawcett, J. W., O'Leary, D. D. M., and Cowan, W. M. (1984). Activity and the control of ganglion cell death in the rat retina. *Proc. Natl. Acad. Sci. USA* **81**, pp. 5589–93.

Fraser, S. E. (1983). Fiber optic mapping of the Xenopus visual system: shift in the retinotectal projection during development. *Dev. Biol.* **95**, pp. 505–11.

Frost, D. O. (1984). Axonal growth and target selection during development: retinal projections to the ventrobasal complex and other 'nonvisual' structures in neonatal syrian hamsters. *J. Comp. Neurol.* **230**, pp. 576–92.

Frost, D. O. and Schneider, G. E. (1979). Postnatal development of retinal projections in Syrian hamsters: a study using autoradiographic and anterograde degeneration techniques. *Neuroscience* **4**, pp. 1649–77.

Fujisawa, H., Thanos, S., and Schwarz, U. (1984). Mechanisms in the development of retinotectal projections in the chick embryo studied by surgical deflection of the retinal pathway. *Dev. Biol.* **102**, pp. 356–67.

Gaze, R. M., Keating, M. J., Ostberg, A., and Chung, S. H. (1979). The relationship between retinal and tectal growth in larval Xenopus. Implications for the development of the retinotectal projection. *J. Embryol. exp. Morphol.* **53**, pp. 103–43.

Ginsburg, K. S., Johnsen, J. A., and Levine, M. W. (1984). Common noise in the firing of neighbouring ganglion cells in goldfish retina. *J. Physiol. (Lond.)* **351**, pp. 433–51.

Grant, S. and Keating, M. J. (1986). Ocular migration and the metamorphic and post metamorphic maturation of the retinotectal system in Xenopus laevis: an autoradiographic and morphometric study. *J. Embryol. exp. Morphol.* **92**, pp. 43–69.

Green, L. and Shooter, E. (1981). Nerve growth factor: biochemistry, synthesis and mechanism of action. *Ann. Rev. Neurosci.* **3**, pp. 353–402.

Grobstein, P. and Comer, C. (1983). The nucleus isthmi as an intertectal relay for the ipsilateral oculotectal projection in the frog, Rana Pipiens. *J. Comp Neurol.* **216**, pp. 54–74.

Gruberg, E. R. and Lettvin, J. Y. (1980). Anatomy and physiology of a binocular system in the frog Rana pipiens. *Brain Res.* **192**, pp. 313–25.

Harris, W. A. (1980). The effects of eliminating impulse activity on the development of the retinotectal projection in salamanders. *J. Comp. Neurol.* **194**, pp. 303–17.

Hebb, D. O. (1949). *The organization of behavior.* Wiley, New York.

Holt, C. E. (1984). Does timing of axon outgrowth influence initial retinotectal topography in Xenopus. *J. Neurosci.* **4,** pp. 1130–52.

Holt, C. E. and Harris, W. A. (1983). Order in the initial retinotectal map in Xenopus: a new technique for labelling growing nerve fibres. *Nature* **301,** pp. 13–19.

Holt, C. E. and Thompson, I. A. (1984). The effects of Tetrodotoxin on the development of hamster retinal projections. *J. Physiol. (Lond.)* **357,** p. 24P.

Innocenti, G. M. (1981). Growth and reshaping of axons in the establishment of visual callosal connections *Science* **212,** pp. 824–7.

Insausti, R., Blakemore, C., and Cowan, W. M. (1984). Ganglion cell death during development of the ipsilateral retinocollicular projection in the golden hamster. *Nature* **308,** pp. 362–5.

Jeffery, G. (1984). Retinal ganglion cell death an terminal field retraction in the developing rodent visual system. *Dev. Brain Res.* **13,** pp. 81–96.

Jeffery, G. and Perry, V. H. (1982). Evidence for ganglion cell death during development of the ipsilateral retinal projection in the rat. *Dev. Brain Res.* **2,** pp. 176–90.

Lamb, A. H. (1984). Motoneuron death in the embryo. *CRC critical reviews in clinical neurobiology* **1,** pp. 141–79.

Land, P. W. and Lund, R. D. (1979). Development of the uncrossed retinotectal pathway, and its relation to plasticity studies. *Science* **205,** pp. 698–700.

LeVay, S., Stryker, M. P., and Shatz, C. J. (1978). Ocular dominance columns and their development in layer VI of the cat's visual cortex: a quantitative study. *J. Comp. Neurol.* **179,** pp. 223–44.

LeVay, S., Wiesel, T. N., and Hubel, D. H. (1981). In *The organization of the cerebral cortex* (eds. G. O. Schmitt, F. G. Worden, G. Adelman and S. G. Dennis), pp. 29–45. MIT Press, Cambridge, MA.

Levi-Montalcini, R. (1982). Developmental biology and natural history of nerve growth factor. *Ann. Rev. Neurosci.* **5,** p. 341–62.

Levine, R. L. and Jacobson, M. (1975). Discontinuus mapping of retina with tectum innervated by both eyes. *Brain Res.* **98,** pp. 172–6.

Martin, P. R., Sefton, A. J., and Dreher, B. (1983). The retinal location and fate of ganglion cells which project to the ipsilateral superior colliculus in neonatal albino and hooded rats. *Neurosci. Lett* **41,** pp. 219–26.

Mastronarde, G. (1983). Correlated activity of cat retinal ganglion cells. I. Spontaneously active inputs to X and Y cells. *J. Neurophysiol.* **49,** pp. 303–15.

McCaffrey, M. R., Bennet, M. R., and Dreher, B. (1982). The survival of neonatal rat retinal ganglion cells in vitro is enhanced in the presence of appropriate part of the brain. *Exp. Brain Res.* **48,** pp. 377–86.

McLoon, S. C. (1982). Alterations in the precision of the crossed retinotectal projection during tectal development. *Science* **215,** pp. 1418–20.

McLoon, S. C. (1985). Evidence for shifting connections during the development of the chick retinotectal projection. *J. Neurosci.* **5,** pp. 2570–80.

Meyer, R. L. (1982). Tetrodotoxin blocks the formation of ocular dominance columns in goldfish. *Science* **218,** pp. 589–91.

Meyer, R. L. (1983). Tetrodotoxin inhibits the formation of refined retinotopography in the goldfish. *Dev. Brain. Res.* **6,** pp. 293–8.

O'Leary, D. D. M. and Cowan, W. M. (1983). Topographic organisation of certain tectal afferent and efferent connections can develop normally in the absence of retinal input. *Proc. Natl. Acad. Sci. USA*. **80,** pp. 6131–5.

O'Leary, D. D. M., Fawcett, J. W., and Cowan, R. M. (1983). The early postnatal restriction of the ipsilateral retinocollicular projection is due to cell death rather than collateral elimination. *Soc. Neurosci. Abstr*. **9,** p. 856.

O'Leary, D. D. M., Fawcett, J. W., and Cowan, W. M. (1986). Topographic targeting errors in the retinocollicular projection and their elimination by selective ganglion cell death. *J. Neurosci*. **6,** pp. 3692–705.

O'Leary, D. D. M., Stanfield, B. B., and Cowan, W. M. (1981). Evidence that the early postnatal restriction of the cells of origin of the callosal projection is due to the elimination of axon collaterals rather than to the death of neurons. *Dev. Brain Res*. **1,** pp. 607–17.

Oppenheim, R. and Chu-Wang, I. W. (1983). In *Somatic and autonomic nerve muscle interactions* (eds. G. Burnstock, and G. Vrobova), pp. 57–107. Elsevier, Amsterdam.

Rager, G. and Rager, U. (1978). Systems matching by degeneration. 1, A quantitative electron microscopic study of the generation and degeneration of ganglion cells in the chicken. *Exp. Brain. Res*. **33,** pp. 65–78.

Reh, T. A. and Constantine-Paton, M. (1984). Retinal ganglion cell terminals change their projection sites during larval development of Rana pipiens. *J. Neurosci*. **4,** pp. 442–57.

Reh, T. A. and Constantine-Paton, M. (1985). Eye specific segregation requires neural activity in 3 eyed Rana pipiens. *J. Neurosci*. **5,** pp. 1132–43.

Rusoff, A. C. (1984). Patterns of axons in the visual system of perciform fish and implications of these paths for rules governing axonal growth. *J. Neurosci*. **4,** pp. 1414–28.

Sachs, G. M., Jacobson, M., and Caviness, V. S. (1986). Postnatal changes in arborization patterns of murine retinocollicular axons. *J. Comp. Neurol*. **246,** pp. 395–408.

Sanes, D. H. and Constantine-Paton, M. (1985). The sharpening of frequency tuning curves requires patterned activity during development in the mouse, *Mus musculus*. *J. Neurosci*. **5,** pp. 1152–6.

Sawcenko, P. E. and Swanson, L. W. (1981). A method for tracing biochemically defined pathways in the central nervous system using combined fluorescence, retrograde transport and immunohistochemical techniques. *Brain Res*. **210,** pp. 31–51.

Schmidt, J. T. (1987). Activity-dependent sharpening of the retinotopic projection on the tectum of goldfish in regeneration and development. In *The making of the nervous system* (eds. J. G. Parnavelas, C. D. Stern, and R. V. Stirling), pp. 380–94. Oxford University Press, Oxford.

Schmidt, J. T. and Edwards, D. L. (1983). Activity sharpens the map during the regeneration of the retinotectal projection in goldfish. *Brain Res*. **268,** pp. 28–39.

Schmidt, J. T. and Eisele, L. E. (1985). Stroboscopic illumination and dark rearing block the sharpening of the regenerated retinotectal map in goldfish. *Neuroscience*. **14,** pp. 535–46.

Schmidt, J. T., Cicerone, C. M., and Easter, S. S., Jr. (1978). Expansion of the half retinal projection to the tectum in goldfish: an electrophysiological and anatomical study. *J. Comp. Neurol*. **177,** pp. 257–78.

Schneider, G. E., Rava, L., Sachs, G. M., and Jhaveri, S. (1981). Widespread branching of retinotectal axons: transient in normal development and anomalous in adults with neonatal lesions. *Soc. Neurosci. Abstr.* **7**, p. 732.

Sengelaub, D. R. and Finlay, B. L. (1982). Cell death in the mammalian visual system during normal development. 1. Retinal ganglion cells. *J. Comp. Neurol.* **204**, pp. 311–17.

Stent, G. S. (1973). A physiological mechanism for Hebb's postulate of learning. *Proc. Natl. Acad. Sci. USA.* **70**, pp. 997–1001.

Straznicky, C., Gaze, R. M., and Horder, T. J. (1979). Selection of appropriate medial branch the optic tract by fibres of ventral retinal origin during development and regeneration: and autoradiographic study in Xenopus. *J. Embryol. exp. Morphol.* **50**, pp. 253–67.

Stryker, M. P. (1981). Late segregation of geniculate afferents to the cat's visual cortex after recovery from binocular impulse blockade. *Soc. Neurosci. Abstr.* **7**, p. 842.

Stryker, M. P. and Strickland, S. L. (1984). Physiological segregation of ocular dominance columns depends on the pattern of afferent electrical activity. *Invest. Ophthalmol.* **25** (Suppl), p. 278.

Stuermer, C. A. and Easter, S. S., Jr. (1984). Rules of order in the retinotectal fascicles of goldfish. *J. Neurosci.* **4**, pp. 1045–51.

Swindale, N. V. (1981). Absence of ocular dominance patches in dark reared cats. *Nature* **290**, p. 332–3.

Thoenen, H. and Edgar, D. (1985). Neurotrophic factors. *Science* **228**, pp. 238–42.

Turner, J. E. (1985). Promotion of neurite outgrowth and survival in dissociated fetal rat retinal cultures by a fraction derived from a brain extract. *Dev. Brain Res.* **18**, pp. 265–74.

Udin, S. B. (1983). Abnormal visual input leads to development of abnormal axon trajectories in frogs. *Nature* **301**, pp. 336–8.

Udin, S. B. and Gaze, R. M. (1983). Expansion and retinotopic order in the goldfish retinotectal map after large retinal lesions. *Exp. Brain. Res.* **50**, pp. 347–52.

Udin, S. B. and Keating, M. J. (1983). Plasticity in a central nervous pathway in Xenopus: anatomical changes in the isthmotectal projection after larval eye rotation. *J. Comp. Neurol.* **203**, pp. 575–94.

Woo, H. H., Jen, L. S., and So, K. F. (1985). The postnatal development of retinocollicular projections in normal hamsters and in hamsters following neonatal mononuclear enucleation: an HRP tracing study. *Brain Res.* **352**, pp. 1–13.

PART V

Differentiative events

Introduction

We began this volume by asking how cell diversity is generated. We must now return to this question to ask how the neurons generated by the processes outlined in the previous chapters consolidate their fates as distinct phenotypes. How do they produce the multitude of neurotransmitter types and morphological types found in the adult nervous system? How is the pattern made functional? In parallel with the development of definitive connections between neurons is the synthesis of their transmitters and receptors, the moulding of the shape of their receiving areas—the dendritic tree—and their output areas—the axonal arborizations. Recent advances in neuropharmacology have yielded a plethora of transmitters. The four chapters in this section stress the complexity of the system and the difficulties inherent in the study of the genesis of this complexity. With the advent of accessible techniques in molecular biology and their judicious use by researchers in this field, perhaps the next few years will see some of these problems resolved.

Classical cell biologists have long recognized the importance of the cytoskeleton in determining both cell shape and the position of cellular components such as hormone and growth factor receptors, as well as cellular movements. These movements include cell migrations as seen in early development as well as subcellular movements of cytoplasm and organelles, such as those seen in axoplasmic transport and cytoplasmic streaming, which are important in distributing nutrients and other components to remote parts of the cell anatomy. Neuronal asymmetry is essential for their functional compartmentalization. For example, if a dendrite with many arbors receives inputs from several other neurons, each of which releases a different neurotransmitter, it is important for the correct receptors to be present at the appropriate synapses. The cytoskeleton could control the position of synaptic assemblies that are connected to it directly or indirectly. It probably also controls cell shape by controlling the position of adhesive sites in the cell membrane into which it is inserted.

This section begins with a review of components of the tubulin cytoskeleton and their roles in neuronal morphogenesis. Chapters 22 and 23 then review some of the developmental changes that lead to the diversification of neurotransmitters and their receptors in cells of the central and peripheral nervous systems. Finally, Chapter 24 considers some of the factors that are important in determining the shape of dendritic arbors.

21

Microtuble-associated proteins and neuronal morphogenesis

ANDREW MATUS

MOLECULAR APPROACHES TO NEURONAL MORPHOGENESIS

The characteristic dendritic and axonal fields of different types of neurons play a major role in determining the pathways available for signal transmission in the mature brain. Comparing the neighbouring Purkinje cell and granule cell neurons of the cerebellar cortex provides a good illustration of the profound influence that dendritic form can have on synaptic connectivity. The extensively branched dendrites of each Purkinje cell allow the integration of inputs from many thousands of synapses that converge upon them. The granule cell dendrites are, by comparison, short and poorly branched and several may share one mossy fibre axon terminal so that they act as a point of divergence of afferent signals (Eccles, Ito, and Szentagothai 1967; Palay and Chan-Palay 1974). Similar examples of patterns of connectivity depending upon appropriately formed axonal and dendritic fields occur throughout the brain (Sheperd 1974; Szentagothai and Arbib 1974) and one of the goals of cellular neurobiology is to understand how this diversity of form is generated and controlled during neuronal differentiation in the developing nervous system.

Several kinds of observations suggest that many of the fundamental characteristics of neuronal form are intrinsic to the class of neuron. For example, hippocampal pyramidal cells can still produce their characteristic multipolar dendrites, even when abnormal histogenesis leaves them 'upside down' with respect to the surrounding tissue (van der Loos 1965), and these cells also develop their characteristic shapes when grown in culture independent of contacts with other cells (Banker and Cowan 1977; Seiffert, Ranscht, Fink, Forster, Beckh, and Muller 1984). However, this may not be true for all neuronal cell types. Cerebellar granule cells grown in culture retain the size and shape of their cell body and make axon-like processes but produce nothing that resembles the dendrites that develop *in vivo* (Messer 1977; Privat, Marson, and Drain 1979). More important, it is clear that the details of dendritic and axonal form are not fixed but are 'plastic', because they may be altered by a variety of extrinsic circumstances including tissue damage (Lynch and Cotman 1975) and environmental input (Rakic 1974; Lund 1978). It is generally believed that developmental plasticity is regulated by patterns of activity in the developing nervous system arising from external stimuli. Presumably they exert their influence via the molecular mechanisms that regulate axon and dendrite growth. However, before this can be studied the basic molecular mechanisms involved in the growth of neuronal processes must be discovered and characterized.

MICROTUBULES ARE IMPLICATED IN NEURITE EXTENSION

Electron microscopy has shown that axons and dendrites are extremely rich in microtubules (Peters, Palay, and Webster 1976) and their importance for the generation and maintenance of neuronal processes has been demonstrated by experiments using drugs, such as colchicine, that cause microtubules to depolymerize. When such drugs are applied to either neuroblastoma cells (Seeds, Gilman, Amano, and Nirenberg 1970; Yamada, Spooner, and Wessels 1970) or primary neurons (Bray, Thomas, and Shaw 1978; Matus, Bernhardt, Bodmer, and Alaimo 1986) growing in tissue culture the inevitable consequence is that the neurites shrink back into the cell body (Fig. 21.1).

Evidently, then, assembled microtubules are essential to the integrity of neuronal processes, but how is the formation of microtubules translated into the growth of an axon or dendrite? Some clues have been gained from the observation of cultured cells, which has suggested that the morphological stability of neurites depends on their content of stable assembled microtubules, because one of the earliest effects microtubule depolymerizing drugs have on neurites is the loss of cylindrical form and the appearance of lateral filopodia (Bray *et al.* 1978; Anglister, Farber, Shahar, and Grinvald 1982; Matus *et al.* 1986; also see Fig. 21.1). Recent experiments have shown that microtubules in interphase non-neuronal cells are in a state of dynamic instability, growing rapidly toward the periphery from centrally located initiator sites while at the same time being subject to sudden collapse (Schulze and Kirschner 1986). It seems unlikely that cells whose microtubules are in such a state of flux could produce a stable axon or dendrite. Thus in looking for molecules that transform microtubule formation into process outgrowth, stabilization of the microtubules will be of major importance. However, stabilization by itself is insufficient to explain the character of axonal and dendrite growth, because one of its most striking properties is its plasticity. This has been demonstrated recently by direct observations of neuronal morphology in young growing animals, which showed that the developing dendrites possess a high degree of structural plasticity (Purves, Hadley, and Voyvodic 1986).

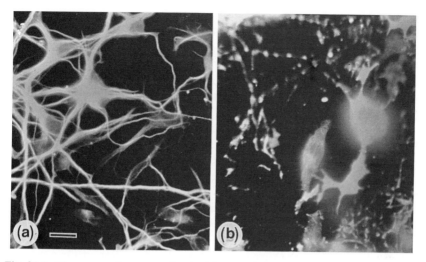

Fig. 21.1. Hippocampal neurons that had been maintained in dissociated cell culture for seven days. (a) shows a control culture, fixed and stained with monoclonal antibodies against the microtubule-associated protein MAP2 as described by Matus *et al.* (1986). (b) shows a culture from the same set that had been exposed to the tubulin depolymerizing drug nocodazole at 0·25 μg/ml for two hours prior to fixation. Note that in addition to retracting, the cell processes have an irregular outline after nocodazole. Scale bar: 20 μm.

MICROTUBULE-ASSOCIATED PROTEINS MAY REGULATE MICROTUBULE FORMATION

From the above considerations it is obviously of interest to identify molecular components in neurons that regulate microtubule formation, and particularly those that might influence the balance between plasticity and stability. One obvious place to look for such molecules is in the microtubules themselves. This has been done by examining microtubules repolymerized from brain and it has found that, in addition to the structural subunit, tubulin, they contain other proteins known as microtubule-associated proteins (MAPs). Several of these have now been purified and shown to promote tubulin polymerization *in vitro* (e.g. MAP2 and tau: Herzog and Weber 1978; MAP1: Kuznetsov, Rodionov, Gelfand, and Rosenblat 1981; MAP3: Huber, Pehling, and Matus 1986).

The idea that these proteins might be involved in the growth of axons and dendrites has been further stimulated by the recent discovery that antibodies against several of them selectively stain different microdomains of the neuronal cytoplasm (Cumming and Burgoyne 1983; Matus, Huber, and Bernhardt 1983). The different patterns of compartmentalization shown by the various MAPs are very striking. The first to be discovered was MAP2, which throughout the brain is selectively associated with the dendrites of neurons (Bernhardt and Matus 1984; Caceres, Birder, Payne, Bender, Rebhun, and Steward 1984; De Camilli, Miller, Nauone, Theurkauf, and Vallee 1984). More recently tau MAP has been found to be associated with axons (Binder, Frankfurter, and Rebhun 1985). Other MAPs show more complex patterns. For example, MAP1 is present in both axons and dendrites (Bloom, Schonfield, and Vallee 1984; Huber and Matus 1984) but, in adult brain, dendrites are more intensely stained by anti-MAP1 than are axons (Huber and Matus 1984). MAP5 appears to be neuron specific and present at similar levels in both axons and dendrites (Riederer, Cohen, and Matus 1986). MAP3 shows a more complicated pattern, being present in astroglial cells and neurons, but in the adult brain its neuronal distribution is limited to neurofilament-rich axons (Huber, Alaimo-Beuret, and Matus 1985).

More subtle differences in cellular location also occur for molecules whose distributions overlap. An example of such a phenomenon is provided by MAP1 and MAP2 in Purkinje cell dendrites. Examination of the cerebellar cortex at low magnification shows that anti-MAP1 staining is much stronger in the molecular layer than in the granular layer [Fig. 21.2(a)], whereas the opposite is true for anti-MAP2 staining [Fig. 21.2(b)]. The myelinated axon tracts of the white matter also react differently, there being weak staining by anti-MAP1 but absolutely no reaction with anti-MAP2. The difference in staining of the granular layer is also clear at higher magnifications where the granule cells and their process are revealed as the major site of MAP2 staining [Fig. 21.3(b); also see Bernhardt and Matus 1984]. Differences in the patterns of Purkinje cell staining by the two antibodies are also revealed. Anti-MAP1 strongly stains the cell bodies and initial axon segments [Fig. 21.3(a)] whereas anti-MAP2 staining is significantly weaker in Purkinje cell bodies than more distally in the dendritic tree [Fig. 21.3(b); also see Huber and Matus 1984].

These observations raise some interesting questions: Are the different levels of expression of MAP1 and MAP2 in granule and Purkinje cells related to the morphological differences between them? Does the difference in distribution between MAP1 and MAP2 mean that there are different classes of microtubules, of different chemical composition, within the same neuron? Finally, as a somewhat radical consideration, could it be that despite their strong association with microtubules *in vitro*, the distributions of these proteins in living cells are determined by binding to something other than microtubules?

DEVELOPMENTAL REGULATION

Various MAPs undergo simultaneous changes in expression during brain maturation

Microtubule-associated proteins undergo striking changes in form and abundance in developing brain that also implicates them in neuronal

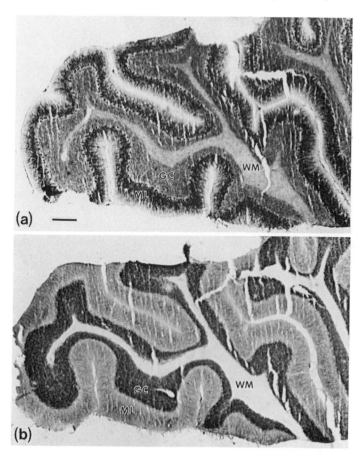

Fig. 21.2. Comparison of anti-MAP1 (a) and anti-MAP2 (b) staining patterns in adult rat cerebellum. These acetone-fixed cryostat sections were cut from the same block of tissue and prepared as described in Huber and Matus (1984). GC, granular layer; ML, molecular layer; WM, white-matter axon tracts. Scale bar: 500 μm.

morphogensis. In the case of MAP1 the change is marked by a steady increase in level from barely detectable in embryonic day 19 (E19) rat brain to being one of the most prominent MAPs in adults (Riederer *et al.* 1986). Tau MAP proteins also change, from two predominant components in the neonate to five or six bands in the adult (Mareck, Fellous, Francon, and Nunez 1980), and the high molecular weight components of MAP2 change from a single component (b) before postnatal day 10 (P10) to two components (a and b) by P20 (Binder, Frankfurter, Kim, Caceres, Payne, and Rebhun 1984; Burgoyne and Cumming 1984). A smaller (70 kD) protein which reacts with some monoclonal antibodies against MAP2 undergoes a dramatic drop in abun-

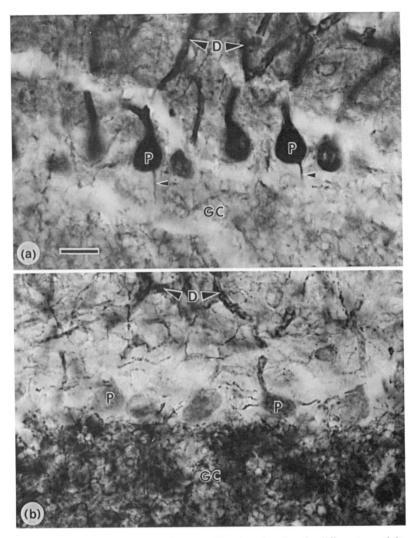

Fig. 21.3. The same material at higher magnification showing the different reactivity of granule cells (GC) and Purkinje cells (P) with anti-MAP1 (a) and anti-MAP2 (b). In (a) initial axon segments of Purkinje cells are indicated by arrow-heads. Note that for anti-MAP2 dendrites stain more strongly in the upper molecular layer (D) than close to the cell body (P), whereas for anti-MAP1 the intensity is comparable in cell body and dendrites. Scale bar: 30 μm.

dance over the same period (Reiderer and Matus 1985). We have recently shown that this protein is an independently expressed fragment of MAP2 which we call MAP2c (Garner, Brugg, and Matus, submitted for publication).

The recently discovered proteins MAP1 (X) (Calvert and Anderton 1985),

MAP3 (Reiderer and Matus 1985), and MAP5 (Reiderer *et al.* 1986) are all substantially more abundant in juvenile brain than in adult (from five- to ten-fold). In each case the large drop in level occurs between P10 and P20 in rat brain. Prior to this time each of these MAPs is transitorily expressed in neuronal compartments from which it is absent in adult brain (Bernhardt, Huber, and Matus 1985; Calvert and Anderton 1985; Riederer *et al.* 1986). In the case of MAP3 this is particularly striking because in the cerebral cortex of neo-natal animals it is present in the cell bodies and processes of all neurons whereas in the adult it only occurs in glial cells (Riederer and Matus 1985). One of the most intriguing features of these developmental changes in MAP expression is the similarity in their time courses. For all the MAPs that have been investigated, the change from the neo-natal to the adult pattern in rat brain is accomplished by the end of the third post-natal week, which coincides with the time at which axons and dendrites reach their adult form (Berry 1982).

MAP2 distribution in developing Purkinje cells suggests a role in dendrite formation

During rat Purkinje cell development MAP2 becomes increasingly localized within the dendrites. At birth it is present in the cell bodies and becomes concentrated in patches beneath the surface membrane (Bernhardt and Matus 1982). As the apical dendrites begin to grow out, anti-MAP2 staining is strongest at a position distal, but not terminal, within the developing processes [Fig. 21.4(a)]. As the dendrites elongate, the restricted localization of the MAP2 becomes progressively more pronounced so that the cell body and proximal portion of the apical dendrite are relatively lightly stained compared to the region of the dendrites in the outer molecular layer [Fig. 21.4(b),(c)]. This partitioning of MAP2 within the dendritic cytoplasm is particularly marked in Purkinje cells. One further observation suggests that the characteristic morphology of the Purkinje cell, with its exclusively apical dendritic tree and the relatively remote location of afferent synapses with respect to the cell body, may influence MAP2 distribution. During early stages of development MAP2 is found in somatic spines, short protrusions from the cell body which are transitorily post-synaptic to climbing fibres. When these retract, anti-MAP2 staining disappears from the cell body.

Because MAP2 promotes tubulin polymerization *in vitro* one might expect that its presence in the developing Purkinje cell dendrites would be associated with the formation of stable microtubules. However, the situation is not so straight forward. In the developing cerebellar cortex the granule cell axons (parallel fibres) stain more strongly with anti-tubulin than the neighbouring Purkinje cell dendrites, and in electron microscopic preparations we found well-preserved microtubules in parallel fibre axons, but in Purkinje cell dendrites next to them microtubules appeared to be lacking (Bernhardt and

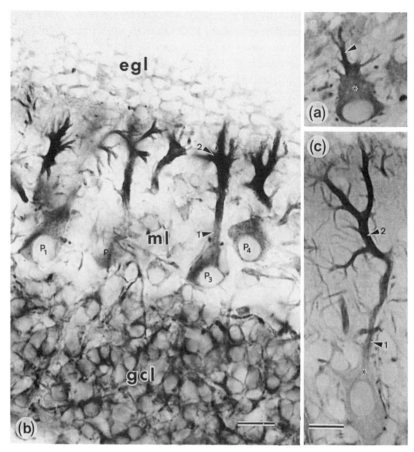

Fig. 21.4. The distribution of MAP2 in developing Purkinje cells. Brain from 3-day (a), 7-day (b), and 15-day (c) rat cerebellum was fixed and stained as described in Bernhardt and Matus (1984). Note the relative weak staining of the cell body cytoplasm [asterisks in (a) and (c)] and the difference in staining intensity between the proximal and distal region of the apical dendrite (respectively labelled 1 and 2 in (b) and (c). ml, molecular layer; gcl, granule cell layer; egl, external granule cell layer; P, Purkinje cells. Scale bars: (a) and (c): 20 μm; (b) 25 μm.

Matus 1982). This suggests either that tubulin is less abundant than MAP2 in developing Purkinje cell dendrites or that highly abundant MAP2 (and perhaps other MAPs) mask tubulin epitopes. Both explanations may hold. The absence of observable microtubules in dendrites while neighbouring axons contain them may indicate that the dendritic tubulin is unassembled, perhaps because its concentration is too low to initiate polymerization even in the presence of abundant MAP2. Alternatively microtubules in developing Purkinje cell dendrites may be unstable and difficult to fix. Even this last, rather technical, explanation suggests that significant differences in microtubule stability occur in different neuronal compartments of the developing brain.

MAP expression in neurons developing in culture

Cultured neurons are an attractive subject for studying the relationship between changes in microtubule proteins and neuronal differentiation, both because cultured cells are readily manipulated and because they can be observed continuously. An important preliminary question is whether neurons differentiating in culture can achieve the morphology they exhibit in the brain. The evidence suggests that they can to a partial degree. For example, in hippocampal slice cultures the cell bodies of pyramidal cells form a single layer and develop recognizable apical and basal dendrites, which are correctly oriented, whereas in cerebellar slices the Purkinje cells have multiple dendrites which are stunted compared to the profusely branched single apical dendrite they develop in brain (Gahwiler 1981).

In dissociated cell cultures different types of neurons express their morphological potential to varying degrees. As in slice cultures, hippocampal pyramidal cells exhibit all of their fundamental morphological characteristics (Banker and Cowan 1977), whereas the differentiation of cerebellar granule cells in culture is less complete than it is in the brain. In dissociated cell cultures from neo-natal rat cerebellum, granule cell neurons retain their characteristic size and round cell body and over a period of a week to 12 days they extend a long, thin process that forms few branches and is of axon-like appearance (Messer 1977; Privat *et al.* 1979; Alaimo-Beuret and Matus 1985). They do not make any processes resembling the short, club-ended dendrites that characterize these cells in the brain (Palay and Chan-Palay 1974). In these cultured granule cells tubulin is present throughout the cell body and processes whereas MAP2 is restricted to the cell body and an initial varicose segment of the processes (Alaimo-Beuret and Matus 1985). MAP2 is absent from granule cell axons in the brain (Bernhardt and Matus 1984), so its absence from the processes that these cells make in culture appears to confirm their identification as axons. On the other hand, the presence of MAP2 in the initial portion of these processes indicates that, even within a single neuronal process, MAP2 and tubulin can be differently distributed.

Hippocampal pyramical cells in culture are multipolar, extending several processes that are recognizably dendritic and usually one that has axonal morphology (Banker and Cowan 1977). All these processes contain tubulin, but in the differentiated cells MAP2 is absent from the axons except in their initial portion (Caceres, Banker, Steward, Binder, and Payne 1984; Matus *et al.* 1985). Thus in both cerebellar granule cells and hippocampal pyramidal cells the cut-off point for MAP2 lies within the axon. A further interesting feature that has emerged from observing cultured cells is that during development MAP2 is present throughout all the processes both of granule cells (Alaimo-Beuret and Matus 1985) and of pyramidal cells (Caceres, Banker, and Binder 1986). Only later does its distribution within axons become restricted.

PROSPECTS FOR FUNCTIONAL STUDIES

Despite the large number of biochemical and cytological studies on MAPs that have appeared over the past few years we still have only the most rudimentary knowledge of their functions in living neurons. It is generally presumed that the MAPs promote tubulin polymerization and function as linkers between microtubules and other elements of the cytoskeleton, but this notion is supported only by *in vitro* experiments. To discover what MAPs contribute to neuronal morphogenesis will require the design of experiments that address functional questions directly. The best prospects at the moment appear to come from the use of cultured neurons, and especially from experiments in which individual MAPs or antibodies against them are introduced into cells and the consequence for neurite growth are studied. Another potentially rich source of information is the use of cloned DNA. The isolation of cDNA probes for MAPs has only recently begun. These have already proved their value in demonstrating that tau and MAP2 are the products of unique genes and that cDNAs for these molecules do not readily cross-hybridise with other brain messenger RNAs (Drubin, Caput, and Kirschner 1984; Lewis, Villasante, Sherline, and Cowan 1986). Such data, and the sequence information on MAP primary structure that will shortly become available, should provide a major advance in our understanding of possible relationships between the different MAPs, particularly with respect to their tubulin binding sites.

REFERENCES

Alaimo-Beuret, D. and Matus, A. (1985). Changes in the cytoplasmic distribution of microtubule-associated protein 2 during the differentiation of cultured cerebellar granule cells. *Neuroscience* **14**, pp. 1103–15.
Anglister, L., Farber, I., Shahar, I. C., and Grinvald, A. (1982). Localization of voltage-sensitive calcium channels along developing neurites: their possible role in regulating neurites elongation. *Dev. Biol.* **94**, pp. 351–65.
Banker, G. A. and Cowan, M. (1977). Rat hippocampal neurons in dispersed cell culture. *Brain Res.* **126**, pp. 397–425.
Bernhardt, R. and Matus, A. (1982). Initial phase of dendrite growth: evidence for the involvement of high molecular weight microtubule-associated protein (HMWP) prior to the appearance of tubulin. *J. Cell Biol.* **92**, pp. 589–93.
Bernhardt, R. and Matus, A. (1984). Light and electron microscopic studies on the

distribution of microtubule-associated protein 2 in rat brain: a difference between dendritic and axonal cytoskeletons. *J. Comp. Neurol.* **226**, pp. 203–19.

Bernhardt, R., Huber, G., and Matus, A. (1985). Differences in the development patterns of three microtubule-associated proteins in the rat cerebellum. *J. Neurosci.* **5**, pp. 977–91.

Berry, M. (1982). Cellular differentiation: development of dendritic arborizations under normal and experimentally altered conditions. *Neurosci. Res. Prog. Bull.* **20**, pp. 451–61.

Binder, L. I., Frankfurter, A., and Rebhun, L. I. (1985). The distribution of tau in the mammalian central nervous system. *J. Cell Biol.* **101**, pp. 1371–8.

Binder, L., Frankfurter, A., Kim, H., Caceres, A., Payne, M. R., and Rebhun, L. I. (1984). Heterogeneity of microtubule-associated protein 2 during rat brain development. *Proc. Natl. Acad. Sci. USA.* **81**, pp. 5613–17.

Bloom, G. S., Schonfield, T. A., and Vallee, R. B. (1984). Widespread distribution of the major polypeptide component of MAP1 (microtubule-associated protein 1) in the nervous system. *J. Cell Biol.* **98**, pp. 320–30.

Bray, D., Thomas, C., and Shaw, G. (1978). Growth cone formation in cultures of sensory neurons. *Proc. Natl. Acad. Sci. USA* **81**, pp. 5613–29.

Burgoyne, R. D. and Cumming, R. (1984). Ontogeny of microtubule-associated protein 2 in rat cerebellum: differential expression of the doublet polypeptides. *Neuroscience* **11**, pp. 157–67.

Caceres A., Banker, G. A., and Binder, L. (1986). Immunocytochemical localization of tubulin and microtubule-associated protein 2 during the development of hippocampal neurons in culture. *J. Neurosci.* **6**, pp. 714–22.

Caceres, A., Banker, G., Steward, O., Binder, L., and Payne, M. (1984). MAP2 is localized to the dendrites of hippocampal neurons which develop in culture. *Dev. Brain Res.* **13**, pp. 314–8.

Caceres, A., Binder, L. I., Payne, M. R., Bender, P., Rebhun, L., and Steward, O. (1984). Differential subcellular localization of tubulin and microtubule-associated protein MAP2 in brain tissue as revealed by immunocytochemistry with monoclonal antibodies. *J. Neurosci.* **4**, pp. 394–410.

Calvert, R. and Anderton, B. H. (1985). A microtubule-associated protein (MAP1) which is expressed at elevated levels during development of the rat cerebellum. *EMBO J.* **4**, pp. 1171–6.

Cumming, R. and Burgoyne, R. D. (1983). Compartmentalization of neuronal cytoskeleton *Biosci. Reports* **3**, pp. 997–1006.

De Camilli, P., Miller, T. E., Navone, F., Theurkauf, W. E., and Vallee, R. B. (1984). Distribution of microtubule-associated protein 2 in the nervous system of the rat studied by immunofluorescence. *Neuroscience* **11**, pp. 819–46.

Drubin, D. G., Caput, D., and Kirschner, M. W. (1984). Studies on the expression of the microtubule-associated protein, tau, during mouse brain development, with newly isolated complementary DNA probes. *J. Cell Biol.* **98**, pp. 1090–7.

Eccles, J., Ito, M., and Szentagothai, J. (1967). *The cerebellum as a neuronal machine.* Springer-Verlag, Berlin.

Gahwiler, B. (1981). Morphological differentiation of nerve cells in thin organotypic cultures derived from rat hippocampus and cerebellum. *Proc. R. Soc. Lond. B* **211**, pp. 2897–90.

Herzog, W. and Weber, K. (1978). Fraction of brain microtubule-associated proteins. *Eur. J. Biochem.* **92**, pp. 1–8.

Huber, G. and Matus, A. (1984). Differences in the cellular distributions of two microtubule-associated proteins, MAP1 and MAP2, in rat brain. *J. Neurosci.* **4**, pp. 151–60.

Huber, G., Alaimo-Beuret, D., and Matus, A. (1985). MAP3: characterization of a novel microtubule-associated protein. *J. Cell Biol.* **100**, pp. 496–507.

Huber, G., Pehling, G., and Matus, A. (1986). The novel microtubule-associated protein MAP3 contributes to the in vitro assembly of brain microtubules. *J. Biol. Chem.* **261**, pp. 2270–3.

Kuznetsov, S. A., Rodionov, V. I., Gelfand, V. I., and Rosenblat, V. A. (1981). Microtubule-associated protein MAP1 promotes microtubule assembly in vitro. *FEBS Letters* **135**, pp. 241–4.

Lewis, S. A., Villasante, A., Sherline, P., and Cowan, N. J. (1986). Brain-specific expression of MAP2 detected using a cloned cDNA probe. *J. Cell Biol.* **102**, pp. 2098–105.

Lund, R. D. (1978). *Developmental and plasticity of the brain.* Oxford University Press, New York.

Mareck, A., Fellous, A., Francon, J., and Nunez, J. (1980). Changes in the composition and activity of microtubule-associated proteins during brain development. *Nature (Lond.)* **284**, pp. 353–5.

Matus, A., Huber, G., and Bernhardt, R. (1983). Neuronal microdifferentiation. *Cold Spring Harb. Symp. Quant. Biol.* **48**, pp. 775–82.

Matus, A., Bernhardt, R., Bodmer, R., and Alaimo, D. (1985). Microtubule-associated protein 2 and tubulin are differently distributed in the dendrites of developing neurons. *Neuroscience* **17**, pp. 371–89.

Messer, A. (1977). The maintenance and identification of cerebellar granule cells in monolayer cultures. *Brain Res.* **130**, pp. 1–12.

Palay, S. L. and Chan-Palay, V. (1974). *Cerebellar cortex.* Springer-Verlag, New York.

Peters, A., Palay, S. L. and Webster, H. deF. (1976). *The fine structure of the nervous system.* W. B. Saunders, Philadelphia, PA.

Privat, A., Marson, A. M., and Drain, M. J. (1979). In vitro models of neural growth. *Progr. Brain Res.* **51**, pp. 335–56.

Purves, D., Hadley, R. D., and Voyvodic, J. T. (1986). Dynamic changes in the dendritic geometry of individual neurons visualized over periods of up to three months in the superior cervical ganglion of living mice. *J. Neurosci.* **6**, pp. 1051–60.

Rakic, P. (1974). Intrinsic and extrinsic factors influencing the shape of neurons and their assembly into neuronal circuits. In *Frontiers in neurology and neuroscience research* (eds. P. Seeman and G. Brown), pp. 112–32. University of Toronto Press, Toronto.

Riederer, B. and Matus, A. (1985). Differential expression of distinct microtubule-associated proteins during brain development. *Proc. Natl. Acad. Sci. USA.* **82**, pp. 6006–9.

Riederer, B., Cohen, R., and Matus, A. (1986). MAP5: a novel brain microtubule-associated protein under strong devlopmental regulation. *J. Neurocytol.* **15**, pp. 763–75.

Schulze, E. and Kirschner, M. (1986). Microtubule dynamics in interphase cells. *J. Cell Biol.* **102**, pp. 1020–31.

Seeds, N. W., Gilman, A. G., Amano, T., and Nirenberg, M. W. (1970). Regulation of axon formation by clonal cell lines of a neuronal tumor. *Proc. Natl. Acad. Sci. USA* **60**, pp. 160–7.

Seiffert, T., Ranscht, B., Fink, H., Forster, H., Beckh, S., and Muller, H. W. (1984). Development of hippocampal pyramidal cells in tissue culture: a molecular approach. In *Neurobiology of the hippocampus* (ed. W. Seiffert), pp. 109–33. Academic Press, New York.

Sheperd, G. M. (1974). *The synaptic organization of the brain. An introduction.* Oxford University Press, New York.

Szentagothai, J. and Arbib, M. A. (1974). Conceptual models of neural organization. *Neurosci. Res. Prog. Bull.* **12,** pp. 370–510.

Van der Loos, H. (1965). The 'improperly' oriented pyramidal cells in the cerebral cortex and its possible bearing on problems of growth and cell orientation. *Bull. John Hopkins Hosp.* **117,** pp. 228–50.

Yamada, K. M., Spooner, B. S., and Wessels, N. K. (1970). Axon growth: roles of microfilaments and microtubules. *Proc. Natl. Acad. Sci. USA* **66,** pp. 1206–12.

22

Neurotransmitter differentiation in cortical neurons

MARION E. CAVANAGH AND JOHN G. PARNAVELAS

We are interested in the differentiation of neurochemically defined neuronal types. We have used the development of somatostatin (somatotropin-release-inhibiting factor, SRIF) containing neurons in the rat visual cortex as a model system. However, to appreciate the significance of this study it is necessary to know about the structure of the adult cortex and about some of the earlier studies of its development.

CYTOLOGY OF ADULT RAT VISUAL CORTEX

The cortex is divided into areas which were originally defined in terms of their cytological differences and later discovered to serve different functions. Figure 22.1 shows a dorsal view of the rat brain. The primary visual cortex is area 17 which is surrounded by areas 18 and 18a, the visual association cortex (Krieg 1946). The adult rat cortex is conventionally described in terms of six layers. Layer I is the distinct relatively cell-free layer beneath the pial surface. In the rat, layers II and III are not usually divided. Layer IV contains small- and medium-sized neurons and is thicker in the primary visual cortex than in the association cortex on either side. Layer V contains the largest neurons of the cortex, with axons projecting the greatest distances. Layer VI can be subdivided into an upper part (VIa) and a lower part (VIb), the latter consisting largely of horizontally aligned cells forming the border of the cortex with the white matter (Peters 1985).

Neuronal types in the cortex are principally divided on morphological grounds into pyramidal and non-pyramidal neurons. The majority of neurons are pyramidal of various sizes, but with few exceptions are in the classic shape of a rather tapered pear with an apical dendrite forming a tuft in layer I and an axon descending from a broad base. Non-pyramidal neurons are of a multitude of forms, as revealed by Golgi studies, but can be divided into three main groups, namely bipolar, bitufted, or multipolar (Feldman and Peters 1978). Functionally, pyramidal cells are projection neurons, i.e. their axons project outside the cortex, whereas non-pyramidal neurons are local circuit

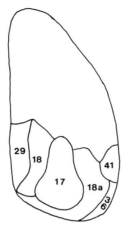

Fig. 22.1. Dorsal view of the right hemisphere of the rat brain showing the primary visual cortex, area 17, and the visual association cortex, areas 18 and 18a. (Redrawn after Krieg 1946.)

neurons or interneurons, making their connections locally within the cortex. This is a broad generalization to which there may be a few exceptions.

TRANSMITTERS

The major transmitters of pyramidal neurons are believed to be glutamate and aspartate. Pyramidal neurons have been labelled by retrograde axonal transport, mainly after injection of D-[³H] aspartate but also of D-[³H] glutamate into the appropriate projection areas (Streit 1984). There is relatively little direct immunocytochemical evidence for the presence of transmitters in pyramidal cells because it is difficult to raise antibodies to single amino acids, but they have been raised to glutamate conjugated to bovine serum albumin (Ottersen and Storm-Mathisen 1984), and also to aspartate (Campistron, Buijs, and Geffard 1986), and have been used to demonstrate pyramidal neurons in the cortex.

The major transmitter of non-pyramidal neurons is γ-amino butyric acid (GABA). The localization of GABA has been studied either by uptake of [³H]-GABA (Hökfelt and Ljungdahl 1972; Somogyi, Freund, and Kisvárday 1984), by using antibodies to the GABA synthesizing enzyme, glutamic acid decarboxylase (GAD) (Ribak 1978), or by antibodies to conjugated GABA (Ottersen and Storm-Mathisen 1984; Hodgson, Penke, Erdei, Chubb, and Somogyi 1985). GABAergic cells are found throughout the visual cortex but with a higher concentration in layer IV (Lin, Lu, and Schmechel 1986), and this is confirmed by a recent study which measured GAD levels in cortical layers and found a peak in layer IV (McDonald, Speciale, and Parnavelas 1987).

Four neuropeptides have so far been localized unequivocally in non-pyramidal neurons of the visual cortex. They are: SRIF, neuropeptide-Y (NPY), originally located with an antibody to avian pancreatic polypeptide (APP) (Di Maggio, Chronwall, Buchanan, and O'Donohue 1985), cholecystokinin (CCK), and vasoactive intestinal polypeptide (VIP). SRIF comprises about 3 per cent of all cortical neurons and is found throughout layers II–VI, although there are very few SRIF neurons in layer IV but rather more SRIF neurons in layers II/III than in layers V and VI (McDonald, Parnavelas, Karamanlidis, Brecha, and Koenig 1982*d*; Lin *et al.* 1986). There are about half the number of NPY-positive cells as SRIF-postive cells (McDonald, Parnavelas, Karamanlidis, and Brecha 1982*b*). CCK-positive neurons are very few in number, representing only about 1 per cent of the total neuronal population (McDonald, Parnavelas, Karamanlidis, Rosenquist, and Brecha 1982*c*). There are approximately the same percentage (3 per cent) of VIP cells as SRIF cells (McDonald, Parnavelas, Karamanlidis, and Brecha 1982*a*).

Acetylcholine (ACh) neurons have been identified by means of an antibody to choline acetyltransferase (ChAT) in the rat visual cortex (Eckenstein and Thoenen, 1983), whereas previously only cholinergic terminals had been shown to be present. These cholinergic neurons are mostly present in layers II/III, making up about 2 per cent of all cortical neurons.

DEVELOPMENT OF RAT VISUAL CORTEX

On the twelfth day of gestation (E12) in the rat, the forebrain (telencephalon) consists of a fluid-filled vesicle bounded by a thin 'skin' of pseudostratified neuroepithelium. This 'skin' thickens by cell division and migration to form the layered structure of the adult cortex.

The modern era in the study of cortical development began with the [^{3}H]-thymidine studies of Angevine and Sidman (1961) in the mouse. The first autoradiographic study of the developing rat cortex was made by Berry and Rogers in 1965. Although the process of cortical development had been described previously, and it had been appreciated not only that cell division took place solely at the ventricular surface but also that migration of cells was involved, earlier authors had misinterpreted the cellular movements. The autoradiographic studies established beyond doubt that the cortex was formed by an 'inside-out' process, that is to say that the innermost cellular layers of the cortex are formed first and the outermost last. After the initial autoradiographic studies, the self-appointed Boulder Committee of 1970 set out a new terminology for developing cortex which took account of the new ideas and attempted to clarify the 'inconsistent and inaccurate' language currently in use.

Figure 22.2 summarizes the five stages in the development of the cortex as defined by the Boulder Committee (1970): stage (a), ventricular zone, the

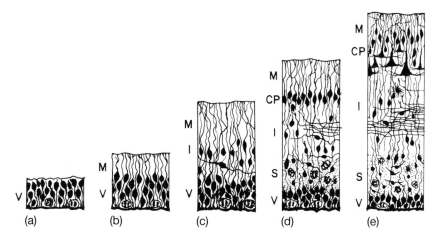

Fig. 22.2. Schematic drawing of the five stages [(a)–(e)] in the development of the vertebrate cortex. CP, cortical plate; I, intermediate zone; M, marginal zone; S, subventricular zone; V, ventricular zone. [Reproduced from Boulder Committee (1970) by kind permission of Alan R. Liss, Inc., New York.]

original proliferative zone; stage (b), a ventricular zone and a marginal zone, establishing a polarity; stage (c), a ventricular zone separated from the marginal zone by an intermediate zone, the future white matter; stage (d), the formation of the cortical plate below the marginal zone and of the subventricular zone, a second proliferative layer internal to the ventricular zone; and stage (e), a more advanced stage with the cortical plate increasing in thickness and the intermediate zone acquiring more axons both efferent and afferent. This process of division and migration continues with the newest cells migrating right to the top of the cortical plate and the earliest formed cells sinking down to form layer VIb.

This relatively simple scheme has been modified subsequently by various authors who after more detailed studies in various species have introduced new concepts and new terms. The major new concept is that put forward both by Marin-Padilla (1978) and by Rickmann, Chronwall, and Wolff (1977). Marin-Padilla proposed that the marginal zone should be considered as the primordial plexiform layer while Rickmann and colleagues suggested that the marginal zone should be considered as the pallial anlage or forerunner of the whole cortex. Essentially these proposals are similar and they mean that the cortical plate forms within the marginal zone and not beneath it. The evidence for this is the finding of cells 'born' before the earliest cells of the cortical plate both in the marginal zone (layer I of the adult) and in the adult subcortical white matter. Thus, in the rat, cells produced at E13 are located in layers I and the white matter, while neurons produced during E14–21 are found in layers VI to II.

Golgi studies of developing neurons in rat visual cortex show that they only begin to elaborate processes after having reached their final position in the cortex (Berry and Rogers 1965). This means that the first appearance of neurons with dendrites and axons is in layer VI and these are already present at birth. Postnatal development continues with growth of axons and dendrites in layers VI–II taking place during the first two weeks in an inside-out sequence. Although dendritic and axonal branching continues to the fourth postnatal week, by the end of the second week all neurons are sufficiently well developed to be morphologically distinct. The non-pyramidal neurons reach an equivalent state of maturity to the pyramidal cells at about the same time in all layers (Parnavelas, Bradford, Mounty, and Lieberman 1978). These observations are in conflict with the generally accepted notion that local circuit neurons are the last to appear and differentiate (Jacobson 1975).

A STUDY OF THE MIGRATION AND NEUROCHEMICAL DIFFERENTIATION OF PEPTIDE-CONTAINING NEURONS IN RAT OCCIPITAL CORTEX

Our study was designed to take a fresh look at the development of peptide-containing cells by combining the techniques of immunocytochemistry and autoradiography. The aim was to discover whether these cells were co-generated in layers with the bulk of the pyramidal cells or whether they were a separate population of cells which distributed throughout the cortex as suggested by the hypothesis that local circuit neurons are generated later than projection neurons.

Experimental design and methods

The strategy of the experiment was as follows: since the majority of cortical cells are generated from E14 until birth at E22, time-mated pregnant Sprague-Dawley rats were used and one was injected with [³H]-thymidine on each of the days E14 to E22. These were allowed to develop normally and gave birth at E22 or E23. From each litter the brains of pups were fixed at birth and at two-day intervals up to two weeks. With some of the larger litters, a few pups were allowed to survive to five weeks. The animals were fixed by perfusion with Bouin's fluid, which we have found to be best for preserving antigenicity when the tissue is to be subsequently embedded in paraffin wax. The study was performed on wax embedded material, firstly to preserve all the [³H]-thymidine material and secondly to enable relatively thin sections (10 μm) to be cut for autoradiography, since with thick sections little of the low-energy tritium would reach the emulsion.

From each brain, serial sections were cut throughout the occipital region in order to cover the visual cortex (area 17). Two sections were mounted per slide. Every tenth slide was stained with toluidine blue to allow morphological identification of areas and layers. The overall plan was to stain immuno-cytochemically 10 per cent of the slides for each of the peptides SRIF, VIP, CCK, and NPY, and then to stain a further 10 per cent for each of the peptides and combine this with autoradiography. The remaining 10 per cent would be prepared as straight autoradiographs. This scheme allowed double-labelled (i.e. immunocytochemistry and autoradiography) sections to be compared with either technique alone to control for interference between the two techniques. Unfortunately, at present, we are not yet able to present the results of this complete scheme but have concentrated on SRIF-containing cells in the first two weeks of life and, accordingly, slides designated for SRIF alone, SRIF plus autoradiography, and autoradiography alone have been processed.

The immunocytochemistry was carried out with anti-SRIF as used by McDonald *et al.* 1982*d*. This is a polyclonal antibody raised against the synthetic tetradecapeptide. The procedure was the peroxidase–anti-peroxi-dase method of Sternberger and the peroxidase was visualized using 3-3′-diaminobenzidine (DAB) as a substrate. When combining immunocyto-chemistry with autoradiography the slides were given two additional washes in distilled water and air dried as there is a risk of a chemical reaction between excess DAB and the photographic emulsion. For autoradiography (ARG) slides were coated with Ilford K2 emulsion and exposed for a month, after which the slides were developed in Kodak D19.

Assessment of results

The preparations were examined under bright field and dark field illumination and the distribution of SRIF-positive, SRIF-positive plus ARG-labelled, and ARG-labelled cells plotted by means of a drawing tube attachment. To assess which cells were double-labelled, only nuclei with at least 10 grains were counted (see Fig. 22.3). This criterion was based on the fact that the heaviest labelled cells had about 20 grains over their nuclei and had presumably only divided once since incorporation of [^{3}H]-thymidine, and that, since cell turnover time is 11–19 hours (von Waechter and Jaensch 1972), cells with 10 or more grains would have made only one more division and therefore would have been born within 24 hours of the injection of [^{3}H]-thymidine. Also, since double-labelled cells were not particularly numerous, only one half of the brain was drawn, but all the double-labelled cells from both sections of the slide were plotted on it. This method resulted in drawing four-times the density of double-labelled cells. All cells from the midline to the rhinal fissure were plotted. After the double-labelled cells had been plotted individually, the location of the band of the most-heavily-labelled cells was superimposed

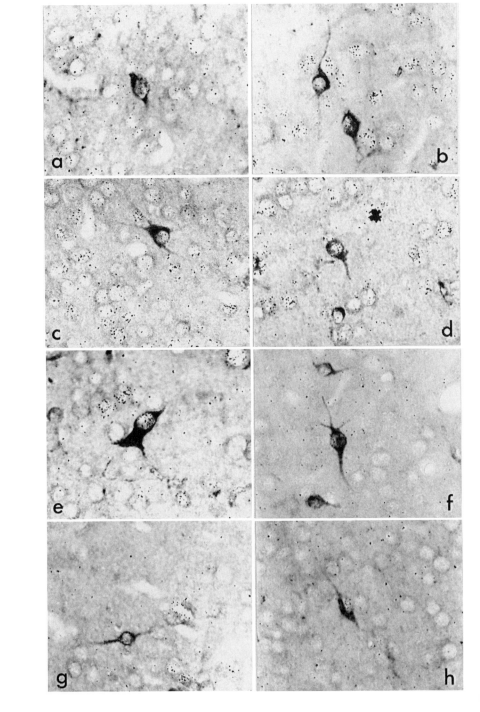

under dark field illumination at low power in order to compare the position of SRIF neurons with the majority of neurons born at the same time (Fig. 22.4).

RESULTS

Autoradiography

Examination of autoradiographs alone from animals injected at E14 to E21 and killed at two weeks postnatal revealed that the number of cells born on each day of gestation gradually increased from day E14 to E17 and declined to E21, and that cells born early and late in this period are distributed in a much narrower band. Thus cells born at E14 are found in the very bottom of layer VI while cells born at E15 and E16 are found throughout layer VI. Cells born at E17 are much more numerous and, although they are centred on the upper part of layer V, they are rather more widely spread. Cells born at E18 are principally found in layer IV while cells born at E19 and E20 are found in layers II and III. Cells born at E21 are very few in number and are found at the border with layer I (Fig. 22.5). Part of this apparent spread is due, of course, to the fact that the neurons of layer V are the largest pyramidal cells of the cortex and are less densely packed than in other layers. There also appears to be a double distribution in area 17, which may be the result of cells originating from the subventricular proliferative layer (Fig. 22.4).

Immunocytochemistry

Examination of the total population of SRIF-positive cells confirmed the previous description (McDonald *et al.* 1982*d*) of a somewhat bimodal distribution with cells principally in layers II/III and layer VI, although the present study showed rather more cells in layer VI than in layers II/III in contrast to the previous study, but this may be due to the fact that we were not looking at a fully mature cortex. It also showed that area 17 was relatively deficient in SRIF-positive cells compared to area 18 and 18a (Fig. 22.4).

Combined immunocytochemistry and autoradiography

The distribution of the double-labelled (SRIF and autoradiography) cells is the crucial new finding from this study. In the first place the distribution plots reveal that SRIF-positive neurons are generated on each day from E14–21. However, they are not generated evenly throughout this period. The day when

Fig. 22.3. Photomicrographs of SRIF-positive cells from two-week-old rats also labelled with [^{3}H]-thymidine at the gestational days indicated. (a) E14; (b) E15; (c) E16; (d) E17 layer VI; (e) E17 layer II; (f) E18; (g) E20; (h) E21. Magnification: × 575.

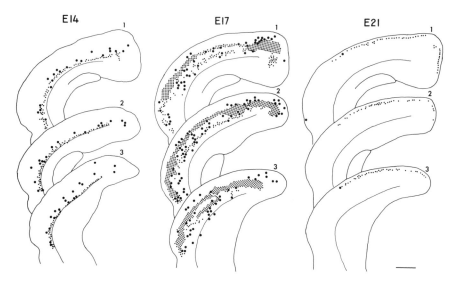

E14   E17   E21

Fig. 22.4. Drawings of a selection from the plots made to count and locate double-labelled neurons. The hemisections are all from the occipital cortex of two-week-old rats. The first section is the most rostral and the third the most caudal in which counts were made. Small dots represent the heaviest [³H]-thymidine-labelled cells in the hemisphere shown. Large dots represent the SRIF-positive cells with 10 or more grains over the nucleus from both hemispheres of two adjacent sections. The age at which each rat was injected with [³H]-thymidine is shown above. Scale bar: 1 mm.

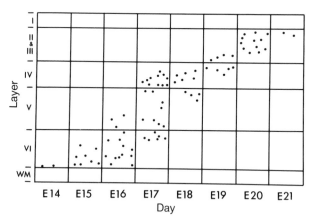

Fig. 22.5. Position of heaviest labelled cells in strips through the visual cortex of two-week-old rats injected with [³H]-thymidine on the days indicated. WM: white matter.

most SRIF-positive cells are born is E17, as for neurons in general, but proportionately more are born early rather than late. If we take the cells plotted as described above, the average number of double-labelled cells per 10 μm section throughout the occipital region (average of 20 sections per brain) is 10 at E14, 18 at E15, 12 at E16, 30 at E17, 8 at E18, 3 at E19, 1 at E20, and less than 1 at E21. Thus although there are some SRIF-positive cells generated throughout the period of cortical formation (E14–21), most are generated at or before E17, i.e. in the first half of this period. There is also an indication of a gradient throughout the occipital region with high numbers of double-labelled cells per section in the more rostral sections (Fig. 22.4).

Differentiation of SRIF-positive neurons from birth to two weeks

This brings us to the question of how SRIF-positive neurons develop between their generation and their adult form. At two weeks of age it is relatively easy to identify a SRIF-positive cell. Although it has been shown that non-pyramidal neurons continue to grow and increase their dendritic and axonal arborizations after that time (Parnavelas *et al.* 1978), by the end of the second week the numbers and distribution of SRIF-positive cells are the same as in the adult (McDonald *et al.* 1982*d*) and so it can be reasonably assumed that no more SRIF-positive cells reveal themselves after that time. In 10 μm sections it is not possible to make the morphological classifications of these neurons that can be made in Golgi preparations or in thicker immunocytochemical preparations. Nevertheless, it is possible to see that most of these cells have a clear nucleus surrounded by SRIF-positive cytoplasm and the beginnings of dendrites. One also finds stained processes which would appear to be dendrites, and fine fibres, often beaded, suggestive of axons. As one moves backwards in time it becomes progressively more difficult to identify SRIF-positive neurons with absolute certainty. This is due to three factors: (1) the SRIF content of individual cells is lower; (2) they have less cytoplasm; and (3) the background staining is higher. Background staining remains relatively high during the first postnatal week but then fades rapidly so that it has disappeared by about 10 days of age.

   The previous study (McDonald *et al.* 1982*d*) of the postnatal development of SRIF-containing neurons in the rat visual cortex was performed on fixed but unembedded free-floating 40 μm sections, a method which is probably marginally more sensitive than the post-embedding method used here for detecting the very low levels of SRIF present in neurons when they first appear. In spite of lower sensitivity we have been able to detect a very few SRIF-positive cells in layer VIb at birth or at one day of age (23 days *post-coitum*, PC) and these were labelled with [^{3}H]-thymidine from injection at E14. These cells contain very little SRIF because, in the same sections, strongly staining SRIF-positive cells were seen in other parts of the brain (e.g. olfactory cortex) so that faint staining is not due to a technical failure.

At 2–3 days of age (25PC) there is a slight increase in SRIF-positive neurons. They are all in layer VI, and double-labelled cells can be seen from E14, E15, and E16. At 5–7 days of age (27–29 PC), although the numbers of SRIF-positive neurons have increased, there are no double-labelled neurons from E17. All the SRIF-positive neurons in 5- and 7-days-old cortices labelled at E17 are totally devoid of silver grains and must therefore have been born before E17. At 9 days of age (31PC) the first SRIF-positive neurons labelled with grains from E17 appear. The first double-labelled neurons from E18 appear at 10 days of age (33PC), and at 12–13 days of age (35PC) the first double-labelled cells from E19, E20 and E21 appear.

Leaving aside the phenomenon of transient expression (see below) this suggests that neurons begin to express SRIF between 9 and 14 days after their 'birth', with earlier generated neurons beginning to synthesize SRIF sooner than those generated later. However, the first neurons have less distance to migrate than the last, since the cortex is considerably thinner at E14 than at E21, so that neurons would seem to require at least 8 days after migration before they begin to express SRIF. There is no evidence that the diffusely distributed neurons, i.e. those born at E17 or E18 but which end up together with those born at E14–16 in layer VI, begin to express SRIF any earlier than those located in layers IV and V. This suggests that they have gone through the full migrational pathway.

As our studies were entirely postnatal it is not possible to say how long before the birth of the animal the SRIF-positive neurons born at E14 were detectable. A prenatal study on the development of SRIF-positive neurons (Eadie and Parnavelas 1987) has shown that a few SRIF-positive neurons can be detected as early as E17 in the subplate (future layer VI). Their study was made on free-floating 50–100 μm sections, which is most probably a more sensitive method than the post-embedding method used by us, and can therefore detect lower levels of SRIF. However these SRIF-positive neurons were only present in every small numbers (one cell per 100 μm section). It is possible that, if we had used thicker free-floating sections, we would have been able to detect more SRIF-positive cells earlier, but because of the low energy of tritium we would have decreased the number of [³H]-thymidine-labelled cells and thus the number of double-labelled cells.

Comparison with previous double-labelled studies

Two other groups of workers have used a similar approach to study the same basic problem. They have both looked at the birth dates of GABAergic cells in the visual cortex of the rat. Wolff, Balcar, Zetzsche, Böttcher, Schmechel, and Chronwall (1984*b*) and Miller (1985) both showed that GABAergic non-pyramidal cells are generated throughout the period E14–21 in the rat, although Miller (1985) showed that they are distributed with pyramidal cells born at the same time, while Wolff *et al.* (1984*b*) considered that they were diffusely distributed in the cortex irrespective of their birth dates.

Our data show that SRIF-positive non-pyramidal cells are generated throughout the period E14–21, thus agreeing with both Miller (1985) and Wolff *et al.* (1984*b*). As to the final distribution of these cells it would seem that our results fall somewhere between the two. Wolff and his colleagues used an antibody against GAD to identify GABAergic non-pyramidal neurons and they looked at the thirtieth postnatal day, having labelled cells with [³H]-thymidine on each of days E15–20. They stated that: 'Most of the [³H]-labelled, GAD-positive neurons were found outside the main intensely [³H]-labelled, band of GAD-negative (mainly pyramidal) neurons and there were also a few diffusely positioned strongly [³H]-labelled and GAD-negative neurons. Consequently it seems that most of the GABAergic neurons follow the diffuse rather than the inside-to-outside mode of positioning and, vice versa, most of the diffusely positioned neurons are GABAergic'. This description fits to some extent the patterns that we have seen. Many of the ³H-labelled SRIF-positive neurons were found outside the main intensely ³H-labelled band of cells. However, most of them were in a band slightly behind (i.e. nearer to the pial surface), which could be accounted for by the fact that we were counting both fully labelled and half-labelled cells. On the other hand there were cells which were way out of line which could not be explained in this manner, some half-labelled cells from E17 being found in layer VIb.

Miller's (1985) experiment was more sophisticated. He used an antibody to GABA on cells born on days E14, E15, E17, E18, and E20. In addition he looked at the position of pyramidal neurons projecting to the contralateral cortex which he identified by retrograde labelling with wheatgerm agglutinin conjugated horseradish peroxidase (WGA–HRP) and which had been born on the same days (Fig. 22.6). This method showed that the GABA-positive non-pyramidal and WGA-HRP-positive pyramidal neurons occupied the same layers in the cortex, and that, for both, although there is a clear peak, the spread is wider than one might anticipate. However, it is noteworthy that for cells born at E17 the band of lightly labelled GABA-positive cells extends below the main band to a greater extent than the WGA-HRP-labelled cells. These are cells which will have been born after E17 and which therefore would be expected to be in the upper layers of the cortex.

The most recent paper by Miller (1986) on the migration of GABA-immunoreactive neurons showed a shorter delay between the completion of migration and the onset of expression of GABA than the delay that we have shown in SRIF expression. This and other evidence (see below) suggests that GABA is the first non-pyramidal neurochemical to be expressed.

CO-EXISTENCE OF NEUROTRANSMITTERS IN NON-PYRAMIDAL NEURONS

To what extent can SRIF-positive neurons be compared with GABA- or

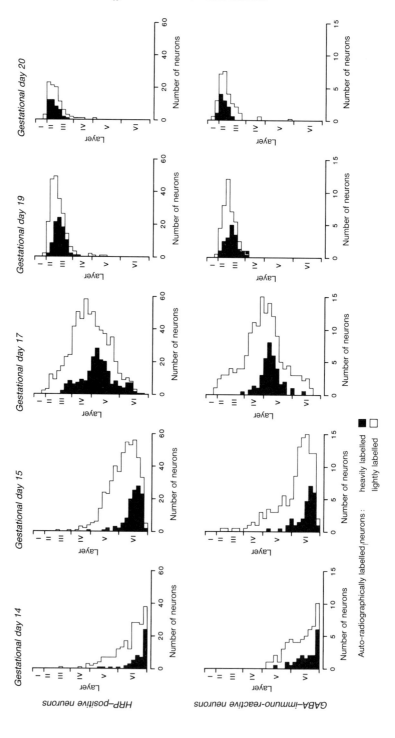

GAD-positive neurons? GABAergic neurons are found in all layers of the cortex and display a wide variety of non-pyramidal morphologies. In fact it is believed that most of the non-pyramidal cells of the cortex are GABAergic (Jones and Hendry 1986). It has also been shown that a proportion of GAD-positive cells are also SRIF-positive (Schmechel, Vickey, Fitzpatrick, and Elde 1984; Lin *et al.* 1986). In rat visual cortex, although 15 per cent of neurons are GAD-positive and 2–3 per cent of neurons are SRIF-positive, most SRIF-positive cells are GAD-positive. It is estimated that only 15 per cent of SRIF-positive neurons are not GAD-positive. It could be that SRIF-positive neurons form a specific sub-population of GABAergic cells which are born early in the week of cortical development.

Other neuropeptides have also been shown to co-exist with GABA. NPY has been shown to co-exist both with GABA and with SRIF (Chronwall, Chase, and O'Donohue 1984). CCK has been shown to co-exist with GABA (Somogyi, Hodgson, Smith, Nunzi, Gorio, and Wu 1984). CCK has also been shown to co-exist with VIP (Kosaka, Kosaka, Tateishi, Hamaoka, Yanai-hara, Wu, and Hama 1985) and since almost all CCK neurons contain GABA, then, by inference, VIP may co-exist with GABA but it has definitely been shown to co-exist with ChAT (Eckenstein and Baughman 1984). It has also been shown at the electron microscope level that the somata of ChAT-positive and VIP-positive cells have a very similar ultrastructural morphology which is quite different from that of SRIF-positive cells (Parnavelas 1986). The very latest information is that SRIF co-exists with both VIP and CCK (Papado-poulos, unpub. obs). Fig. 22.7 is an attempt to summarize these combinations in a simple scheme.

DEVELOPMENT OF OTHER TRANSMITTERS

There have been no studies of the development of pyramidal cell transmitters. Immunocytochemical studies of the development of GAD activity in rat visual cortex show that the first cell bodies staining positively for GAD appear before birth in layer I and the subplate which will become layer VI. After birth GAD-positive neurons appear in a sequence mainly in layers VI and V during the first week and in layers IV and II/III during the second week, although

---

Fig. 22.6. Distributions of double-labelled neurons. The numbers of HRP-positive and GABA-immunoreactive neurons double-labelled by a prenatal injection of tritiated thymidine are plotted. Double-labelled neurons with many silver grains over their nuclei (heavily labelled neurons) and those with a few silver grains over their nuclei (lightly labelled neurons) are noted by solid bars and clear bars, respectively. Each group is based on the mean data from two animals. From each animal, the distribution of double-labelled neurons in four vertical strips of cortex, each 375 μm in width, were compiled. [Reproduced from Miller (1985) by kind permission of Elsevier, Amsterdam.]

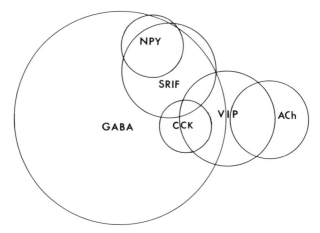

Fig. 22.7. Co-existence of GABA with four peptides and ACh. The areas of the circles are roughly proportional to the numbers of neurons containing the indicated neurochemical.

some increase in number and elaboration at dendrites and axons continues up to the end of the fourth postnatal week (Wolff, Böttcher, Zotzsche, Oertel, and Chronwall 1984a). This is in agreement with a recent study of measurements of GAD activity in individual layers of developing rat visual cortex which showed a great increase in GAD activity between days 8 and 18 (McDonald *et al.* 1987).

SRIF-positive neurons first appear at birth in layer VI, and throughout the first two postnatal weeks the neurons appear in successively higher layers until they have attained their adult distribution, although they do continue to grow for at least another week (McDonald *et al.* 1982d). NPY-positve neurons follow a similar path (McDonald *et al.* 1982b). CCK-positive neurons do not appear until the third postnatal day but develop rapidly thereafter, being found throughout the cortex by day 8 (McDonald *et al.* 1982c). VIP-positive neurons do not appear until a little later. According to Emson, Gilbert, Loren, Fahrenkrug, Sundler, and Schaffalitzky de Muckadell (1979), they first appear in layers V and VI at day 7, containing only a low amount of VIP. However, by postnatal days 14–21 they are present in all layers, particularly layers II–VI. They interpret this as a migration of these cells during the period 7–14 days, but, as we have seen, it is more likely to reflect the inside-out maturation of the cortex. McDonald *et al.* (1982a) reported the first VIP-positive neurons at post-natal day 4 or 5 in layers V and VI, but concentrated in layers II/III by 8 days. Confirmation of the late development of VIP comes from radioimmunoassay of SRIF and VIP in developing rat brain (Nobou, Bessen, Rostene, and Rosselin 1985) which showed that SRIF was found before birth in rat cortex while VIP first appeared after birth. This would suggest that the obvious next step in our study is to look at the birth dates of VIP-positive cells. Since they are found predominantly in the upper layers (II/III) of the cortex it might suggest that VIP-positive neurons are born late in the week of cortical neuron development, at the time when the production of SRIF-positive neurons is in decline.

ChAT-positive neurons, which develop even later, do not appear until the eleventh postnatal day, but increase rapidly during the next few days until the end of the third week. Thereafter, a more gradual development brings the picture to that of the adult (Dori, Parnavelas, and Eckenstein 1985). These immunocytochemical results have been confirmed by measurement of ChAT levels in the developing cortex (McDonald *et al.* 1987).

TRANSIENT APPEARANCE OF TRANSMITTERS DURING BRAIN DEVELOPMENT

We have not looked at prenatal brains in this study, but in some of the new-born and one of the two-day-old brains we have found small patches of SRIF-positive pyramidal cells in the cortical plate in the rostral part of area 18. It has been reported previously that SRIF-positive cells are found in various parts of the prenatal rat central visual pathway (Laemle, Feldman, and Lichtenstein 1982). Noteworthy in the present context is that SRIF-immunoreactivity is present throughout the cortical plate at E20 in presumptive areas 17, 18, and 18a, so that the few positive cells that we have found could be the tail-end of a transient expression of SRIF. This transient appearance of neuroactive substances would seem to be a fairly widespread phenomenon in development. In our laboratory, ChAT-positive cells were found in the cortex at E17 when, in postnatal life, ACh has not been demonstrated until about eleven days after birth (Parnavelas and Dori 1986). Furthermore, some of these early ChAT-positive cells also seemed to have pyramidal morphology despite the fact that ACh is a non-pyramidal cell transmitter in postnatal life.

Another example is furnished by the very extensive and thorough study of Woodhams, Allen, McGovern, Allen, Bloom, Balazs, and Polak (1985) which documents the ontogeny of the NPY system throughout the whole rat brain from E13. This shows that NPY-positive pyramidal neurons are found maximally developed in the cortex at E20 with axons in the corpus callosum, but that they have disappeared by postnatal day 4. Other substances such as plasma proteins (Cavanagh and Møllgård 1985; Cavanagh and Warren 1985) have also been shown to make a transient appearance in the developing cortex of several species, all of which have been suggested as playing a role in development. This would suggest, perhaps, that the transient appearance of transmitters, especially at times before there is any significant synaptogenesis (Blue and Parnavelas 1983), has nothing to do with transmission or modulation, but is concerned with some form of cell recognition or guidance. However, as yet, there have been no experiments that can test suggestions of this kind.

CONCLUSIONS

One type of non-pyramidal neuron in the occipital cortex of the rat, the SRIF-positive neuron, is generated throughout the period of cortical formation (E14–21) along with pyramidal cells; however, it does not end up distributed as precisely in layers as pyramidal cells. We have also demonstrated that most of these cells are born early rather than late in this period, contradicting the theory that local circuit neurons are generated after projection neurons. Additionally, we have shown that these neurons do not express their adult chemical specificity until several days (eight or more) after they have reached their final position in the cortex.

The age at which neurons begin to express adult chemical identity varies with the transmitter, ranging from before birth for GABA to eleven days after birth for ACh. Whether this expression is a response to events in the environment of the neuron, such as the arrival of incoming axons, or is entirely genetically specified is a question which has not yet been addressed.

ACKNOWLEDGEMENTS

Our thanks are due to the Medical Research Council which supported this work, to James Cope and Amy Cavanagh who assisted with the histology, to Eva Franke who mounted hundreds of autoradiographs, and to Shihan Jayasuriya who typed the manuscript.

REFERENCES

Angevine, J. B. and Sidman, R. L. (1961). Autoradiographic study of cell migration during histogenesis of cerebral cortex in the mouse. *Nature* **192,** pp. 766–8.

Berry, M. and Rogers, A. W. (1965). The migration of neuroblasts in the developing cerebral cortex. *J. Anat.* **99,** pp. 691–709.

Blue, M. E. and Parnavelas, J. G. (1983). The formation and maturation of synapses in the visual cortex of the rat. I. Qualitative analysis. *J. Neurocytol.* **12,** pp. 599–616.

Boulder Committee (1970). Embryonic vertebrate central nervous system: revised terminology. *Anat. Rec.* **166,** pp. 257–62.

Campistron, G., Buijs, R. M., and Geffard, M. (1986). Specific antibodies against aspartate and their immunocytochemical application in the rat brain. *Brain Res.* **365,** pp. 179–84.

Cavanagh, M. E. and Møllgård, K. (1985). An immunocytochemical study of the distribution of some plasma proteins within the developing forebrain of the pig with special reference to the neocortex. *Dev. Brain Res.* **17**, pp. 183–94.

Cavanagh, M. E. and Warren, A. (1985). The distribution of native albumin and foreign albumin injected into lateral ventricles of prenatal and neonatal rat forebrains. *Anat. Embryol.* **172**, pp. 347–51.

Chronwall, B. M., Chase, T. N., and O'Donohue, T. L. (1984). Co-existence of neuropeptide Y and somatostatin in rat and human cortical and rat hypothalamic neurons. *Neurosci. Lett.* **52**, pp. 213–7.

Di Maggio, D. A., Chronwall, B. M., Buchanan, K., and O'Donohue, T. L. (1985). Pancreatic polypeptide immunoreactivity in rat brain is actually neuropeptide Y. *Neuroscience* **15**, pp. 1149–57.

Dori, I., Parnavelas, J. G., and Eckenstein, F. (1985). The postnatal development of the cholinergic system in the rat visual cortex. *Neurosci. Lett. Suppl.* **22**, p. S354.

Eadie, L. A. and Parnavelas, J. G. (1987). Development of ultrastructural features of somatostatin-immunoreactive neurons in embryonic and postnatal visual cortex of the rat. *J. Neurocytol.* (in press).

Eckenstein, F. and Baughman, R. W. (1984). Two types of cholinergic innervation in cortex, one co-localized with vasoactive intestinal polypeptide. *Nature* **309**, pp. 153–5.

Eckenstein, F. and Thoenen, H. (1983). Cholinergic neurons in the rat cerebral cortex demonstrated by immunohistochemical localization of choline acetyltransferase. *Neurosci. Lett.* **37**, pp. 211–5.

Emson, P. C., Gilbert, R. F. I., Loren, I., Fahrenkrug, J., Sundler, F., and Schaffalitzky de Muckadell, O. B. (1979). Development of vasoactive intestinal polypeptide (VIP) containing neurones in the rat brain. *Brain Res.* **117**, pp. 437–44.

Feldman, M. L. and Peters, A. (1978). The forms of non-pyramidal neurons in the visual cortex of the rat. *J. Comp. Neurol.* **179**, pp. 761–94.

Hodgson, A. J., Penke, B., Erdei, A., Chubb, I. W., and Somogyi, P. (1985). Antisera to γ-aminobutyric acid. I. Production and characterization using a new model system. *J. Histochem. Cytochem.* **32**, pp. 229–39.

Hökfelt, T. and Ljungdahl, A. (1972). Autoradiographic identification of cerebral and cerebellar cortical neurons accumulating labelled Gamma-aminobutyric acid (^{3}H-GABA). *Exp. Brain Res.* **14**, pp. 354–62.

Jacobson, M. (1975). Polymorphism of LCN's and the evolution of the central nervous system. *Neurosci. Res. Prog. Bull.* **13**, pp. 415–6.

Jones, E. G. and Hendry, S. H. C. (1986). Co-localization of GABA and neuropeptides in neocortical neurons. *Trends Neurosci.* **9**, pp. 71–6.

Kosaka, T., Kosaka, K., Tateishi, K., Hamaoka, Y., Yanaihara, N., Wu, J. -Y., and Hama, K. (1985). GABAergic neurons contain CCK-8-like and/or VIP-like immunoreactivities in the rat hippocampus and dentate gyrus. *J. Comp. Neurol.* **239**, pp. 420–30.

Krieg, W. J. S. (1946). Connections of the cerebral cortex. I. The albino rat. A. Topography of the cortical areas. *J. Comp. Neurol.* **84**, pp. 221–76.

Laemle, L. K., Feldman, S. C., and Lichtenstein, E. (1982). Somatostatin-like immunoreactivity in the central visual pathway of the prenatal rat. *Brain Res.* **251**, pp. 365–70.

Lin, C. -S., Lu, S. M., and Schmechel, D. E. (1986). Glutamic acid decarboxylase and somatostatin immunoreactivity in rat visual cortex. *J. Comp. Neurol.* **244,** pp. 369–83.

Marin-Padilla, M. (1978). Dual origin of the mammalian neocortex and evolution of the cortical plate. *Anat. Embryol.* **152,** pp. 109–26.

McDonald, J. K., Speciale, S. G., and Parnavelas, J. G. (1987). The laminar distribution of glutamate decarboxylase and choline acetyltransferase in the adult and developing visual cortex of the rat. *Neuroscience* **21,** pp. 825–32.

McDonald, J. K., Parnavelas, J. G., Karamanlidis, A. N., and Brecha, N. (1982*a*). The morphology and distribution of peptide-containing neurons in the adult and developing visual cortex of the rat. II. Vasoactive intestinal polypeptide. *J. Neurocytol.* **11,** pp. 825–37.

McDonald, J. K., Parnavelas, J. G., Karamanlidis, A. N., and Brecha, N. (1982*b*). The morphology and distribution of peptide-containing neurons in the adult and developing visual cortex of the rat. IV. Avian pancreatic polypeptide. *J. Neurocytol.* **11,** pp. 985–95.

McDonald, J. K., Parnavelas, J. G., Karamanlidis, A. N., Rosenquist, G., and Brecha, N. (1982*c*). The morphology and distribution of peptide containing neurons in the adult and developing visual cortex of the rat. III. Cholecystokinin. *J. Neurocytol.* **11,** pp. 881–95.

McDonald, J. K., Parnavelas, J. G., Karamanlidis, A. N., Brecha, N., and Koenig, J. I. (1982*d*). The morphology and distribution of peptide-containing neurons in the adult and developing visual cortex of the rat. I. Somatostatin. *J. Neurocytol.* **11,** pp. 809–24.

Miller, M. W. (1985). Cogeneration of retrogradely labelled corticocortical projection and GABA-immunoreactive local circuit neurons in cerebral cortex. *Dev. Brain Res.* **23,** pp. 187–92.

Miller, M. W. (1986). The migration and neurochemical differentiation of γ-aminobutyric acid (GABA). Immunoreactive neurons in rat visual cortex as demonstrated by a combined immunocytochemical–autoradiographic technique. *Dev. Brain Res.* **28,** pp. 41–6.

Nobou, F., Besson, J., Rostene, W., and Rosselin, G. (1985). Ontogeny of vasoactive intestinal polypeptide and somatostatin in different structures of the rat brain: effects of hypo- and hypercorticism. *Dev. Brain Res.* **20,** pp. 296–301.

Ottersen, O. P. and Storm-Mathisen, J. (1984). Glutamate- and GABA-containing neurons in the mouse and rat brain, as demonstrated with a new immuncytochemical technique. *J. Comp. Neurol.* **229,** pp. 374–92.

Parnavelas, J. G. (1986). Morphology and distribution of peptide containing neurons in the cerebral cortex. *Progr. Brain Res.* **66,** pp. 119–34.

Parnavelas, J. G. and Dori, I. (1986). A transient population of cholinergic neurons in the developing rat cerebral cortex. *Neurosci. Lett. Suppl.* **24,** p. S47.

Parnavelas, J. G. and Lieberman, A. R. (1979). An ultrastructural study of the maturation of neuronal somata in the visual cortex of the rat. *Anat. Embryol.* **157,** pp. 311–28.

Parnavelas, J. G., Bradford, R., Mounty, E. J., and Lieberman, A. R. (1978). The development of non-pyramidal neurons in the visual cortex of the rat. *Anat. Embryol.* **155,** pp. 1–14.

Parnavelas, J. G., Kelly, W., Franke, E., and Eckenstein, F. (1986). Cholinergic neurons and fibres in the rat visual cortex. *J. Neurocytol.* **14,** pp. 329–36.

Peters, A. (1985). The visual cortex of the rat. In *Cerebral cortex. Vol. 3. Visual cortex* (eds. A. Peters and E. G. Jones), pp. 19–80. Plenum Press, New York.

Ribak, C. E. (1978). Aspinous and sparsely-spinous stellate neurons in the visual cortex of rats contain glutamic acid decarboxylase. *J. Neurocytol.* **7**, pp. 461–78.

Rickmann, M., Chronwall, B. M., and Wolff, J. R. (1977). On the development of non-pyramidal neurons and axons outside the cortical plate: the early marginal zone as a pallial anlage. *Anat. Embryol.* **151**, pp. 285–307.

Schmechel, D. E., Vickey, B. G., Fitzpatrick, D., and Elde, R. P. (1984). GABAergic neurons of mammalian cerebral cortex: widespread subclass defined by somatostatin content. *Neurosci. Lett.* **47**, pp. 227–32.

Somogyi, P., Freund, T. F., and Kisvárday, Z. F. (1984). Different types of [^{3}H]-GABA accumulating neurons in the visual cortex of the rat. Characterization by combined autoradiography and Golgi impregnation. *Exp. Brain Res.* **54**, pp. 45–56.

Somogyi, P., Hodgson, A. J., Smith, A. D., Nunzi, M. G., Gorio, A., and Wu, J. -Y. (1984). Different populations of GABAergic neurons in the visual cortex and hippocampus of cat contain somatostatin- or cholecystokinin-immunoreactive material. *J. Neurosci.* **4**, pp. 2590–603.

Streit, P. (1984). Glutamate and aspartate as transmitter candidates for systems of the cerebral cortex. In *Cerebral cortex. Vol. 2. Functional properties of cortical cells* (eds. E. G. Jones and A. Peters), pp. 119–43. Plenum Press, New York.

von Waecher, R. and Jaensch, B. (1972). Generation times of the matrix cells during embryonic brain development: an autoradiographic study in rats. *Brain Res.* **46**, pp. 235–50.

Wolff, J. R., Böttcher, H., Zetzsche, T., Oertel, W. H., and Chronwall, B. M. (1984*a*). Development of GABAergic neurons in rat visual cortex as identified by glutamate decarboxylase-like immunoreactivity. *Neurosci. Lett.* **47**, pp. 207–12.

Wolff, J. R., Balcar, V. J., Zetzsche, T., Böttcher, H., Schmechel, D. E., and Chronwall, B. M. (1984*b*). Development of the GABAergic system in rat visual cortex. In *Gene expression and cell–cell interactions in the developing nervous system* (eds. J. M. Lauder and P. Nelson), pp. 215–34. Plenum Press, New York.

Woodhams, P. L., Allen, Y. S., McGovern, J., Allen, J. M., Bloom, S. R., Balazs, R., and Polak, J. M. (1985). Immunohistochemical analysis of the early ontogeny of the neuropeptide Y system in the rat. *Neuroscience* **15**, pp. 173–202.

23

The development of neurotransmitter receptors

S. P. HUNT

Our views on the development of neurotransmitter receptors in the central nervous system (CNS) and of the relationship of the receptor to the pre-synaptic axon terminal have largely been shaped by the extensive observations made at the neuromuscular junction, particularly of the nicotinic acetylcho-line receptor (AChRn) on skeletal muscle and, to a lesser extent, the β-adrenergic and muscarinic receptors on cardiac and smooth muscle. However, direct comparison of these model peripheral systems to the CNS is, primarily for technical reasons, extremely difficult. Identification and analysis at the single cell level is hampered by the small size of post-synaptic neurons, particularly during development, compared to muscle cells, the difficulty of studying single cells without disrupting the local environment, and a lack of receptor ligands which bind irreversibly and can therefore be studied at the ultrastructural level. To compound these difficulties, our views on the relationship between receptors and their presumed endogenous ligands have become increasingly vague (Iversen 1984). The traditional idea of focal synaptic action coupled to the morphological concept of the synapse, has become one end of a spectrum of mechanisms extending to a diffuse and non-synaptic action of some neurotransmitter substances, particularly the neuro-peptides, but also monoamine neurotransmitters and acetylcholine at the muscarinic subclass of cholinergic receptors (AChRm). Many of these diffuse actions are thought to be mediated by receptors coupled to second messenger systems, such as cyclic adenosine monophosphate (cAMP), calcium, diacylg-lycerol and inositol triphosphate, and to have a rather slower physiological action than the rapid focal events in which neurotransmitter substances act directly on ion channels.

In many ways the concept of diffuse neurotransmitter action within the CNS is highly speculative and requires experimental verification. Purely on anatomical grounds, it is clear that most putative neurotransmitter substances are located at morphologically defined synapses, yet there is little evidence to suggest that neurotransmitter receptors are restricted to the post-synaptic density (see below).

In the following account peripheral mechanisms of neurotransmitter receptor development and regulation are briefly reviewed, and the extent to which these mechanisms can be detected in the CNS is evaluated.

DEVELOPMENT OF NEUROTRANSMITTER RECEPTORS AT THE NEUROMUSCULAR JUNCTION

Skeletal muscle

The analysis of muscle AChRn has been made considerably easier by the discovery that the snake toxin, α-bungarotoxin, binds selectively and with high affinity to muscle receptors and blocks nicotinic cholinergic transmission. Using this tool, AChRn has been detected on the surface of muscle cells before synaptogenesis, but is diffusely distributed. During the development of the neuromuscular junction, AChRn receptor collects under the motor nerve terminal, probably under the control of an 'aggregating' factor released by the nerve (Bevan and Steinbach 1967; Dennis 1981, Ziskind-Conhaim, Geffen, and Hall 1984). As the animal develops, extrajunctional receptor is lost and mature junctional receptor appears. The adult form of the receptor is physiologically and biochemically distinct from the extrajunctional receptor, probably due to a change in the protein subunit structure of the cholinergic receptor (Mishina, Takai, Imoto, Noda, Takahashi, Numa, Methfessel, and Sakmann 1986). Adult bovine receptor is a pentameric structure made up from four basic subunits: two α-, β-, ε-, and δ. The α-subunit is responsible for most of the α-bungarotoxin binding, while two acetylcholine molecules binding to the α-subunits (but in the presence of the other subunits) are required to initiate channel opening and the influx of sodium ions (Sakmann, Methfessel, Mishina, Takahashi, Takai, Kurasaki, Fukuda, and Numa 1985). At the extrajunctional receptor, γ-subunit is found in place of the ε-subunit. Molecular reconstruction of the two forms of the receptor has demonstrated that the mean channel-opening time becomes shorter and the conductance longer when the γ-subunit is replaced by the ε-subunit, replicating more or less exactly the sequence of events seen *in vivo* over the first two or three post-natal weeks in the rat (Mishina *et al.* 1986).

Muscle cells are polynucleate, diaphragm cells having as many as 500 nuclei spread evenly along the length of the cell and with some evidence that those nuclei immediately beneath the muscle end-plate are specialized to synthesise the mature form of the acetylcholine receptor proteins (Merlie and Sanes 1985). Extrajunctional receptor synthesis is inhibited by activity in the muscle and reappears in mature muscle following denervation (Lomo and Jansen 1980), although levels of junctional receptor remain constant.

In summary, the distribution and synthesis of mature AChRn is directed by the innervating motor axon terminal, a process that can be, in part, recapitulated by denervation and re-innervation of the muscle. The extrajunctional form of the receptor appears diffusely before innervation and is suppressed following synaptogenesis.

Cardiac muscle

Cardiac muscle is innervated both by post-ganglionic parasympathetic cholinergic fibres and by autonomic adrenergic axons, whose effects are mediated through muscarinic cholinergic and β-adrenergic receptors, respectively (Loffleholz and Pappano 1985). During ontogenesis, the neurotransmitter receptors appear before pre-synaptic components can be detected in the heart (Galfer, Klein, and Catterall 1977; Chen, Yamamura, and Roeske 1979). Mapping of receptors using autoradiography and physiological methods implied that, during development and in the adult muscle, receptors are diffusely distributed over the cell surface (Lane, Sastre, Law, and Salpeter 1977; Hartzell 1980). Loffleholz and Pappano (1985) have described this arrangement as one of neurotransmitter being 'bath applied' to the muscle, it being theoretically possible to calculate that neurotransmitter released from a varicosity could diffuse over distances of up to 100 μm in diameter. The action of acetylcholine is not directly on the ion channel but is mediated via a guanosine triphosphate (GTP) binding protein, resulting in both the inhibition of the noradrenergic stimulation of adenylate cyclase activity and the generation of inositol triphosphate (Brown and Brown 1984), while the noradrenergic action is mediated by the intracellular generation of cAMP (Pappano 1977; Chen et al, 1979).

It is also possible to manipulate the levels of β-adrenergic receptors experimentally suggesting a regulatory role for the pre-synaptic component on post-synaptic receptor density. It has been demonstrated that for the β-adrenergic receptor there is an inverse relationship between receptor density, and the degree of receptor occupancy by an agonist (Harden 1983; Sibley and Lefkowitz 1985). Guanethidine treatment over five weeks, which reduced the noradrenaline content of the heart, produced a significant increase in the number of cardiac β-adrenoreceptors (Glaubiger, Tsai, Lefkowitz, Weiss, and Johnson 1978). This was reflected in the increased accumulation of cAMP. In contrast, chronic infusion of catecholamines into the rat reduced the number of cardiac adrenoreceptors (Chang, Klein, and Kunos 1982). While such an affect has not been demonstrated for muscarinic cholinergic receptors in the adult, the developmental control of receptor density by pre-synaptically released agonists could be a potent control mechanism in the developing animal (see below).

DEVELOPMENT OF NEURONAL NEUROTRANSMITTER RECEPTORS

The cellular localization of receptors in the adult

Two examples have been given of focal and diffuse modes of synaptic interaction in the periphery. Clearly, therefore, one means of deciding upon the most likely mode of interaction is to examine the regional localization of particular neurotransmitter receptors on the cells of the nervous system.

However, ultrastructural study using radioactive receptor ligands is beset with problems of diffusion and resolution, although a number of studies have been attempted, albeit with rather equivocal results. Using [³H]-flunitrazepam, a benzodiazepine, over 50 per cent of silver grains were found over synaptic complexes in the cerebellum and cortex (Mohler, Battersby, and Richards 1980), while with the putative AChRn ligand α-bungarotoxin roughly the same proportion of silver grains was seen over synaptic complexes in the hippocampus of the rat (Hunt and Schmidt 1978a, 1978b). However, within the CNS the α-bungarotoxin binding protein may not be synonymous with the central AChRn. In most cases, α-bungarotoxin does not block synaptic transmission in the CNS, and is topographically distinct from the high-affinity binding sites for acetylcholine and nicotine (Clarke, Schwartz, Paul, Pert, and Pert 1985). However, using [³H]-propylbenzilycholine mustard (PBCM), a selective and irreversible AChRm antagonist, a significant fraction of silver grains were associated with synaptic complexes in the rat hippocampus and cortex (Kuhar, Taylor, Wamsley, Hulme, and Birdsall 1981). The percentage of synaptic binding was only 20–42, leaving a significant proportion over non-synaptic regions. Of particular interest was the result that the iodinated met-enkephalin analogue, FK33–824, labelled only 7 per cent of synaptic junctions in the rat striatum, while 53 per cent of silver grains were over axo-dendritic, 18 per cent over axo-axonic, and 3 per cent over axo-somatic contacts (Hamel and Beaudet 1984). Taken together, these results suggest that neurotransmitter binding sites were as likely, or considerably more likely, to be found extrasynaptically as at morphologically defined synaptic regions.

While the resolution of autoradiographic methods can be criticized, the results of immunohistochemical methods using antibodies raised against putative glycine and γ-amino butyric acid (GABA) receptors have recently been described. Preliminary results using immunocytochemistry at the ultrastructural level claim a receptor localization at the post-synaptic density, but an extensive analysis has not yet been published (Richards, Schoch, Mohler, and Haefely 1980; Schoch, Richards, Haring, Takacs, Stähli, Staehelin, Haefely, and Mohler 1985; Altschuler, Betz, Parakkal, Reeks, and Wenthold 1986). A number of studies at the light microscopic level have indicated that receptor protein can also be found on glial cells and on axons and axon terminals. For example, opiate receptors are found on pituicytes and on certain small sensory neural perikarya and axons (Ninkovic, Hunt, and Gleave 1982; Lightman, Ninkovic, Hunt, and Iversen 1983; Ninkovic and Hunt 1983). Muscarinic receptors, which can mediate the hydrolysis of inositol phospholipids, have been described on cortical astrocytes (Murphy, Pearce, and Morrow 1986), as have adrenergic and histamine receptors on human astrocytoma cells (Clark *et al.* 1971).

A number of physiological studies have suggested that neurons have a differential sensitivity over their surfaces to iontophoretically applied neurotransmitter candidates either in culture or in slice preparations. This was true of GABA, glycine, and glutamate iontophoresed onto cultured mouse spinal neurons, although the cell body was always sensitive (Barker and Ransom 1978; Barker, McBurney, and MacDonald 1982). Differential sensitivity of dendrites to glutamate was also seen in slices of olfactory cortex and hippocampus (Richards 1978; Spencer, Gribkoff, and Lynch 1978), although the presence of pre-synaptic glutamate receptors in these areas complicates interpretation of the data (Monaghan and Cotman 1982). Biochemical evidence would also tend to suggest, however, that certain types of glutamate receptors are localized at isolated synaptic junctions and isolated post-synaptic densities (Fagg and Matus 1984). However, the activation of GABA receptors which depolarize hippocampal pyramidal cells are thought to be on dendrites and extra-synaptic (Alger and Nicoll, 1982), and indeed the majority of GABA-containing axon terminals synapse on pyramidal cell bodies (Mugnaini and Oertel 1985).

Perhaps the most dramatic result was the demonstration that in sympathetic ganglia of the frog a lutenizing-hormone releasing hormone (LHRH)-like peptide can diffuse many microns beyond the axonal site of release to cause a late slow excitatory post-synaptic potentials (EPSP) in distant neurons not normally innervated by LHRH-containing axons and terminals (Jan and Jan 1982). There is also evidence that, in the adult brain, areas with substantial densities of particular receptors may be devoid of the relevant endogenous ligand. For example, β-adrenergic receptors are found in high density in the rat striatum, but little or no noradrenaline (NA) has been found there using immuno-histochemical methods to detect the synthetic enzyme, dopamine β-hydroxylase (Levitt and Moore 1978; Rainbow, Parsons, and Woolfe 1984). Similar examples can be found for most neurotransmitter receptors which have been mapped autoradiographically (Herkenham and McClean 1986). While this 'mismatch' will be discussed more fully below, it is clear that these receptors are unlikely to be located at synapses, as no pre-synaptic element releasing the relevant neurotransmitter is present.

In summary, data concerning receptor localization in the CNS is incomplete and the relationship with the pre-synaptic axon terminal unclear. Neurons, unlike muscles, receive multiple, biochemically diverse inputs, which may require totally different mechanisms for both the insertion of receptor proteins into the neural membrane and their development control. A simple analysis of neurotransmitter actions as 'focal or diffuse' is therefore not possible and indeed may be a gross oversimplification.

The appearance of receptor during development

Kent, Pert, and Herkenham (1982) have described three patterns of opiate receptor expression during development and which can be seen to varying degrees in the generation of most receptor proteins within the CNS. In the first case there is an initial rapid appearance of receptor. Examples include the development of opiate receptor binding and benzodiazepine binding in the rat striatum (Kent *et al* 1982; Schlumpf, Richards, Lichtensteiger, and Mohler 1983). Secondly, it is possible to detect a gradual climb to adult receptor densities. This is the case for most amino-acid transmitter receptors investigated (Zukin, Young, and Snyder 1975; Enna, Yamamura, and Snyder 1976). Finally, there can be an increase of receptor density to supramaximal levels followed by a loss to adult levels. This loss can be either diffuse, as detected by *in vitro* binding assays, or specific to particular brain regions and usually picked up with auto-radiographic methods (Kuhar, de Souza, and Unnerstall 1986). The majority of neuropeptide receptors increase to supramaximal levels soon after birth before decreasing to adult levels (Roth and Beinfield 1985; Dam and Quirion 1985; Blanchard and Barden 1986; Quirion and Dam 1986), as do certain monoamine receptor subtypes (Keshles and Levitski 1984; Lau, Pylypiw, and Ross 1985, Simmons and Jones 1985). The selective disappearance or rearrangement of receptor populations during development has been reported for opiates in the olfactory cortex (Fig. 23.1) (Kent *et al.* 1982) and cerebellum (Tsang, Ho, and Ho 1982), for α-bungarotoxin binding sites in the hippocampus (Fig. 23.2) (Hunt and Schmidt, 1979), for muscarinic receptors in the cerebellum and cortex (Fig. 23.3) (Rotter, Field, and Raisman 1979a), for substance-P receptors in the hind brain of the rat (Dam and Quirion 1985), and for muscarinic cholinergic receptors in the retina (Sugiyama, Daniels, and Nirenberg 1977).

There are a number of possible explanations for these losses of receptor. It has been suggested that peptide receptors, in particular, may be important in phenomena, independent of neurotransmission, such as cell migration (Zagon and McLaughlin 1983, 1986; Zagon, Rhodes, and McLaughlin 1985). Administration of the opiate antagonist, naltrexone, to postnatal rats resulted in a substantial increase in cerebellar size when given chronically, including a 20 per cent increase in glial cell numbers, while temporary receptor blockade inhibited growth (Zagon and McLaughlin 1983). Opioid peptides were also found transiently within the germinative cell layer of the cerebellum (Zagon *et al.* 1985) and correspondingly low levels in the adult (Tsang *et al.* 1982). This suggested a possible trophic role for the opiates in development. The second possibility is that certain peptide receptors might mediate mitogenic effects, as it has been shown that substance-P and substance-K receptors can mediate the stimulation of DNA synthesis in cultured, smooth muscle cells (Nilsson, von Euler, and Dalsgaard 1985). The loss of binding sites may also be the result of the massive cell death which occurs post-natally in the rat. There is also a loss of protospines from differentiating neurons and a reduction in the polyinnervation that can occur in some systems (Lund 1978; Cowan, Fawcett, O'Leary, and Stanfield 1984).

The physiologically or biochemically measured response of neurons to exogenously applied ligand develops predictably after the appearance of the

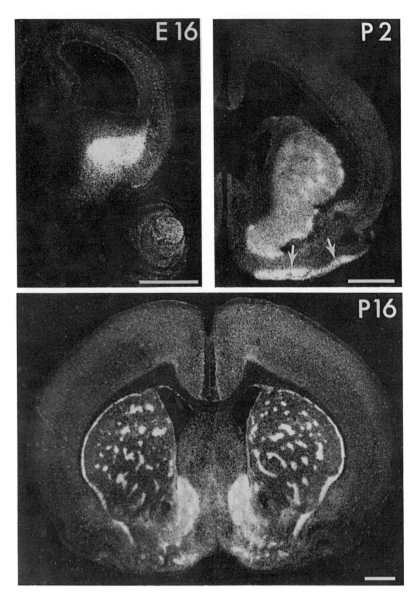

Fig. 23.1. Dark field photomicrographs of developing rat brain at embryonic stage 16 (E16), postnatal day 2 (P2) and P16. The [³H]-naloxone binding appears as white areas. Densely labelled areas at P2 are the striatum, palaeocortex and olfactory tubercle. Labelling of the lateral olfactory tract and olfactory tubercle (arrows) decreases substantially by P16. Scale bar: 1 mm. [Reproduced from Kent *et al.* (1982) by kind permission of Elsevier, Amsterdam.]

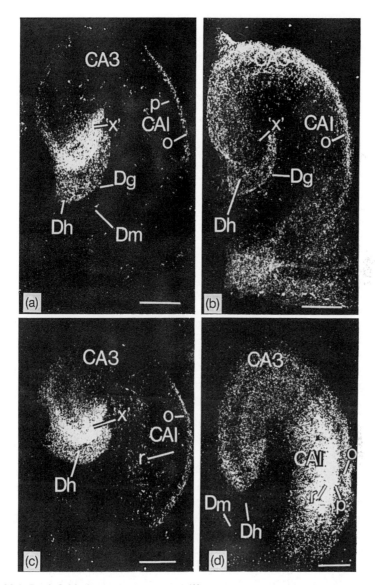

Fig. 23.2. Dark field photomicrographs of [^{125}I]-alpha-bungarotoxin binding in the rat hippocampus in the adult (a), at postnatal day 4 (d), and in the adult following a neonatal lesion of the cholinergic septal pathway (c). The septal pathway was traced into the hippocampus following tritiated amino-acid injections into the septum and axoplasmic transport of label to the hippocampus (b). A patch of intense receptor labelling is seen during development within field CA1 (d) and disappears in the adult [(a),(c)]. The pattern of binding is not affected by septal denervation at birth (c). Abbreviations: Dg, dentate granule cells; Dm, molecular layer of dentate gyrus; Dh, hilus of dentate gyrus; o, stratum oriens; p, pyramidal cell layer; r, stratum radiatum; 'x', region of intence labelling in the adult. Scale bars: (a)–(c), 1 mm; (d), 0·5 mm. [Reproduced from Hunt and Schmidt (1979) by kind permission of Pergamon Press, Oxford.]

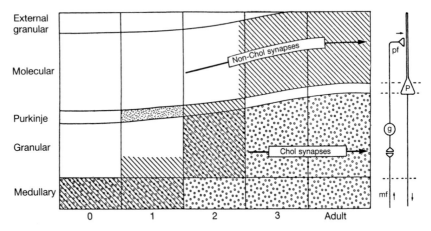

Fig. 23.3. The development of muscarinic receptor binding (striped area), acetylcholi-nesterase-containing Purkinje cells (dotted area), and acetylcholinesterase-containing mossy fibres (circled areas) in the various layers of the vestibulo-cerebellum during the first three weeks (1, 2, 3) after birth (0). Purkinje cells (P) transiently express acetylcholinesterase perhaps because of a temporary cholinergic mossy fibre (mf) input. Cholinergic markers begin to disappear at about 10 days of age. Muscarinic receptors in the molecular layer may be associated with Purkinje cell dendrites as a 'histogenic memory'. g = granule cells, pf = parallel fibres. [Reproduced from Rotter *et al* (1979a) by kind permission of Elsevier, Amsterdam.]

relevant binding site (Harden, Woolfe, Sporn, Perkins, and Molinoff 1977*a*; Harden, Mailman, Stueller, and Breese 1979; Minneman, Pittman, and Molinoff 1981; Keshles and Levitski 1984; Lau *et al*. 1985; Simmons and Jones 1985; Chalazonitis and Crain 1986). The development of the inositol triphosphate second messenger system (Berridge and Irvine 1984) occurs later than the receptor mediated stimulation of adenylate cyclase and may be linked to the differentiation of neurons (Weiss, Pin, Sebben, Kemp, Sladeczek, Gabrion, and Bockaert 1986). Pre-synaptic components usually develop, biochemically, at approximately the same time (Coyle and Axelrod 1971; Coyle and Enna 1976; Enna *et al*. 1976; Harden *et al*. 1977*a*; Keshles and Levitski 1984) or just after the first indications of a post-synaptic binding site are found. Rarely do pre-synaptic markers make an appearance before post-synaptic receptors (e.g. glycine; see Zukin *et al*. 1975), suggesting that at least the initial expression of receptor protein is independent of synaptogenesis or pre-synaptic influence (Harden, Woolfe, Sporn, Ponlos, and Molinoff 1977*b*).

The experimental manipulation of receptor density and distribution

Levels of catecholamine receptors can be modulated by treatments which vary the concentration of agonist available to the post-synaptic cell. In the adult, intraventricular treatment with 6-hydroxydopamine resulted in an increase in the number of cortical β_1-adrenergic receptors and striatal dopamine receptors. In contrast, a decrease in cortical β_1-adrenoreceptors has been reported following the administration of the uptake inhibitor, desmethylimipramine, producing an excess of NA at the receptor (Minneman, Pittman, and Molinoff 1981). Neurotensin receptors on dopamine-containing neurons of the substantia nigra pas compacta have also been shown to increase in density following long-term neuroleptic treatment (Uhl and Kuhar 1984), and substance-P receptors increase in the cortex following striatal lesions with kainic acid (Mantyh and Hunt 1986). A similar lesion caused an increase in density of benzodiazepine and muscimol (GABA) receptors in the substantia nigra pars reticulata (Penney, Pan, Young, Frey, and Dauth 1981; Lo, Niehoff, Kuhar, and Snyder 1983) and striatum (Campochiaro, Schwarz, and Coyle 1977). In contrast, several investigations of cholinergic pathways, involving sectioning of cholinergic afferents to the pons or hippocampus (Fig. 23.2) and deafferentation of sympathetic ganglia, failed to produce any evidence for changes in AChRm and AChRn numbers as a consequence of the treatment (Burt 1978; Hunt and Schmidt 1979; Rotter *et al.* 1979b).

Manipulations in the early post-natal rat, involving the destruction of descending serotoninergic (5-hydroxytryptamine, 5-HT) and adrenergic fibre systems to the spinal cord, resulted in a 50 per cent increase in 5-HT-binding in cord tissue one week after lesion and twice normal levels at four weeks (Lau *et al.* 1985). A similar pattern was also seen for the α-adrenergic receptor. However, β-adrenergic receptors were unaffected, although numbers could be increased by treatment with triiodothyronine. Increase of β-adrenergic receptors is seen, however, in the spinal cord of adult animals and in the cortex of neonatal animals treated with 6-hydroxydopamine (Harden *et al.* 1977b; Jones, Alcantara, and Adecne 1984).

In summary, the experimental manipulation of receptor density has not been described for all neurotransmitter receptors. However, it does suggest a mechanism by which the density of some neurotransmitter receptors could be modulated during development.

CAN THE DEVELOPMENTAL REGULATION OF RECEPTORS EXPLAIN THE MISMATCH BETWEEN RECEPTOR AND TRANSMITTER LOCALIZATION IN THE BRAIN?

There is now a considerable volume of literature to suggest that mismatch between neurotransmitter levels and density of receptor binding sites is not an exceptional event, but one which is found for virtually all endogenous receptor ligands. Muscarinic acetylcholine receptor binding sites are found over the granule cells of the cerebellum where no acetylcholine is found (Rotter *et al.* 1979*b*); similarly, substance-P levels are highest in the substantia nigra pars reticulata, yet virtually no tachykinin receptors are found there (Mantyh and Hunt 1986). Neurotensin receptors in the cat striatum are found in the matrix compartment while the majority of neurotensin immunoreactivity is located in the striosomal compartment (Goedert, Mantyh, Emson, and Hunt 1984). There are many other examples which have recently been extensively reviewed by Herkenham and McLean (1986). In essence these authors conclude that mismatch between receptor and ligand levels, while probably not a methodological artefact, does reflect the diffuse action of putative neurotransmitter substances at a distance from the site of release. While this may indeed be the case within the local neuronal circuitry, it is difficult to accept that the hypothesis is generalizable to areas where the agonist levels and putative receptor levels are virtually inversely related. This suggests an active relationship between the agonist and receptor such that the level of ligand may set the density of a particular receptor during development. Before this idea is considered further, two alternative but not exclusive developmental hypotheses will be considered—that receptor mismatch is in part a legacy of transient events taking place during ontogeny and that receptor proteins are expressed in groups or families, only some members of which may be appropriate.

Receptors without ligand are a memory trace of developmental events

Several studies have suggested that binding sites for neurotransmitters seen in the adult are reflections of events taking place during ontogeny and which become redundant in the adult. Opioid peptides and opiate binding sites are seen transiently in the developing cerebellum, perhaps playing some trophic role (Tsang *et al.* 1982; Zagon and McLaughlin 1986), while it has been suggested that opiate binding sites on dorsal root ganglion cells become 'uncoupled' during development and that the opioid receptor is present finally only on axon terminals of these neurons in the spinal cord and periphery (Chalazonitis and Crain 1986). In an attempt to explain the persistence of muscarinic acetylcholine receptors in the molecular layer of the cerebellum, it has been suggested that Purkinje cells pass through a cholinoceptive phase receiving a transient cholinergic input (Fig. 23.3). A high-affinity choline uptake mechanism is present in the neonatal rat cerebellum and disappears at about ten days of age. Adult Purkinje cells are sensitive to acetylcholine, and it was suggested that this muscarinic receptor may be a 'histogenic' memory of a transient developmental stage (Rotter *et al.* 1979*a*).

Linked receptor genes and co-existence of neurotransmitters

A recent hypothesis put forward to explain receptor–ligand mismatch has suggested that receptor genes are expressed in groups, and that these groupings were predetermined by the co-existence of neuropeptides and neurotransmitter substances within various neurons (Schultzberg and Hök-felt 1986). The example given is of neuropeptide tyrosine (NPY) and NA. The authors suggest that because NA and NPY coexist in many neurons, that in many post-synaptic neurons there is an automatic expression of α_2- and NPY receptors, even in areas where the pre-synaptic neurons contain only one of the ligands. Examples of neurotransmitter co-existence are so widespread within the nervous system that it is at present difficult to assess this hypothesis. It is, however, extremely probable that receptors are expressed in groups which may be invariant.

REGULATION OF RECEPTOR DENSITY

It was suggested above that regulation of receptor density during development by levels of agonist was possibly an extremely potent force in shaping the receptor maps of the adult brain. Herkenham and McLean (1986) suggest that mismatch can be resolved by invoking the diffusion of neurotransmitter over considerable distances. However, while this may be the case for local neural circuits, the extent of mismatch of ligand and receptor is such as to suggest an active suppression of receptor density by ligand concentration. For example, in the amygdala there is an inverse relationship between β-adrenergic receptors and levels of dopamine β-hydroxylase, and other inversse relationships are seen in the hippocampus and thalamus (Rainbow *et al.* 1984). Similarly, for α_1-adrenoreceptors inverse relationships exist in the thalamus and substantia nigra (Jones, Ganger, and Davis 1984). It is unlikely that this type of regulation extends to all receptor types, although it could be argued that families of neuropeptide receptors are linked to monoamine receptors. An attempt to uncover down-regulated substance-P receptors in the adult substantia nigra by kainic acid lesions of the adult rat striatonigral pathway— hence removing substance-P from the substantia nigra—was unsuccessful (Mantyh and Hunt 1986). However, in this case there may well be other tachykinins and tachykinin receptors involved in the circuit (Mantyh, Maggio, and Hunt 1984). There may also be sensitive periods during development such that dramatic changes in receptor density are limited to early stages in the ontogeny of the nervous system. In neo-natal animals treated with the neurotoxin 6-hydroxydopamine there was both a noradrener-gic denervation of the cerebral cortex and a noradrenergic hyperinnervation of the cerebellum. This resulted in an increase in β-adrenergic receptor density in the cortex and a decrease in receptor density in the cerebellum (Harden *et al.* 1977*b*, 1979).

The effects of prenatal deafferentation on receptor distribution in the CNS mapped using receptor autoradiography has not been directly studied.

Nevertheless, a recent study by Isacson, Dawbarn, Brundin, Gage, Emson, and Björklund (1987) may provide some insights into the developmental mechanisms of receptor density control. Embryonic striatal tissue transplanted into adult host lesioned striatum showed areas or striosomes of high dopmine receptor binding (using [^{3}H]-spiroperidol). This is never seen in the adult or during normal development (Murrin, Gibbens, and Ferrer 1985) and may reflect the absence of a substantial dopamine-rich innervation to the graft. The dopamine projection does appear concentrated in islands within the striatum during development (Graybiel, Pickel, Joh, Reis, and Ragsdale 1981; Edley and Herkenham 1984) and may down-regulate dopamine receptors on neurons in these histochemically discrete striosomal regions, so producing the diffuse picture seen in the adult.

CONCLUSIONS

1. The expression of neurotransmitter receptor protein in the CNS appears to occur before, and to be independent of, innervation.
2. The position of receptor proteins on the cell membrane is largely unknown, but is likely to be both diffuse and focal, depending on the neurotransmitter receptor under study and the nature of synaptic transmission. In some cases the receptor may be clustered at the post-synaptic density or on parts of the dendritic tree, but until high-resolution techniques become available the data remain equivocal.
3. During development, receptors may play roles unrelated to neurotransmission.
4. It is not known whether innervation affects the distribution of receptor on a particular neuron during development. However, it is suggested that, in many cases, regulation of receptor density by agonist levels may be an important force in shaping the final adult map of receptor densities.

ACKNOWLEDGEMENTS

My thanks to Dr Anne Stephenson for reading and criticizing the manuscript and to Mary Wynn and Jackie Nethercott for typing the manuscript.

REFERENCES

Alger, B. E. and Nicoll, R. A. (1982). Pharmacological evidence for two kinds of GABA receptor on rat hippocampal pyramidal cells studied *in vitro*. *J. Physiol. (Lond.)* **328,** pp. 125–41.
Altschuler, R. A., Betz, H., Parakkal, M. H., Reeks, K. A., and Wenthold, R. J. (1986).

Identification of glycinergic synapses in the cochlear nucleus through immunocyto-chemical localisation of the postsynaptic receptor. *Brain Res.* **369**, pp. 316–20.

Barker, J. L. and Ransom, B. R. (1978). Amino-acid pharmacology of mammalian central neurons grown in tissue culture. *J. Physiol. (Lond.)* **280**, pp. 331–54.

Barker, J. L., McBurney, R. W., and Macdonald, J. R. (1982). Fluctuation analysis of neutral amino-acid responses in cultured mouse spinal neurons. *J. Physiol. (Lond.)* **332**, pp. 365–87.

Berridge, M. J. (1986). The molecular basis of communication within the cell. *Scientific American* **253**, pp. 124–35.

Berridge, M. J. and Irvine, R. F. (1984). Inositol triphosphate, a novel second messenger in cellular signal transduction. *Nature* **312**, pp. 315–21.

Bevan, S. and Steinbach, J. H. (1967). The distribution of α-bungarotoxin binding sites on mammalian skeletal muscle developing *in vivo*. *J. Physiol. (Lond.)* **267**, pp. 195–213.

Blanchard, L. and Barden, N. (1986). Ontogeny of receptors for thyrotropin-releasing hormone in the rat brain. *Dev. Brain Res.* **24**, pp. 85–8.

Brown, J. H. and Brown, S. L. (1984). Agonists differentiate muscarinic receptors that inhibit cyclic AMP formation from those that stimulate phophoinositide metab-olism. *J. Biol. Chem.* **259**, pp. 3777–81.

Burt, D. R. (1978). Muscarinic receptor binding in rat sympathetic ganglia unaffected by denervation. *Brain Res.* **143**, pp. 573–9.

Campochiaro, P., Schwarz, R., and Coyle, J. T. (1977). GABA receptor binding in rat striatum: localization and effects of denervation. *Brain Res.* **136**, pp. 501–11.

Chalazonitis, A. and Crain, S. M. (1986). Maturation of opioid sensitivity of fetal mouse dorsal root ganglion neuron perikarya in organotypic cultures: regulation by spinal cord. *Neuroscience* **17**, pp. 1181–98.

Chang, H. Y., Klein, R. M., and Kunos, G. (1982). Selective desensitization of cardiac β-adrenoceptors by prolonged *in vivo* infusion of catecholamines in rats. *J. Pharm. Exp. Ther.* **221**, pp. 784–9.

Chen, F. C., Yamamura, H. I., and Roeske, W. R. (1979). Ontogeny of mammalian myocardial β-adrenergic receptors. *Eur. J. Pharm.* **58**, pp. 255–64.

Clark, R. D. and Perkins J. P. (1971) Regulation of adenosine 3′,,5′-cyclic monophos-phate concentration in cultured human astrocytoma cells by catecholamines and histamine. *Proc. Natl. Acad. Sci. USA* **68**, pp. 2757–60.

Clarke, P. B. S., Schwartz, R. D., Paul, S. M., Pert, C. B., and Pert, A. (1985) Nicotinic binding in rat brain: autoradiographic comparison of [^{3}H] acetylcholine, [^{3}H] nictoine and [^{125}I] α-bungarotoxin. *J. Neurosci.* **5**, pp. 1307–15.

Cowan, W. M., Fawcett, J. W., O'Leary, D. D. M., and Stanfield, B. B. (1984). Regressive events in neurogenesis. *Science* **225**, pp. 1258–65.

Coyle, J. T. and Axelrod, J. (1971). Development of the uptake and storage of L-[^{3}H]-norepinephrine in rat brain. *J. Neurochem.* **18**, pp. 2061–75.

Coyle, J. T. and Enna, S. J. (1976). Neurochemical aspects of the ontogenesis of GABAergic neurons in the rat brain. *Brain Res.* **111**, pp. 119–33.

Dam, T. V. and Quirion, R. (1985). Ontogeny of substance P receptors in rat brain. *Soc. Neuroscience Abstr.* **11**, p. 10.

Dennis, M. J. (1981). Development of the neuromuscular junction: inductive interactions between cells. *Ann. Rev. Neurosci* **4**, pp. 43–68.

Edley, S. M. and Herkenham, M. (1984). Comparative development of opiate receptors and dopamine revealed by autoradiography and histofluoresence. *Brain Res.* **305**, pp. 27–42.

Enna, S. J., Yamamura, H. I., and Snyder, S. H. (1976). Development of muscarinic cholinergic and GABA receptor binding in chick embryo brain. *Brain Res.* **101**, pp. 177–83.

Fagg, G. E. and Matus, A. (1984). Selective association of N-methyl aspartate and quisqualate types of L-glutamate receptor with brain postsynaptic densities. *Proc. Natl. Acad. Sci. USA.* **81**, pp. 6876–80.

Foster, A. C., Mena, E. E., Fagg, G. T., and Cotman, C. W. (1981). Glutamate and asparate binding sites are enriched in synaptic junctions isolated from rat brain. *J. Neurosci.* **1**, pp. 620–5.

Galfer, J. B., Klein, W., and Catterall, W. A. (1977). Muscarinic acetylcholine receptors in developing chick heart. *J. Biol. Chem.* **252**, pp. 8692–9.

Glaubiger, G., Tsai, B. S., Lefkowitz, R. J., Weiss, D., and Johnson, E. M. (1978). Chronic quanethidine treatment increases cardiac β-adrenergic receptors. *Nature* **273**, pp. 240–2.

Goedert, M., Mantyh, P. W., Emson, P. C., and Hunt, S. P. (1984). Inverse relationship between neurotensin receptors and neurotensin-like immunoreactivity in cat striatum. *Nature* **307**, pp. 543–6.

Goedert, M., Mantyh, P. W., Hunt, S. P., and Emson, P. C. (1983). Mosaic distribution of neurotensin-like immunoreactivity in the cat striatum. *Brain Res.* **274**, pp. 176–9.

Goffinet, A. M., Hemmendinger, L. M., and Caviness, V. S. (1986). Autoradiographic study of β_1-adrenergic receptor development in the mouse forebrain. *Dev. Brain Res.* **24**, pp. 187–91.

Graybiel, A. M., Pickel, V. M., Joh, T. H., Reis, D. J., and Ragsdale, C. W. (1981). Direct demonstration of a correspondence between the dopamine islands and acetylcholinesterase patches in the developing striatum. *Proc. Natl. Acad. Sci. USA.* **78**, pp. 5871–5.

Hamel, E. and Beaudet, A. (1984). Electron microscopic autoradiographic localization of opioid receptors in rat neostriatum. *Nature* **312**, pp. 155–7.

Harden, T. K. (1983). Agonist-induced desensitization of the β-adrenergic receptor-linked adenylate cyclase. *Pharm. Rev.* **35**, pp. 5–32.

Harden, T. K., Mailman, R. B., Mueller, R. A., and Breese, G. R. (1979). Noradrenergic hyperinnervation reduces the density of β-adrenergic receptors in rat cerebellum. *Brain Res.* **166**, pp. 194–8.

Harden, T. K., Woolfe, B. B., Sporn, J. R., Perkins, J. P., and Molinoff, P. B. (1977*a*). Ontogeny of β-adrenergic receptors in rat cerebral cortex. *Brain Res.* **125**, pp. 99–108.

Harden, T. K., Woolfe, B. B., Sporn, J. R., Ponlos, B. K., and Molinoff, P. B. (1977*b*). Effects of 6-hydroxydopamine on the development of the β adrenergic receptor/adenylate cyclase system in rat cerebral cortex. *J. Pharm. Exp. Ther.* **203**, pp. 132–43.

Hartzell, H. C. (1980). Distribution of muscarinic acetycholine receptors and presynaptic nerve terminals in amphibian heart. *J. Cell Biol.* **86**, pp. 6–20.

Hays, S. E., Houston, S. H., Beinfeld, M. C., and Pau, S. M. (1981). Post-natal ontogeny of cholecystokinin receptors in rat brain. *Brain Res.* **213**, pp. 237–41.

Herkenham, M. and McLean, S. (1986). Mismatches between receptor and transmitter localisation in the brain. In *Quantitative receptor autoradiography* (eds. C. A. Boast, E. W. Snowhill, and C. A. Alton), pp. 137–71. Alan R. Liss Inc., New York.

Hohmann, C. F., Pert, C. C., and Ebner, F. F. (1985). Development of cholinergic markers in the mouse forebrain. II Muscarinic receptor binding in cortex. *Dev. Brain Res.* **23**, pp. 243–53.

Hunt, S. P. and Schmidt, J. (1979). The relationship of α-bungarotoxin binding activity and cholinergic termination within the rat hippocampus. *Neuroscience.* **4**, pp. 585–92.

Hunt, S. P. and Schmidt, J. (1978a). The electron microscopic autoradiographic localization of α-bungarotoxin binding sites within the central nervous system of the rat. *Brain Res.* **142**, pp. 152–9.

Hunt, S. P. and Schmidt, J. (1978b). Some observations on the binding patterns of α-bungarotoxin in the central nervous system of the rat. *Brain Res.* **157**, pp. 213–32.

Isacson, O., Dawbarn, D., Brundin, P., Gage, F. H., Emson, P. C., and Björklund, A. (1987). Striatal grafts in the ibotenic acid lesioned striatum: striosomal organization as revealed by immunocytochemistry and receptor autoradiography. *Neuroscience* (in press).

Iversen, L. L. (1984). Amino-acids and peptides: fast and slow chemical signals in the nervous system. *Proc. R. Soc. Lond. B.* **221**, pp. 245–60.

Jan, L. Y. and Jan, Y. N. (1982). Peptidergic transmission in sympathetic ganglion of the frog, (Rana Catabiensa). *J. Physiol. (Lond.)* **327**, pp. 219–46.

Jones, D. J., Alcantara, O. F., and Adecne, R. M. (1984). Supersensitivity of the noradrenergic system in the spinal cord following intracisternal injection of 6-hydroxydopamine. *Neurophamacology* **23**, pp. 431–8.

Jones, L. S., Ganger, L. L., and Davis, J. N. (1984). Anatomy of brain α-adrenergic receptors: in vitro autoradiography with [^{125}I]—Heat. *J. Comp. Neurol.* **231**, pp. 190–208.

Kent, J. L., Pert, C. B., and Herkenham, M. (1982). Ontogeny of opiate receptors in rat forebrain: visualization by in vitro autoradiography. *Dev. Brain Res.* **2**, pp. 487–504.

Keshles, O. and Levitzki, A. (1984). The ontogenesis of β-adrenergic receptors and of adenylate cyclase in the developing rat brain. *Biochem. Pharm.* **33**, pp. 2331–3.

Kuhar, M. J., de Souza, E. B., and Unnerstall, J. R. (1986). Neurotransmitter receptor mapping by autoradiography and other methods. *Ann. Rev. Neurosci.* **9**, pp. 27–59.

Kuhar, M. J., Taylor, N., Wamsley, J. K., Hulme, E. L., and Birdsall, N. J. M. (1981). Muscarinic cholinergic receptor localisation in brain by electron microscopic autoradiography. *Brain Res.* **216**, pp. 1–9.

Lane, M. A., Sastre, A., Law, M., and Salpeter, M. (1977). Cholinergic and adrenergic receptors on mouse cardiocytes *in vitro*. *Dev. Biol.* **57**, pp. 254–69.

Lau, C., Pylypiw, A., and Ross, L. L. (1985). Development of serotinergic and adrenergic receptors in the rat spinal cord: effects of neonatal chemical lesions and hyperthyroidism. *Dev. Brain Res.* **19**, pp. 57–66.

Levitt, P. and Moore, R. Y. (1978). Noradrenaline neuron innervation of the neocortex in the rat. *Brain Res.* **139**, pp. 219–31.

Lightman, S. L., Ninkovic, M., Hunt, S. P., and Iversen, L. L. (1983). Evidence for opiate receptors on pituicytes. *Nature* **305**, pp. 235–7.

Lo, M. M. S., Niehoff, D. L., Kuhar, M. J., and Snyder, S. H. (1983). Differential localization of type I and type II benzodiazepine binding sites in substantia nigra. *Nature* **306**, pp. 57–60.

Loffelholz, K. and Pappano, A. J. (1985). The parasympathetic neuroeffector junction of the heart. *Pharm. Rev.* **37**, pp. 1–24.

Lomo, T. I and Jansen, J. K. S. (1980). Requirements for the formation and maintenance of neuromuscular connections. *Curr. Top. Dev. Biol.* **16**, pp. 253–81.

Lund, R. D. (1978). *Development and plasticity of the brain.* Oxford University Press, New York.

Mantyh, P. and Hunt, S. P. (1986). Changes in [³H] substance P receptor binding in the rat brain after kainic acid lesions of the corpus striatum. *J. Neurosci.* **6**, pp. 1537–44.

Mantyh, P. W., Maggio, J. E., and Hunt, S. P. (1984). The autoradiographic distribution of kassinin and substance K binding sites is different from substance P binding sites. *Eur. J. Pharm.* **102**, pp. 361–4.

Mantyh, P. W., Pinnock, R. D., Downes, C.P., Goedert, M., and Hunt, S. P. (1984). Correlation between inositol phospholipid hydrolysis and substance P receptors in rat CNS. *Nature* **309**, pp. 795–7.

Marshall, L. M. (1981). Synaptic localization of α-bungarotoxin binding which blocks nicotinic transmission at frog sympathetic neurons. *Proc. Natl. Acad. Sci. USA* **78**, pp. 3014–18.

Merlie, J. P. and Sanes, J. R. (1985). Concentration of acetylcholine receptor mRNA in synaptic regions of adult muscle fibres. *Nature* **317**, pp. 66–8.

Minneman, K. P., Pittman, R. N., and Molinoff, P. B. (1981). β-adrenergic receptor subtypes: properties, distribution and regulation. *Ann. Rev. Neurosci.* **4**, pp. 419–61.

Mishina, M., Kurosaki, T., and Tobimatsu, T., Morimoto, Y., Noda, M., Yamamoto, T., Terao, M., Lindstrom, J., Takahashi, T., Kuno, M., and Numa, S. (1984). Expression of functional acetylcholine receptor from cloned cDNAs. *Nature* **307**, pp. 604–8.

Mishina, M., Takai, T., and Imoto, K., Noda, M., Takahashi, T., Numa, S., Methfessel, C., and Sakmann B. (1986). Molecular distinction between fetal and adult forms of muscle acetylcholine receptor. *Nature* **321**, pp. 406–11.

Mohler, H., Battersby, M. K., and Richards, J. G. (1980). Benzodiazepine receptor protein identified and visualized in brain tissue by photoaffinity label. *Proc. Natl. Acad. Sci. USA* **77**, pp. 1666–70.

Monoghan, D. T. and Cotman, C. W. (1982). The distribution of [³H] kainic acid binding sites in rat CNS as determined by autoradiography. *Brain Res.* **252**, pp. 91–100.

Mugnaini, E. and Oertel, W. H. (1985). An atlas of the distribution of GABA-ergic neurons and terminals in the rat CNS as revealed by GAD immunohistochemistry. In *Handbook of chemical neuroanatomy vol 4, part I* (eds. A. Björklund and T. Hökfelt), pp. 436–595. Elsevier, Amsterdam.

Murphy, S., Pearce, B., and Morrow, C. (1986). Astrocytes have both M_1 and M_2 muscarinic receptor subtypes. *Brain Res.* **364**, pp. 177–80.

Murrin, L. C., Gibbens, D. L., and Ferrer, J. R. (1985). Ontogeny of dopamine, serotonin and spirodecanone receptors in rat forebrain—an autoradiographic study. *Dev. Brain Res.* **23**, pp. 91–109.

Nicoletti, F., Iadorola, M. J., Wroblewski, J. T., and Costa, E. (1986). Excitatory amino-acids recognition sites coupled with inositol phospholipid metabolism: developmental changes and interaction with α-adrenoreceptors. *Proc. Natl. Acad. Sci. USA* **83**, pp. 1931–5.

Nilsson, J., von Euler, A. M., and Dalsgaard, C. J. (1985). Stimulation of connective tissue cell growth by substance P and substance K. *Nature* **315**, pp. 61–3.

Ninkovic, M. and Hunt, S. P. (1983). α-bungarotoxin binding sites on sensory neurons and their axonal transport in sensory afferents. *Brain Res.* **272**, pp. 57–69.

Ninkovic, M., Hunt, S. P., and Gleave, J. R. W. (1982). Localization of opiate and histamine H₁-receptors in primate sensory ganglia and spinal cord. *Brain Res* **241,** pp. 197–206.

Olson, L., Seiger, A., and Fuxe, K. (1982). Heterogeneity of striatal and limbic dopamine innervation: highly fluorescent islands in developing and adult rats. *Brain Res.* **44,** pp. 283–8.

Palacios, J. M. and Kuhar, M. J. (1982*a*). Neurotensin receptors are located on dopamine containing neurons in rat midbrain. *Nature* **294,** pp. 587–9.

Palacios, J. M. and Kuhar, M. J. (1982*b*). Ontogeny of high-affinity GABA and benzodiazepine receptors in the rat cerebellum: an autoradiographic study. *Dev. Brain Res* **2,** pp. 531–9.

Pappano, A. J. (1977). Ontogenetic development of autonomic neuroeffector transmitter reactivity in embryonic and fetal hearts. *Pharmacol. Rev.* **29,** pp. 3–33.

Pazos, A., Palacios, J. M., Schlumpf, M., and Lichtensteiger, W. (1985). Pre and post-natal ontogeny of brain neurotensin receptors: an autoradiographic study. *Soc. Neurosci. Abstr.* **11,** p. 602.

Penney, J. B., Pan, H. S., Young, A. B., Frey, K. A., and Dauth, G. W. (1981). Quantitive autoradiography of [³H] muscimol binding in the rat brain. *Science* **214,** pp. 1036–8.

Quiron, R. and Dam, T.-V. (1968) Ontogeny of Substance P receptor binding sites in rat brain. *J. Neurosci.* **6,** pp. 2187–99.

Rainbow, T. C., Parsons, B., and Woolfe, B. B. (1984). Quantitative autoradiography of β_1 and β_2 adrenergic receptors in rat brain. *Proc. Natl. Acad. Sci. USA* **81,** pp. 1585–9.

Richards, C. D. (1978). Evidence of localisation of glutamate receptors in layer 1A of the dendritic field of neurons in the prepiriform cortex. In *Iontophoresis and transmitter mechanisms in the mammalian central nervous system* (eds. R. Ryall and J. S. Kelly), pp. 185–7. Elsevier, Amsterdam.

Richards, J. G., Schoch, P., Mohler, H., and Haefely, W. (1980). Benzodiazepine receptors resolved. *Experientia* **42,** pp. 121–6.

Roth, B. L. and Beinfeld, M. C. (1985). The post-natal development of VIP binding sites in rat forebrain and hindbrain. *Peptides* **6,** pp. 27–30.

Rotter, A., Field, P. M., and Raisman, G. (1979*a*). Muscarinic receptors in the central nervous system of the rat. III. Post-natal development of binding of [³H] propylbenzilycholine mustard. *Brain Res. Rev.* **1,** pp. 185–205.

Rotter, A., Birdsall, N. J. M., Burgen, A. S. V., Field, P. M., Smolen, A., and Raisman, G. (1979*b*). Muscarinic receptors in the central nervous system of the rat. IV. A comparison of the effects of axotomy and deafferentation on the binding of [³H] propylbenzilylcholine mustard and associated synaptic changes in the hypoglossal and pontine nuclei. *Brain Res. Rev.* **1,** pp. 207–24.

Sakmann, B., Methfessel, C., and Mishina, M., Takahashi, T., Takai, T., Kurasaki, M., Fukuda, K., and Numa, S. (1985). Role of acetylcholine receptor subunits in gating of the channel. *Nature* **318,** pp. 538–43.

Schlumpf, M., Richards, J. G., Lichtensteiger, W., and Mohler, H. (1983). An autoradiographic study of the prenatal development of benzodiazepine–binding sites in rat brain. *J. Neurosci.* **3,** pp. 1478–87.

Schoch, P., Richards, J. G., Haring, P., Takacs, B., Stähli, C., Staehelin, T., Haefely, W., and Mohler, H. (1985). Colocalization of GABA, receptors and benzodiazepine receptors in the brain shown by monoclonal antibodies. *Nature* **314,** pp. 168–71.

Schultzberg, M. and Hökfelt, T. (1986). The mismatch problem in receptor autoradiography and the coexistence of multiple messengers. *Trends Neurosci.* **9,** pp. 109–10.

Sibley, D. R., and Lefkowitz, R. J. (1985). Molecular mechanisms of receptor desensitization using the β-adrenergic receptor-coupled adenylate cyclase system as a model. *Nature* **317,** pp. 124–9.

Simmons, K. E. and Jones, D. J. (1985). The post-natal development of norepinephrine–stimulated cyclic AMP accumulation in the rat spinal cord. *Dev. Brain Res.* **18,** pp. 306–10.

Spain, J. W., Roth, D. L., and Coscia, C. J. (1985). Differential ontogeny of multiple opioid receptors. *J. Neurosci.* **5,** pp. 584–8.

Spencer, H., Gribkoff, V. K., and Lynch, G. S. (1978). Distribution of acetylcholine, glutamate and aspartate sensitivity over the dendritic fields of hippocampal CA1 neurons. In *Iontophoresis and transmitter mechanisms in the mammalian central nervous system* (eds. R. Ryall and J. S. Kelly), pp. 194–6. Elsevier, Amsterdam.

Sugiyama, H., Daniels, M. P., and Nirenberg, M. (1977). Muscarinic acetylcholine receptors of the developing retina. *Proc. Natl. Acad. Sci. USA* **74,** pp. 5524–8.

Tsang, D., Ng, S. C., Ho, K. P., and Ho, W. K. K. (1982). Ontogensis of opiate binding site and radioimmunoassayable β-endorphin and enkephalin in regions of rat brain. *Dev. Brain Res.* **3,** pp. 637–44.

Uhl, G. R. and Kuhar, M. J. (1984). Chronic neuroleptic treatment enhances neurotensin receptor binding in human and rat substantia nigra. *Nature* **309,** pp. 350–2.

Weiss, S., Pin, J. P., Sebben, M., Kemp, D. E., Sladeczek, F., Gabrion, J., and Bockaert, J. (1986). Synaptogenesis of cultured striatal neurons in serum free medium: a morphological and biochemical study. *Proc. Natl. Acad. Sci. USA* **83,** pp. 2238–42.

Zagon, I. S. and McLaughlin, (1983). Increased brain size and cellular content in infant rats treated with an opiate antagonist. *Science* **221,** pp. 1179–80.

Zagon, I. S. and McLaughlin, P. J. (1986). Opioid antagonist (naltrexone) modulation of cerebellar development: histological and morphometric studies. *J. Neurosci.* **6,** pp. 1424–32.

Zagon, I. S., Rhodes, R. E., and McLaughlin, P. J. (1985). Distribution of enkephalin immunoreactivity in germanitive cells of developing rat cerebellum. *Science* **227,** pp. 1049–51.

Ziskind-Conhaim, L., Geffen, I., and Hall, Z. W. (1984). Redistribution of acetylcholine receptors on developing rat myotubes. *J. Neurosci.* **4,** pp. 2346–9.

Zukin, S. R., Young, A. B., and Snyder, S. H. (1975). Development of the synaptic glycine receptor in chick embryo spinal cord. *Brain Res.* **83,** pp. 525–30.

24

Factors influencing the development of dendritic form

M. BERRY AND M. SADLER

The dendritic trees of neurons are very varied, ranging from unbranched, relatively simple structures to huge, elaborately patterned, complex networks. Despite the plethora of different forms, all dendritic trees share a common function of generating post-synaptic potentials, in response to afferent axonal vollies, which are integrated over the tree and which ultimately influence the spike-generating axon hillock area of the neuron. The frequency of firing is thus a direct translation of these integrated, summed dendritic post-synaptic potentials. Branching patterns may be relevant to integration, since potentials sequentially interact at branch points *en route* to the soma. Dendritic trees also effect spatial dispersion of post-synaptic membrane to facilitate the sampling of activity in neighbouring axonal arrays at varying radial distances from somata. Definitions of the structure of dendritic trees, their development, and plasticity are thus fundamental to an understanding of the function of the neuron and, indeed, the brain as a whole. Because they are branched, dendrites are amenable to topological analysis, which achieves a precise quantitative definition of an arborescence, facilitating a better understanding of growth modes and also of the mechanics of remodelling which underlie plasticity. We have used the Purkinje cell (PC) dendritic tree as the basis for our studies, both because it is a planar structure, and thus can be represented as a two dimensional projection, and also because PC connections are well defined. The latter property facilitates the experimental manipulation of afferent fibres with a view to elucidating the role of environmental factors in growth and remodelling. Moreover, the possibility of discovering the genetics of PC dendritic development is available from studies on the many varieties of mutant mice which exist with defined cerebellar abnormalities. Much of the work relating to the nature/nurture aspects of dendritic form have been reviewed by Berry, McConnell, and Sievers (1980*a*), Berry, Sievers, and Baumgarten (1980*b*, 1980*c*), and Berry, McConnell, Sievers, Price, and Anwar (1981). This article will report on our recent work defining growth and remodelling of PC dendritic fields in normal and mutant (*reeler* (*rl*) and *weaver* (*wv*)) mice.

ANALYTICAL METHODS

Before the advent of modern topological methods, dendritic fields were analysed using a target method, originally devised by Sholl (1953, 1955, 1956) but later modified by Eayrs (1955). Berry, Anderson, Hollingworth, and Flinn (1972*a*) and Berry, Hollingworth, Flinn, and Anderson (1972*b*) showed that the target method was grossly inaccurate, producing artefactual results unrepresentative of actual dendritic tree structure and recommended abandonment in favour of more accurate metrical/topological techniques. Attempts to achieve this latter aim take account of the third dimension using either stereophotogrammetry (Mannen 1968), reconstruction from serial sections (Gough 1968; Wyss 1972; Levinthal and Ware 1972); computer correction (Berry *et al.* 1972*b*), or computer tracking microscopes (Glaser and van der Loos 1965; Garvey, Young, Coleman, and Simon 1973; Lindsay and Scheibel 1976, 1981; Overdijk, Uylings, Kuypers, and Kamstra 1978; Glaser, van der Loos, and Gissler 1979). Most methods rely upon Golgi impregnation which randomly stains neurons (Pappas and Purpura 1961; Smit and Colon 1969; Morest 1969*a*, 1969*b*; Blackstad 1970; Kiernan and Berry 1975; Pasternak and Woolsey 1975). Alternative methods have been developed, including horseradish peroxidase, fluorescent dye, and antibody staining (Caddy, Patterson, and Biscoe 1982; Greenlee and Brashear 1983; Weber and Schachner 1984; de Camilli, Miller, Levitt, Walter, and Greengard 1984) and repeated imaging of the same neuron *in vivo* (Purves and Hadley 1985; Purves, Hadley and Voyvodic 1986; Stirling 1986), but these methods have so far had limited application to quantitative studies. A fundamental prerequisite for estimating both metrical and topological parameters is a numerical definition of all segments using either a centrifugal or a centripetal ordering system. Centrifugal systems are the most commonly used; these assign order 1 to the root dendrite (Coleman and Riesen 1968) and ordering increases sequentially at each new branch point [Fig. 24.1(a)]. All segments of nth order are thus $(n-1)$ orders from the origin and are equivalent in this sense. Proximal ordering is unaffected by either segment additions or resorptions, facilitating studies of growth and plasticity.

Vertex analysis

Vertex analysis (Berry and Pymm 1981; Berry and Flinn 1984) was developed from network analysis (Berry, Hollingworth, Anderson, and Flinn 1975; Hollingworth and Berry 1975; Berry 1976; Berry and Bradley 1976*a*) and the terminology of the method is summarized in Fig. 24.1. Vertices are the points in a network which are interconnected by segments, and are terminal, root, and link. There are three types of dichotomous link vertices [V_d, Fig. 24.1(b)] comprising primary (V_a), secondary (V_b), and tertiary (V_c) vertices; these connect centrifugally with 2 terminal, 1 link and 1 terminal, and 2 link vertices,

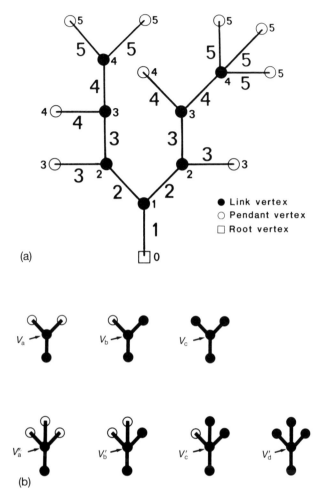

Fig. 24.1. (a) Centrifugal ordering system. Starting at the root-point (axon hillock) all arcs and vertices are ordered successively. Note that each vertex of order *n* is at the *distal* end of a link arc of order *n*. (b) Primary types of dichotomous (Vd) and tichotomous (Vt) vertices (arrowed). Two pendant arcs (and vertices) arise from V_a nodes; one pendant and one link arc arise from V_b and two link arcs from V_c dichotomous vertices. V_t comprise V_a', V_b', V_c', and V_d' and drain $3+0$, $2+1$, $1+2$, and $0+3$ pendant and link arcs, respectively.

respectively. Centripetally all V_d connect with either 1 link or 1 root vertex. Similarly, there are four types of trichotomous link vertices [V_t; Fig. 24.1(b)]. Thus, for a given link vertex draining *n* arcs, there are $(n+1)$ possible link vertex topologies. V_t and V_d are mutually interconnectable within networks. The system of ordering used in vertex analysis is centrifugal [Coleman and

Riesen 1968; see Fig. 24.1(a)]. The mathematical interrelationships between vertices have been defined by Berry and Flinn (1984). In large dichotomous networks, the frequencies of V_a and V_c are almost equal and, so, V_b is the only variable. The ratio of V_a/V_b (the vertex ratio, V_R) thus defines the branching pattern of a given dendritic tree. For example, in networks grown by random terminal growth, $V_R = 1.0$, in networks generated by random segmental growth, $V_R = 0.5$. However, since growth is not constrained to occur according to any of these hypotheses, and since different modes of branching can produce the same topological result, V_R is not a rigid pointer to the type of growth and branching observed.

Computer modelling

Additional criteria for a more sensitive definition of topology may be achieved by computer modelling of networks. By comparison of growth models with observed data, it is possible to test hypotheses against recorded events and discard untenable models of growth accordingly. In practice, the parameter used to compare networks is the ratio, at each order, of the number of terminal vertices/link vertices, and is called the T/L profile of the tree. This parameter has been used to investigate the topology of branched microvascular systems (Ley, Pries, and Gaehtgens 1986) where it has proved to be a sensitive and informative tool.

Adopting the T/L profile, for the definition of a given network, has the advantage, over V_R, of enabling regional variations in the pattern of branching to be investigated within the tree and of incorporating trichotomous and higher order vertices without perturbation of the analysis. Other methods are unable to achieve this and, accordingly, trichotomous nodes present many problems in such cases (Berry, Sadler, and Flinn 1986).

NORMAL GROWTH OF THE PC TREE OF THE MOUSE

Establishment of the tree

Sadler and Berry (1983a, 1983b, 1984) have described the normal growth of the mouse PC tree from birth to 100 days post-natum (dpn) (see Fig. 24.2). By 20 dpn, most segments have been generated [Fig. 24.3(a)] and segment distribution up to the 10th order remains stable throughout development; increases over higher orders occur in the period up to 100 dpn [Fig. 24.3(a)]. Although the distribution of segment lengths is skewed about a peak at 5 μm (Fig. 24.4), a remarkably uniform inter vertex increment of approximately 10 μm/order is established in the mature tree [Fig. 24.5(a)]. V_b terminal segments are consistently 2 μm longer than those of V_a, reaching a maximum mean length by 50 dpn. V_a terminal and link segments reach their maximum length of 9.5 μm and 7.2 μm, respectively, at 100 dpn.

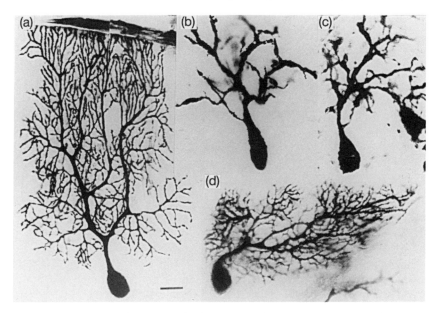

Fig. 24.2. Golgi-Cox stained PCs in both normal and mutant cerebella at various ages: (a) normal PC at 100 dpn; (b) subcortical reeler (**rl**) PC at 20 dpn; (c) weaver (*wv*) PC at 20 dpn; and (d) cortical *rl* PC at 100 dpn. Cortically positioned *rl* PCs are approximately half the height and have shorter segments in a less planar array than normal PCs. Deep *rl* and *wv* resemble each other in that they are both metrically similar with non-planar thick, varicose dendrites. These latter cells show no preferred orientation within the cerebellum. (Scale bar: 20 μm.)

T/L vertex ratio profile

Figure 24.6(a) shows the mean *T/L* profile at each age, together with the projected values for a similar number of trees grown by random terminal branching and containing the same proportion of trichotomy as observed in the real networks. At 7 and 10 dpn, both the observed and projected lines are very close throughout their entire course. At these ages, the V_R values are also similar to projected values for purely random terminal branching (Sadler and Berry 1984), indicating that initial PC growth could have been achieved entirely through random terminal branching. Beyond 10 dpn, all plots depart from the projected line by the 10th order; the maximum deviation occurs at 20 dpn, tending to decrease by 100 dpn. The extent of the deviation of observed from projected values is consistent with the deviation of V_R from its projected values (Sadler and Berry 1984), which is also greatest at 20 dpn.

Computer modelling

Based upon the findings of the metrical and topological data, models were

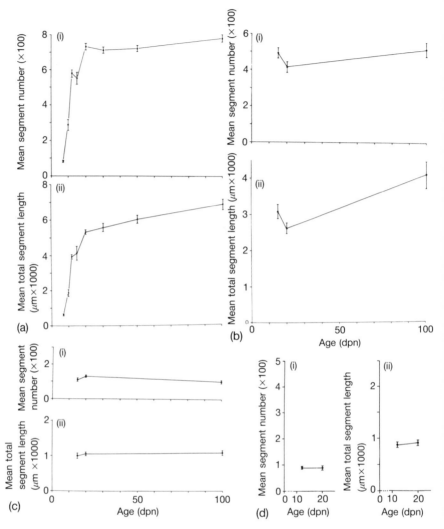

Fig. 24.3. (a) (i) Graph of mean number of segments and (ii) graph of mean total segment length against age, in normal PC dendritic trees. Both plots show the rapid expansion of the networks from 7–20 dpn followed by slight gains up to 100 dpn. (b) (i) Mean number of segments and (ii) mean total segment length against age in cortical *rl* PCs. By 100 dpn, 66 per cent of normal segment number and 59 per cent of normal dendritic length have been elaborated. (c) (i) Mean number of segments and (ii) mean total segment length against age in deep *rl* PCs. These parameters show little significant change over the duration of the study. (d) (i) Mean number of segments and (ii) mean total segment length against age in *wv* PCs. Both *wv* and deep *rl* PCs elaborate approximately 100 segments and 1000 µm of dendritic membrane per cell. Error bars represent standard errors.

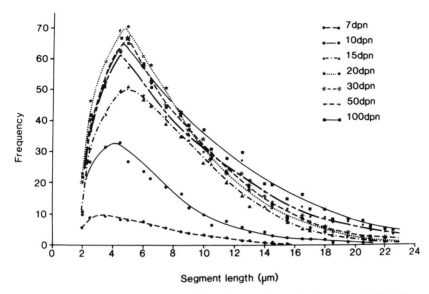

Fig. 24.4. Segment frequency against length at various ages in normal PCs. Here, segments include both terminals and interstitial link arcs. The peak shows a gradual shift towards longer segments reflecting the finding that all segments and terminals are longer in older animals. Moreover, there is an increase in frequency of segments of length 9–24 μm in trees beyond 20 dpn but a loss of segments at the peak frequency length of around 5 μm in the late post-natal period.

constructed which attempt to simulate the observed growth processes. Initially, a small network is established by purely random terminal growth (the approximate size of 7 dpn trees); thereafter, branching is constrained over a growth front. Within the boundaries of this front, branching continues on random terminals, with a small amount of residual random terminal branching behind the front. The best fit [Fig. 24.7(a)] of the modelled to the observed data is obtained by growing a tree entirely by branching on random terminals up to 50 terminals. Then branching is constrained until 90 per cent of the branching occurs within a front comprising the highest 4 orders. This collimation of branching occurred in steps, from a front 10 orders deep, in a tree with 50 terminals, to 5 orders deep, in trees with 110 terminals, and, finally to 4 orders deep, in trees with more than 160 terminals. Behind this front, 10 per cent residual random terminal branching occurs. Figure 24.7(a) compares the T/L profile of this model with that of the observed trees at 12, 20, and 100 dpn.

Between 20 and 100 dpn, remodelling is characterized by an erosion of orders higher than 20 and the generation of new segments over orders 8–18 [Fig. 24.8(a)]. The 20 dpn tree was remodelled by computer simulation of random terminal growth and resorption over specified regions of the tree.

Figure 24.7(a) shows the *T/L* profiles of both observed and computer-generated trees following growth and resorption. Terminals were chosen randomly and the probability of either growth or erosion was set at 0·5; thus modelling simultaneous growth and resorption. The probability that a chosen terminal would branch was set at 0·3 from order 8, rising linearly to 1·00 by order 10; the growth zone was from order 8–18, the probability that a chosen terminal would be resorbed was set at 0·16 at order 16 and increased linearly to 1·00 by order 21; chosen terminals above order 21 were always eroded.

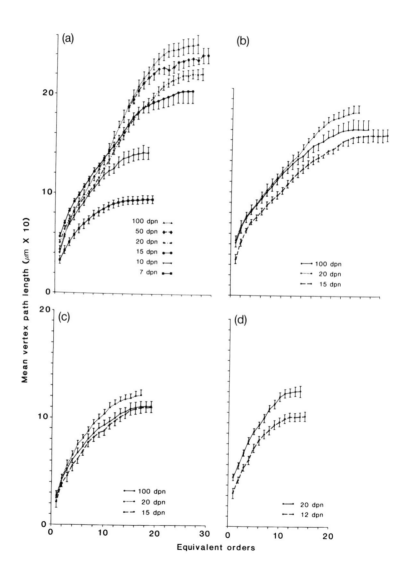

GROWTH OF THE PC TREE IN MUTANT MICE

PC trees of the reeler mouse

Examples of the two types of *rl* PC studied are shown in Fig. 24.2(b) and (d). Cortical *rl* PCs elaborate their dendrites in the superficial molecular layer, and deep *rl* PCs grow in the depths of the cerebellum, outside a normal cortical environment.

Cortical rl *PC trees*

In comparison to control PCs, 89 per cent of normal segment numbers are present by 15 dpn in cortical *rl* PCs, but this subsequently falls to 66 per cent of normal by 100 dpn [Fig. 24.3(b)]. At 15 dpn these cells have also elaborated 75 per cent of normal total dendritic length, which falls to 59 per cent by 100 dpn [Fig. 24.3(b)].

Mean terminal path length demonstrates that, as in normal animals, cortical *rl* cells attain their maximum mean V_p-V_r length by 20 dpn, but have 21–22 per cent shorter path lengths over all ages. There are regions of the trees with very regular inter-vertex path length increments, similar to those seen in control cells [Fig. 24.5(b)]. Interestingly, there is little increase between 20 and 100 dpn plots over most of the tree. As in the normal study, terminals are longer than segments at all ages and V_b terminals have the greatest length of all; by 100 dpn, V_b, V_a, and link segment lengths are respectively 5, 9, and 15 per cent below control values.

The distribution of segments is skewed towards the higher orders, especially marked at 15–20 dpn, and is followed by growth of the tree in the middle orders, but with no segment losses in the highest orders [Fig. 24.9(a)].

Fig. 24.5. (a) Graph of mean vertex path length per order at various ages in normal PCs. Vertex path length is the cumulative length from successive orders of vertices to the root-point of the network. An increasing number of orders are separated by regular inter-vertex increments with age. (b) Mean vertex path length in cortical *rl* PCs at each age. The root segment shows a 52 per cent elongation between 15 and 20 dpn beyond which it remains stable. There is no significant change in the plots at 20 and 100 dpn for most of their length. (c) Mean vertex path length per order at 15, 20, and 100 dpn in deep *rl* PCs. Note that there is no root segment extension during development; it remains approximately 28 μm long, which is similar to the length in 7 dpn normal and 12 dpn *wv* PCs. There is a slight increase in the inter-vertex increments between 15 and 20 dpn, but this decreases by 100 dpn. The 100 dpn plot is not significantly removed from either of those seen at 15 and 20 dpn. (d) Mean vertex path length per order in *wv* PCs. Root segment length shows a significant rise from $31\cdot8\pm5.4$ to $47\cdot5\pm3\cdot5$ μm, a 49 per cent increase. The gradient of both plots is similar, indicating similar inter-vertex increments for the major part of each network at each age. Error bars represent standard errors.

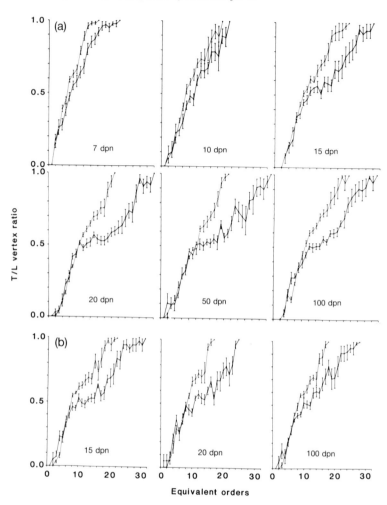

Fig. 24.6. (a) Observed (solid lines) and projected (dashed lines) terminal/link vertex ratios per order, at various ages in normal PCs. The projected T/L profile is based upon entirely random terminal branching and observed values are close throughout their entire length at 7 and 10 dpn. The hypothesis that growth is by random terminal branching at these early ages is also supported by the values of V_R. Beyond 10 dpn, however, the observed lines follow the projected ones up to order 10 and then depart, falling short for the remainder of their course. This discrepancy is maximal at 20 dpn, followed by convergence of the two plots by 100 dpn. (b) T/L vertex ratio profiles for cortical *rl* PCs at 15, 20, and 100 dpn. The observed line departs from the projected (dashed) line (based upon random terminal branching) at around order 8. This is earlier than in the normal study, possibly reflecting increased inhibition to branching caused by the restricted space available to cortically placed *rl* PCs. Beyond order 8, observed T/L vertex ratios are less than expected for a randomly grown network. Error bars represent standard errors.

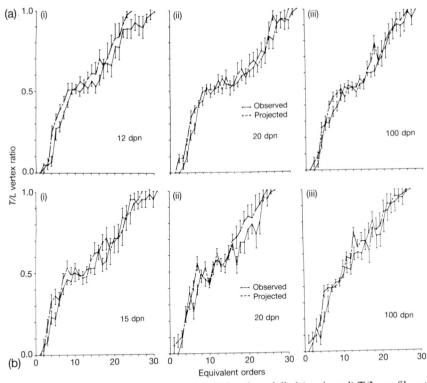

Fig. 24.7. (a) (i) Superimposition of observed and modelled (projected) T/L profiles at 12 dpn in normal PCs. This simulation, at an age between 7 and 20 dpn, demonstrates that the growth model used to generate the 20 dpn trees can also adequately simulate intermediate stages of growth. Observed and projected values of V_R are not significantly different from each other at 0.88 ± 0.04 and 0.84 ± 0.02, respectively. (ii) Superimposition of observed T/L profiles and the computer modelled values at 20 dpn. The model produces a plot which is not significantly removed from the observed values for the majority of its path. V_R for the model is not significantly different from the observed value at 0.82 ± 0.05 and 0.85 ± 0.03, respectively. (iii) Observed and modelled T/L profiles at 100 dpn. Computer generated trees are remodelled versions of networks produced by the model used to grow 20 dpn arbors. Observed V_R is not significantly different from the projected value, at 0.92 ± 0.02 and 0.89 ± 0.02, respectively. (b) Superimposition of observed and computer modelled (projected) T/L vertex ratios per order at 15, 20, and 100 dpn in cortical *rl* PCs. (i) At 15 dpn, trees were simulated by allowing random branching up to 45 terminals, after which growth was collimated into a front of decreasing depth. The front comprised the highest 6 orders and decreased to 5 orders after 65 terminals had been produced and, finally, to 4 orders beyond 115 terminals for the remainder of the tree. Terminals behind the growth front had a 10 per cent chance of branching. Observed and simulated V_R values are not significantly different at 0.86 ± 0.03 and 0.84 ± 0.03, respectively. (ii) Starting from the network produced above, remodelling was simulated, causing growth of terminals from orders 7–13 and resorptions above order 12. Observed and simulated V_R values are not significantly different at 0.87 ± 0.05 and 0.93 ± 0.04, respectively. (iii) Starting from the network in (i), remodelling was exactly as above, but branching of terminals was continued until trees 100 dpn in size were created. Observed and simulated V_R values are both 0.85 ± 0.03. Error bars represent standard errors.

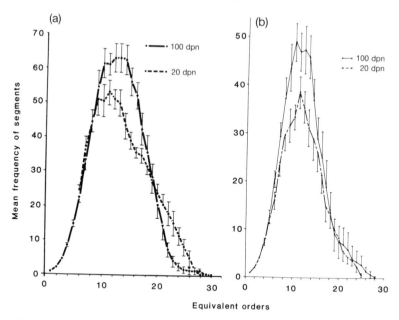

Fig. 24.8. (a) Superimposition of frequency of segments against orders at 20 and 100 dpn in normal PCs. This graph clearly demonstrates the region of segment elaboration between orders 8 and 18 and of segment erosion beyond order 20. (b) Superimposition of segment frequency plots of cortical *rl* PC trees at 20 and 100 dpn demonstrates segment elaboration over the mid-orders (7–14) of the network. There are no further segments eroded from the upper orders beyond 20 dpn. Error bars represent standard errors.

However, there is evidence for early loss of segments, by 20 dpn, in the highest orders, followed by attainment of the very narrow, peaked distribution of segments seen at 100 dpn [Fig. 24.8(b)].

The pattern of change of the T/L profile from 15–100 dpn [Fig. 24.6(b)] in cortical *rl* PCs is similar to that seen in normal PCs; i.e. low orders (1–8) appear to be established by random terminal growth. Beyond the 8th order, growth deviates from this pattern, the divergence becoming greater with time. Computer simulation of growth was similar to that used for normal animals, with random terminal branching restricted to specific regions of the expanding network. Figure 24.6(b) demonstrates that cortical *rl* PC T/L vertex ratios deviate from the projected profile earlier than in controls (order 8, rather than order 10). This effect was simulated by producing a more rapid onset of the restricted growth front in *rl* cells. At 15 dpn, the best fit of the observed data was obtained by allowing the formation of an initial tree of 45 terminals (the size of normal 7 dpn networks) entirely by random terminal branching. Following this, 90 per cent of branching was restricted to a front

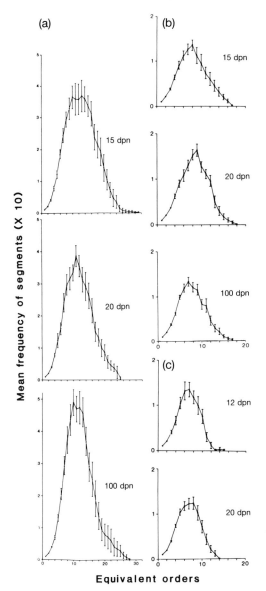

Fig. 24.9. (a) Frequency of segments against order at each age in cortical *rl* PCs. Segment losses occur in the higher orders (>16) between 15 and 20 dpn. (b) Mean frequency of segments per order at 15, 20, and 100 dpn in deep *rl* PCs. Segment distributions are similar at all ages, showing a slight skew towards the higher orders. The distribution in the proximal orders (<9) remains very stable, as it does in all PC types studied. (c) Mean frequency of segments per order at 12 and 20 dpn in *wv* PCs. These distributions display no significant alterations from 12 to 20 dpn. Error bars represent standard errors.

comprising the highest 4 orders, in a series of steps. Initially the front was 6 orders deep until 65 terminals had been produced, and then 5 orders deep up to 115 terminals, beyond which the 4 order front was established. The remaining 10 per cent of branching occurred behind the front [Fig. 24.7(b)].

By 20 dpn, the number of terminals in each tree has declined to 208.7 ± 15.3 from 246.2 ± 16.3 at 15 dpn. Segments are removed from the highest orders, with a slight increase in peak segment production in the middle orders around order 11 [Figs. 24.8(b) and 24.9(a)]. This was simulated by adding segments by random terminal branching across orders 7–13, with the probability of branching on a randomly chosen segment set at 0.3 at order 7, rising to 1.0 by order 9. Terminals were removed above order 12. The probability that a chosen terminal would be eroded started at 0.2 at order 12 and rose linearly to 1.0 by order 16. A total of 37 terminals were resorbed [Fig. 24.7(b)].

Beyond 20 dpn, the networks expand to 261.1 ± 22.4 terminals, the additional 52.4 segments growing in the middle orders. There is no further change to segment frequencies above order 15 [Fig. 24.8(b)]. This was simulated [Fig. 24.7(b)] by using the same model as that used to produce the changes from 15 to 20 dpn, but allowing the networks to expand to 100 dpn levels by random terminal branching over the growth zone from orders 7–13.

Deep rl *PCs*

There is a slight, significant ($p < 0.02$), increase in the mean number of segments between 15 and 20 dpn (108.0 ± 9.1 to 131.5 ± 6.7), succeeded by a decline to 13 per cent of the normal value (101.0 ± 7.6) at 100 dpn [Fig. 24.3(c)]. Mean total segment length shows an insignificant increase from 1014.5 ± 70.1 at 15 dpn to 1090.3 ± 84.0 at 100 dpn [Fig. 24.3(c)]. The mean terminal path lengths show no significant change between 15 and 100 dpn. Thus deep rl cells have attained their maximum V_p-V_r length of around 105 μm by 15–20 dpn (the same time as normal and cortical rl PCs), although this length is only 63 per cent of the normal and 81 per cent of the cortical rl PC values by 100 dpn. As in normal mice, terminals are longer than segments, and V_b terminals are longest overall. All three categories of arc are consistently longer than those of both cortical rl and control PCs at each age. There is no increase in mean root segment length during development of deep rl PCs. From 15 to 20 dpn there is a slight increase in inter-vertex lengths, but, from 20 to 100 dpn, the inter-vertex increments become just significantly decreased beyond order 10 [Fig. 24.5(c)], reflecting the decreased segment frequencies over the same regions of the networks despite increased mean V_a and V_b terminal lengths and slightly raised mean segment lengths of these mature trees. By 100 dpn, the percentage increase for V_b, V_a, and segment lengths compared with cortical and control values are 31, 23, and 34 per cent, and 19, 11, and 23 per cent, respectively. The distribution of mean segment frequencies is unlike that of control and cortical PCs in that there is no apparent erosions of upper-order segments and concomittant growth of the

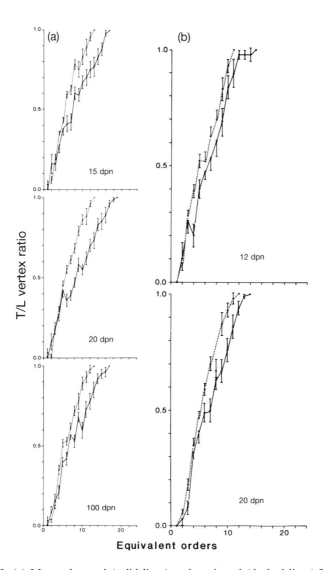

Fig. 24.10. (a) Mean observed (solid lines) and projected (dashed lines) T/L vertex ratios per order at 15, 20, and 100 dpn in deep *rl* PCs. Both projected and observed plots are similar in deep *rl* PCs, especially at 15 and 100 dpn. Deviation from the projected lines is greatest in the distal portion of these diminutive trees, at 20 dpn. (b) Mean observed (solid lines) and projected (dashed lines) T/L profiles against order at 12 and 20 dpn in *wv* trees. Both plots are very similar throughout their whole length at both ages, indicating that *wv* PCs could have grown entirely by random terminal branching. Error bars represent standard errors.

middle orders of the networks; rather segment frequencies over many orders fall during the period from 20 to 100 dpn [Fig. 24.9(b)]. T/L profiles are close to the projected values based upon random terminal growth. The discrepancy between the plots is greatest at 20 dpn [Fig. 24.10(a)].

Wv PC dendritic trees

Mean segment number [Fig. 24.3(d)] is stable at $88·0 \pm 7·0$ [12 per cent of normal at 20 dpn; Fig. 24.3(a)] and mean total segment length shows a slight, but insignificant, increase from $877·0 \pm 58·4$ μm at 12 dpn to $917·3 \pm 67·9$ μm at 20 dpn [Fig. 24.3(d)]. Mean terminal path length, however, rises from $94·7 \pm 4·2$ μm to $113·3 \pm 3·7$ μm over the same period. V_b are the longest of all arcs, followed by V_a and link arcs. While link segments and V_a terminals show no significant change, V_b terminals show a slight, significant ($p < 0·005$) decrease in length. wv arcs are longer, at 20 dpn, than those of the other cell groups studied. At 12 dpn, wv terminals are longer than deep rl PC terminals at 15 dpn, and link arcs are the same length. V_r segment length rises from $31·8 \pm 5·4$ μm to $47·5 \pm 3·5$ μm, an increase in growth of about 49 percent. A large percentage increase in root segment length of about the same magnitude was seen in both normal and cortical rl PCs during early development [Fig. 24.5(a,b,d)]. The gradient of the vertex path length plot is greater than that of the deep rl PCs, reflecting a greater number of longer arcs in wv cells at each age [Fig. 24.5(d)]. The frequency distribution of segments of different order is stable over the period from 12–20 dpn [Fig. 24.9(c)]. The T/L profiles for wv, like those of the deep rl trees, at both 12 and 20 dpn [Fig. 24.10(b)] are close to those calculated on the basis of random terminal growth.

DISCUSSION

Elongation of V_a and V_b terminal segments is probably achieved by persistent growth cone activity, whilst link segment elongation may be effected by interstitial insertion of membrane (Pfenninger and Bunge 1974; Rees, Bunge, and Bunge 1976; Falls and Gobel 1979). The root segment may also increase in length by translocation of the PC nucleus away from the first node (Hendelman and Aggerwal 1980). Lengthening of the root segment occurs in PCs which have attained a definitive polarity with basket cell (BC) invest-ments (Altman 1972c) and climbing fibre (CF) innervation. Increases appear to be independent of parallel fibre (PF) interactions since proximal extensions occur in weaver mutant animals where PFs are totally absent (Bradley and Berry 1978) and in normally positioned reeler PCs (Mariani, Crepel, Mikoshiba, Changeux, and Sotelo 1977) in which PFs are depleted. Similar extension is not seen in culture (Calvet, Calvet, Camacho-Garcia, and Eude 1983) and in the non-polar deep rl PCs. This implies that the processes involved in the attainment of polarity and the initial formation of a major dendritic trunk and its subsequent elongation are interrelated in as yet unknown ways. The reduced probability of V_b terminal segment branching may be related to a reduced interaction with PFs as V_b segments are left behind the advancing growth front of V_a terminals.

Our observation that vertices of the same equivalent order are a similar distance from the root vertex provides support for Rall's (1959) hypothesis that dendrites conduct as simple cables, since a given vertex path length may be considered as an equivalent cylinder, providing the diameters of successive dendritic branch lengths scale in a simple way with the sum of the 3/2 power of all branch diameters (a relationship supported by Lux, Shubert, and Kreutzberg 1970 from *in vivo* measurements of spinal motoneurons). Thus it is likely that vertices with the same path length are separated from the soma by the same electrotonic distance (Rall 1962, 1964, 1970). Such cable properties may be optimized for orthodromic conduction in a branched structure since most of the current entry during synaptic conductance charges the capacitance of the dendritic membrane. Since branching displaces most of the dendritic membrane distally, more charge is stored in the distal tree which generates a steep gradient of electrotonic potential. However, PC dendrites do not behave in an entirely passive cable manner. PC dendritic spines are able to modulate dendritic electrical conductance properties. Recordings *in vivo* (Llinas, Nicholson, and Precht 1969; Pellionisz and Llinas 1977) and spiny dendrite models (Pongracz 1985) show that spines can effectively prevent the antidromic spread of potential throughout the network. The variable diameter of the spine necks amplifies and/or attenuates post synaptic activity (Crick 1982; Perkel 1983; Pongracz 1985). Coupling this with a calcium spike-generating capability in the CF innervated distal tree, and a sodium spike-generating capability in the CF innervated proximal tree (Llinas and Sugimori 1980; Ito and Simpson 1971), the overall integrative capacity of the PC dendritic tree is immense.

The T/L profiles of the normal PC tree shows that, within the first 10 orders, branching patterns follow those of random growth but deviate from this pattern beyond the 10th order. The model that produced the best fit for dendritic growth, up to 20 dpn, is essentially one of random terminal branching, but T/L profiles and V_R (Sadler and Berry 1984) indicate that the tree could not have arisen entirely by random terminal branching. Thus the model incorporates an initial period of random terminal growth establishing a tree of the same size as observed at this early stage. The next phase simulates branching within a collimated front which ascends towards the pial surface. During this period, branching is inhibited both behind the active front, and laterally where adjacent trees meet. Since no spatial information is contained within our computer growth program, border effects and the evolution of a growth front are simulated by reducing the number of orders over which branching occurs in steps from 10 orders, after 50 terminals have been grown, to the highest 4 orders beyond 160 terminals. 90 per cent of branching is concentrated within the frontal zone and 10 per cent throughout the remainder of the network.

This simple model accurately matches the terminal proportions at 20 dpn (and at earlier stages), creating networks in which mean V_R is not significantly different at $0·82 \pm 0·05$ to the observed value of $0·85 \pm 0·03$. Thus, before 20 dpn, each neuron elaborates its dendritic tree to fully occupy its maximum dendritic area by a process of local stochastic interactions between dendrites and newly formed PFs. Beyond 20 dpn, remodelling takes place, the essential features of which are resorption of high-ordered segments and growth of new segments in the middle orders (Sadler and Berry 1984). Our simulation program shows that remodelling could have occurred by purely random resorptions and random new growth of segments, and that the two events probably overlap spatially over the middle orders.

The explanation for remodelling may not be sought in changes in the granule cell (GC)/PC ratio, which is stable beyond 20 dpn (Sadler and Berry 1984), but could be related to an increase in length of subpial PFs (Lauder 1978, Mugnaini 1983) or to PF branching (Chen and Hillman 1982a, 1982b). These events combine to provide modulations in pre-synaptic membrane which might lead to a reorganization of the PC dendritic tree.

It has been established that neurons alter their morphology during development following environmental manipulations such as deafferentation (Jones and Thomas 1962; Sotelo, Hillman, Zamora, and Llinas 1975; Bradley and Berry 1976a; Berry and Bradley 1976c) and changes in the pattern of stimulation (Holloway 1966; Coleman and Riesen 1968; Hubel and Weisel 1970; Volkmar and Greenough 1972; Borges and Berry 1976; Spinelli, Jensen, and Viana di Prisco 1980; Meininger and Baudrimont 1981). Adult plasticity has also been demonstrated in response to environmental enrichment (Uylings, Kuypers, Diamond, and Veltman 1978) and maze training (Greenough, Juraska, and Volkman 1979). Exercise during late post-natal life has been shown to increase the size of mouse PC dendritic trees (Pysh and Weiss 1979), and long-term electrical stimulation has produced dendritic outgrowth in adult cat cortical cells (Rutledge, Wright and Duncan 1974).

Recently it has been possible to study dendrites by repeated imaging of the same neuron *in vivo* (Purves and Hadley 1985; Purves, Hadley, and Voyvodic 1986; Stirling 1986). This has shown that neuronal networks are far more dynamic structures than previously suspected and may undergo a perpetual process of resorption, regrowth, and re-orientation. This study, in common with others, has found that it is the last formed, distal portion of the network which has the greatest potential for change (Berry, Bradley, and Borges 1978; Weiss and Pysh 1978; Dardennes, Jarreau, and Meininger 1984; Leuba and Garey 1984). Proximally, the network remains numerically stable (Berry and Bradley 1976b; Paldino and Purpura 1979, 1979b; Parnavelas and Uylings 1980). Altman (1982) maintains that the PFs of the most superficial region of the molecular layer (ML), which also become the longest (Lauder 1978), have parent GCs with pontine mossy fibre (MF) afferents, whereas GCs supplying shorter PFs in the lower ML have contacts with MFs of spinal origin. The regional changes in the dendritic trees may be related to the phylogenetic age of the two MF systems. The phylogenetically older spinal afferents project to the stable proximal portion of PC dendritic trees, whilst the newer pontine projection is able to effect changes in the network and consequently alter its integrative capacity, thus exerting cerebral modulation of spinal input to cerebellar circuitry. The PC dendritic tree appears to be established largely by stochastic interactions between dendritic growth cone filopodia and PFs at a time when the parent GCs have probably not received afferents (Altman 1972*b*). Remodelling occurs in the post-weaning period when motor skills are improving and refining. It seems reasonable to assume that once meaningful input converges upon the PF/PC system, the PC dendritic network should adapt itself accordingly, in order to produce an appropriately tuned functional network.

Cortical *rl* PC trees are miniature versions of the normal. Their short segment lengths are not correlated with an increased probability of branching since the frequency of V_t is 4 per cent (5–6 per cent in normals) and it is unlikely that the density of PF stacking is greater than normal. The more likely explanation for the stunting of cortical *rl* PC trees is that dendrites elongate at a slower rate than normal. Thus, in the period 20–100 dpn, segment lengths increase by 11 per cent whereas in the normal an increase of 17–18 per cent occurs.

The attainment of polarity by the formation of the root segment is associated with BC investment (Altman 1973; Mariani *et al.* 1977; Anderson and Stromberg 1977). BC *pinceux* can be indentified around both cortical *rl* PCs and those PCs which are embedded in the granular layer (GL). However, BC axons do not penetrate to the central cerebellar mass (Mariani *et al.* 1977) and no root segment extension occurs on deep *rl* PCs. Furthermore, wv cells, which display V_r segment growth, are in a cortical position and have a good supply of BC fibres ramifying about them (Sotelo 1975).

T/L profiles of cortical *rl* PC trees demonstrate a deviation from random terminal growth at 8 orders rather than at 10 orders as in normal PCs. This probably reflects increased border interaction between adjacent trees constraining the available space of each dendritic field.

Remodelling in cortical *rl* PCs begins earlier than in normal trees and involves absorption of high-ordered segments and new growth in the middle orders. Computer modelling of growth shows that cortical *rl* PC trees probably grow in a similar fashion to normal but saturate the confined space quicker by random terminal growth. Remodelling could also be simulated using the same criteria as adopted for the normal tree. Cortical *rl* PCs receive a normal distribution of afferents (Mariani *et al.* 1977; Goffinet, So, Yamamoto, Edwards, and Caviness 1984), are electrophysiologically normal

(Mariani *et al.* 1977; Dupont, Gardette, and Crepel 1983), and, from this quantitative study, develop a normal, but cramped, dendritic tree. Both the metrical and topological results demonstrate differences between cortical *rl* and control trees that are predictable within the framework of the filopodial attachment hypothesis, operating within a restricted dendritic field area.

Despite forshortening errors in the extensively non-planar deep *rl* and *wv* PC trees, both are very similar in size and cortical dimensions. They elaborate a similar number of segments as cortical PCs at 7 dpn; *wv* cells add no more segments thereafter, although deep rl PCs do branch until 15–20 dpn but regress thereafter. In both cell types, all segment lengths are longer than normal. The subcortical position of deep *rl* PCs places them in the path of afferent fibres that run on into the cortex, but removes them from all PFs (Mariani *et al.* 1977). Besides the normal distribution of MFs and CFs to the *GL* and to cortical *rl* PCs (Goffinet *et al.* 1984; Mikoshiba, Nagaike, Kohsaka, Takamatsu, Aoki, and Tsukada 1984), deep *rl* PCs attract an abundance of hererotopic spinal MFs (Wilson, Sotelo, and Caviness 1981; Goffinet *et al.* 1984; Mikoshiba *et al.* 1984), as well as an increased density of CFs (Mariani *et al.* 1977; Caviness and Rakic 1978; Dupont *et al.* 1983) which could initiate dendritic branching, but without subsequent synapse formation, growth is short-lived and opportunistic branching is resorbed.

These findings support the contention that since both *wv* and deep *rl* PCs develop without PFs (Sotelo 1975; Mariani *et al.* 1977), there is no secondary induction of dendritic branching (Berry *et al.* 1978, 1981; Bradley and Berry 1978, 1979). Accordingly, no new segments are added and thus the dendritic arbor may grow only by interstitial extension of existing segments. Initially, primary induction causes the production of a rudimentary dendritic tree seen at 7 dpn, before PF deposition in normal PCs (Sievers, Berry, and Baumgarten 1981). Normally, adhesive interaction, which controls branching frequency and directs PC dendritic growth, is followed by a wave of PF/PC synaptogenesis (Larramendi 1969; Mugnaini 1969; Altman 1972*a*), even if PF numbers are greatly reduced (Berry *et al* 1980*a*, 1980*b*, 1980*c*), which stabilizes segments. If synapses are removed from adult PC dendritic trees by lesioning of PFs, there is a reorganization of the arbor resulting in a loss of spines and terminal dendrites (Mouren-Mathieu and Colonnier 1969; Chen and Hillman 1982*a*, 1982*b*). However, PC segment losses are not incurred by adult CF lesions, but, instead, the proximal segments vacated by CFs become spiny and contacted by PFs (Sotelo *et al.* 1975; Bradley and Berry 1976*b*). Thus maintenance of the spiny distal PC dendritic tree is probably dependent upon continuity of appropriate synaptic contacts. This lends further support to the idea, stated above, that initial control of branching, and subsequent synaptogenesis and branch retention, are independent.

Heterologous synapses between MFs and deep *rl* PC dendritic spines are more frequent (Wilson *et al.* 1981; Goffinet *et al.* 1984) than in *wv* cells (Sotelo 1975; Rakic 1976; Caviness and Rakic 1978), and CF synapses are more extensive than normal, both in number (Mariani *et al.* 1977; Mariani 1982; Dupont *et al.* 1983) and also in extent, spreading onto the normally PF-contacted large dendritic spines (Mariani *et al.* 1977; Wilson *et al.* 1981; Goffinet *et al.* 1984). However, the majority of deep *rl* PC dendritic spines are unattached and remain so throughout development (Rakic 1976; Mariani *et al.* 1977; Caviness and Rakic 1978; Landis and Landis 1978).

wv PCs are normally positioned within the cerebellar cortex. They are multiply CF innervated (Crepel and Mariani 1975; Crepel, Mariani, and Delhaye-Bouchaud 1976; Puro and Woodward 1977; Mariani 1982), with CFs heterotopically synapsing on large dendritic spines, normally supplied by PFs (Sotelo 1975; Landis and Reese 1977; Landis and Landis 1978). Rare heterologous MF axospinous synapses are found (Sotelo 1975; Landis and Reese 1977; Caviness and Rakic 1978). *wv* PCs do not have a similar abundance of surrounding afferent fibres to trigger further branching as do deep *rl* PCs. Thus *wv* dendrites may be able to extend more freely (Rakic and Sidman 1973*a*, 1973*b*) without possible contact inhibitory forces acting to constrain their growth.

Topological parameters for both *wv* and deep *rl* PCs and also for 7 dpn normal trees indicate that all three could have arisen by random terminal branching, although the factors which initiate and control this phase of dendritic growth are unknown. Occasional PFs have been noted in the immediate perinatal period (Altman 1972*b*), and synapses between PC apical sprouts and fibres of unknown origin have been observed at embryonic stage 19 (E19) in rat cerebella (West and del Cerro 1976). These very early contacts may be monoaminergic (MA) since these are the first extrinsic fibres to invade the cerebellum, at E16–17 in the rat (Yamamoto, Ishikawa, and Tanaka 1977; Sievers, Kleman, Jenner, Baumgarten, and Berry 1980) and ultimately synapsing with PC dendrites and somata (Bloom, Hoffer, and Siggins 1971; Lindvall and Bjorklund 1978). Serotoninergic (5-HT) fibres are also distributed to GL and ML and, as collaterals, to the deep cerebellar nuclei (Chan-Palay 1977). Both types of fibre also produce T-shaped axons which run in the ML as PFs (Mugnaini and Dahl 1975; Yamamoto *et al.* 1977; Chan-Palay 1977), although such 5-HT PFs do not synapse with PC dendrites (Chan-Palay 1977). MA fibres throughout the cerebellum have many unattached varicosities along their length. Release of MA from these varicosities could act as a neurohumour (Lauder and Krebs 1976; Chan-Palay 1977). The early appearance of MA fibres in many brain regions suggests a role in the regulation of proliferation, migration, and differentiation of neuronal systems (Maeda, Tohyama, and Shimizu 1974; Lauder and Krebs 1976; Schumpf, Shoemaker, and Bloom 1977; Pettigrew and Kasamatsu 1978; Berry *et al.* 1978, 1980*a*, 1980*b*, 1980*c*). However, direct testing of this hypothesis has not implicated MA fibres in postnatal cerebellar development (Berry *et al.* 1980*a*, 1980*b*, 1980*c*; Sievers *et al.* 1981), despite results to the contrary (Maeda *et al.* 1974; Lauder and Krebs 1976). However, since both *wv* and *rl* cerebella have a qualitatively normal complement of MA afferents (Siggins, Hoffer, and Bloom 1971; Landis and Bloom 1975; Landis, Shoemaker, Schlumpf, and Bloom 1975), it is reasonable to suppose that MA interactions could establish the dendritic trees seen in these animals. The absence of PFs converging on wv and deep *rl* PCs prevents the transition to PF-dependent branching in these cells.

CONCLUSIONS

Our more recent findings of growth and remodelling of normal, *rl* and *wv* PC dendritic trees has led to new insights into the factors shaping dendritic fields. Following induction (Berry *et al.* 1980*a*, 1980*b*, 1980*c*), elongation of one major apical dendrite proceeds at the terminally located growth cone. Branching is also a function of the growth cones and is probably effected by adhesion of dendritic growth cone filopodia to specific sites in the primitive neuropil. Growth over the inductive phase establishes a rudimentary tree with a random terminal pattern of dendritic branching which is probably reflected in the *wv*, deep *rl*, and normal 7 dpn trees. At this stage, PFs induce normal and cortical *rl* cells to embark on a second phase of growth in which the rate of advancement of growth cones through the neuropil is constant throughout this period of development. *wv* and deep *rl* dendritic growth is arrested since no PFs contact the trees of these mutant cells. Adhesive interaction between PFs and dendritic growth cones of cortical *rl* and normal trees establishes a random terminal branching pattern. Branching frequency and segment lengths are directly correlated to the number of adhesive contacts made. The topology of the trees deviates from a random terminal pattern as the boundaries of the field are established by inhibitory interactions between adjacent trees. Similarly, constraints to growth also occur within the tree so that dendrites do not overlap. Thus a growth front is established over the highest ordered terminals and is directed towards the subpial part of the ML in which new PFs are being deposited. The secondary growth phase terminates at about 20 dpn, when PF deposition ceases and when dendritic growth cones have reached the pial surface. The third, or remodelling, phase of dendritic field growth then begins and has been monitored until 100 dpn. This period is characterized by the random removal of high-ordered terminal segments from the tree and the random growth and branching of middle-ordered segments. Spatially, the reorganization of the dendritic tree occurs in the subpial area of the ML where PFs of corticopontine origin tend to continue growing and may organize regrowth according to functional criteria.

REFERENCES

Altman, J. (1972*a*). Postnatal development of the cerebellar cortex in the rat. II. Phases in the maturation of the Purkinje cell and of the molecular layer. *J. Comp. Neurol.* **145**, pp. 399–464.

Altman, J. (1972*b*). Postnatal development of the cerebellar cortex in the rat. III. Maturation of the components of the granular layer. *J. Comp. Neurol.* **145**, pp. 464–514.

Altman, J. (1973). Experimental reorganisation of the cerebellar cortex. III. Regeneration of the external granular layer and granule cell ectopia. *J. Comp. Neurol.* **149**, pp. 153–80.

Altman, J. (1982). Morphological development of the rat cerebellum and some of its mechanisms. In *The cerebellum: new vistas* (eds. S. L. Palay and V. Chan-Palay), pp. 8–49. Springer-Verlag, Berlin.

Anderson, W. J. and Stromberg, W. M. (1977). Effects of low-level X-irradiation on cat cerebella at different post-natal intervals. III. Changes in the morphology of interneurons in the molecular layer, *J. Comp. Neurol.* **171**, pp.51–64.

Berry, M. (1976). Topological analysis of dendritic trees. *Proc. Fourth Int. Cong. Stereol.* pp. 49–54.

Berry, M. and Bradley, P. (1976*a*). The application of network analysis to the study of branching patterns of large dendritic fields. *Brain Res.* **109**, pp. 111–32.

Berry, M. and Bradley, P. (1976*b*). The growth of the dendritic trees of Purkinje cells in the cerebellum of the rat. *Brain Res.* **112**, pp. 1–35.

Berry, M. and Bradley, P. (1976*c*). The growth of the dendritic trees of Purkinje cells in irradiated agranular cerebellar cortex, *Brain Res.* **116**, pp. 361–87.

Berry, M. and Flinn, R. M. (1984). Vertex analysis of Purkinje cell dendritic trees in the cerebellum of the rat. *Proc. R. Soc. Lond. B.* **221**, pp. 321–48.

Berry, M. and Pymm, D. (1981). Analysis of neural networks. In *Neural communication and control* (ed. J. Szekely), pp. 155–69. Akademiai Kiado, Budapest.

Berry, M., Bradley, P., and Borges, S. (1978). Environmental and genetic determinants of connectivity in the central nervous system—an approach through dendritic field analysis. *Progr. Brain Res.* **48**, pp. 113–146.

Berry, M., McConnell, P., and Sievers, J. (1980*a*). Dendritic growth and the control of neuronal form. In *Current topics in developmental biology* (eds. R. K. Hunt and A. A. Moscona), pp. 67–101. Academic Press, New York.

Berry, M., Sadler, M., and Flinn, R. M. (1986). Vertex analysis of neural tree structures containing trichotomous nodes. *J. Neurosci Meth.* **18**, pp. 167–74.

Berry, M., Sievers, J., and Baumgarten, H. G. (1980*b*). The influence of afferent fibres on the development of the cerebellum. In *A multidisciplinary approach to brain development* (eds. C. di Benedetta, R. Balasz, G. Gambos, and G. Porcellati), pp. 91–106. North-Holland Biomedical Press, Amsterdam).

Berry, M., Sievers, J., and Baumgarten, H. G. (1980*c*). Adaptation of the cerebellum to deafferentation. *Prog. Brain Res.* **53**, pp. 65–92.

Berry, M., Anderson, E. M., Hollingworth, T., and Flinn, R. M. (1972*a*). A computer technique for the estimation of the absolute three dimensional array of basal dendritic fields using data from projected histological sections. *J. Microsc.* **95**, pp. 257–67.

Berry, M., Hollingworth, T., Anderson, E. M., and Flinn, R. M. (1975). Application of network analysis to the study of the branching patterns of dendritic fields. *Adv. Neurol.* **12**, pp. 217–45.

Berry, M., Hollingworth, T., Flinn, R. M., and Anderson, E. M (1972*b*). Dendritic field analysis—a reappraisal. *T.-I.-T. J. Life Sci.* **2**, pp. 129–40.

Berry, M., McConnell, P., Sievers, J., Price, S., and Anwar, A . (1981). Factors influencing the growth of cerebellar neural networks. *Bibl. Anat.* **19**, pp. 1–51.

Blackstad, T. W. (1970). Electron microscopy of Golgi preparations for the study of neuronal relations. In *Contemporary research methods in neuroanatomy* (eds. W. J. H. Nauta and S. O. E. Ebbesson), pp. 186–217. Springer-Verlag, Berlin.

Bloom, F. E., Hoffer, B. J., and Siggins, G. R. (1971). Studies on norepinephrine-containing afferents to Purkinje cells of rat cerebellum. I. Localisation of the fibres and their synapses. *Brain Res.* **25,** pp. 501–21.

Borges, S. and Berry, M. (1976). Preferential orientation of stellate cell dendrites in the visual cortex of the dark reared rat. *Brain Res.* **112,** pp. 114–47.

Bradley, P. M. and Berry, M. (1976*a*). The effects of reduced climbing and parallel fibre input on Purkinje cell dendritic growth, *Brain Res.* **109,** pp. 133–51.

Bradley, P. M. and Berry, M. (1976*b*). Quantitative effects of climbing fibre deafferentation on the adult Purkinje cell dendritic tree. *Brain Res.* **112,** pp. 133–40.

Bradley, P. and Berry, M. (1978). The Purkinje cell dendritic tree in mutant mouse cerebellum. A quantitative Golgi study of weaver and staggerer mice. *Brain Res.* **142,** pp. 135–41.

Bradley, P. and Berry, M. (1979). Effects of thiophen on the Purkinje cell dendritic tree: a quantitative Golgi study. *Neuropathol. Appl. Neurobiol.* **5,** pp. 9–16.

Caddy, K. W. T., Patterson, D. L. and Biscoe, T. J. (1982). Use of the UCHT1 monoclonal antibody to explore mouse mutants and development. *Nature* **300,** pp. 441–3.

Calvet, M. -C., Calvet, J., Camacho-Garcia, R., and Eude, D. (1983). The dendritic tree of Purkinje cells: a computer assisted analysis of HRP labelled neurons in organotypic cultures of kitten cerebellum. *Brain Res.* **280,** pp. 199–215.

Caviness, V. S., Jr. and Rakic, P. (1978). Mechanisms of cortical development: a view from mutations in mice. *Ann. Rev. Neurosci.* **1,** pp. 297–326.

Chan-Palay, V. (1977). Serotonin afferents from raphe nuclei to the cerebellum. *Exp. Brain Res. Suppl.* **1,** pp. 20–5.

Chen, S. and Hillman, D. E. (1982*a*). Plasticity of the parallel fibre-Purkinje cell synapse by spine takeover and new formation in the adult rat. *Brain Res.* **240,** pp. 205–20.

Chen, S. and Hillman, D. E. (1982*b*). Marked reorganisation of Purkinje cell dendrites and spines in adult rat following vacating of synapses due to deafferentation. *Brain Res.* **245,** pp. 131–5.

Coleman, P. D. and Riesen, A. H. (1968). Environmental effects on cortical dendritic fields. I. Rearing in the dark. *J. Anat.* **102,** pp. 363–74.

Crepel, F. and Mariani, J. (1975). Anatomical, physiological and biochemical studies of the cerebellum from mutant mice. I. Electrophsiological analysis of cerebellar cortical neurons in the staggerer mouse. *Brain Res.* **98,** pp. 135–47.

Crepel, F., Mariani, J., and Delhaye-Bouchaud, N. (1976). Evidence for a multiple innervation of Purkinje cells by climbing fibres in the immature rat cerebellum. *J. Neurobiol.* **7,** pp. 567–78.

Crick, F. (1982). Do dendritic spines twitch? *Trends Neurosci.* **5,** pp. 44–6.

Dardennes, R., Jarreau, P. H., and Meininger, V. (1984). A quantitative Golgi analysis of postnatal maturation of dendrites in the central nucleus of the inferior colliculus of the rat. *Dev. Brain Res.* **16,** pp. 159–69.

De Camilli, P., Miller, P. E., Levitt, P., Walter, V., and Greengard, P. (1984). Anatomy of cerebellar Purkinje cells in the rat determined by a specific immunohistochemical marker. *Neuroscience* **11,** pp. 761–817.

Dupont, J. -L., Gardette, R., and Crepel, F. (1983). Biochemical properties of cerebellar Pukinje cells in reeler mutant mice. *Brain Res.* **274**, pp. 350–3.

Eayrs, J. T. (1955). The cerebral cortex of normal and hypothyroid rats. *Acta. Anat. (Basel)* **25**, pp. 160–83.

Falls, W. and Gobel, S. (1979). Golgi and EM studies of the formation of dendritic and axonal arbors: the interneurons of the *substantia gelatinosa* of Rolando in newborn kittens. *J. Comp. Neurol.* **187**, pp. 1–18.

Garvey, C. F., Young, J. H., Coleman, P. D., and Simon, W. (1973). Automated three-dimensional dendritic tracking system. *Electroenceph. Clin. Neurophysiol.* **35**, pp. 199–204.

Glaser, E. M. and van der Loos, H. (1965). A semi-automatic computer microscope for the analysis of neuronal morphology. *IEEE Trans. Biomed. Eng.* **12**, pp. 22–31.

Glaser, E. M., van der Loos, H., and Gissler, M. (1979). Tangential orientation and spatial order in dendrites of cat auditory cortex: a computer microscope study of Golgi-impregnated material. *Exp. Brain Res.* **36**, pp. 411–31.

Goffinet, A. M., So, K. -F., Yamamoto, M., Edwards, M., and Caviness, V. S., Jr. (1984). Architectonic and hodological organisation of the cerebellum in reeler mutant mice. *Dev. Brain Res* **16**, pp. 263–76.

Gough, N. G. (1968). A method for the accurate location and orientation of stuctures studied by the use of serial microscopical sections. *J. Microsc.* **88**, pp. 291–300.

Greenlee, J. E. and Brashear, H. R. (1983). Antibodies to cerebellar Purkinje cells in patients with paraneoplastic cerebellar degeneration and ovarian carcinoma. *Ann. Neurol.* **14**, pp. 609–13.

Greenough, W. T., Juraska, J. M., and Volkmar, F. R. (1979). Maze training effects on dendritic branching in occipital cortex of adult rats. *Behav. Neural. Biol.* **26**, pp. 287–97.

Hendelman, W. J. and Aggerwal, A. S. (1980). The Purkinje neuron: I. A Golgi study of its development in the mouse and in culture. *J. Comp. Neurol.* **193**, pp. 1063–79.

Hollingworth, T. and Berry, M. (1975). Network analysis of dendritic fields of pyramidal cells in neocortex and Purkinje cells in the cerebellum of the rat. *Phil. Trans. R. Soc. Lond. B.* **270**, pp. 227–64.

Holloway, R. L., Jr. (1966). Dendritic branching—some preliminary results of training and complexity in rat visual cortex. *Brain Res.* **2**, pp. 393–96.

Hubel, D. H. and Wiesel, T. N. (1970). The period of susceptibility to the physiological effects of unilateral eye closure in kittens. *J. Physiol. (Lond.)* **206**, pp. 419–36.

Ito, M. and Simpson, J. I. (1971). Discharges in Purkinje cell axons during climbing fibre activation. *Brain Res.* **31**, pp. 215–19.

Jones, W. H. and Thomas, D. B. (1962). Changes in the dendritic organisation of neurons in the cerebral cortex following deafferentation. *J. Anat.* **96**, pp. 375–81.

Kiernan, J. A. and Berry, M. (1975). Neuroanatomical methods. In *Methods in brain research* (ed. P. B. Bradley), pp. 1–75. John Wiley, Chichester.

Landis, D. M. D. and Landis, S. C. (1978) Several mutations in mice that affect the cerebellum. *Adv. Neurol.* **21**, pp. 85–105.

Landis, D. M. D. and Reese, T. S. (1977). Structure of the Purkinje cell membrane in staggerer and weaver mutant mice. *J. Comp. Neurol.* **171**, pp. 247–60.

Landis, S. C. and Bloom, F. E. (1975). Ultrastructural identification of noradrenergic boutons in mutant and normal mouse cerebellar cortex. *Brain Res.* **96**, pp. 299–305.

Landis, S. C., Shoemaker, W. J., Schlumpf, M., and Bloom, F. E. (1975).

Catecholamines in mutant mouse cerebellum: fluorescence microscopic and chemical studies. *Brain Res.* **93**, pp. 253–66.

Larramendi, L. M. H. (1969). Analysis of synaptogenesis in the cerebellum of the mouse. In *Neurobiology of cerebellar evolution and development* (ed. R. Llinas), pp. 801–43. American Medical Association, Chicago, IL.

Lauder, J. M. (1978). Effects of early hypo and hyperthyroidism on development of rat cerebellar cortex. IV. The parallel fibres. *Brain Res.* **142**, pp. 25–39.

Lauder, J. M. and Krebs, H. (1976). Effects of p-chlorophenylalanine on time of neuronal origin in the rat. *Brain Res.* **107**, pp. 638–44.

Leuba, G. and Garey, L. J. (1984). Development of dendritic patterns in the lateral geniculate nucleus of monkey: a quantitative Golgi study. *Dev. Brain Res.* **16**, pp. 285–99.

Levinthal, C. and Ware, R. (1972). Three dimensional reconstruction from serial sections. *Nature* **236**, pp. 207–10.

Ley, K., Pries, A. R., and Gaehtgens, P. (1986). Topological structure of rat mesenteric microvessel networks. *Microvasc. Res.* **32**, pp. 315–32.

Lindsay, R. D. and Scheibel, A. B. (1976). Quantitative analysis of dendritic branching pattern of granular cells from human dentate gyrus. *Exp. Neurol.* **52**, pp. 295–310.

Lindsay, R. D. and Scheibel, S. B. (1981). Quantitative analysis of dendritic branching pattern of granule cells from adult rat dentate gyrus. *Exp. Neurol.* **73**, pp. 286–97.

Lindvall, O. and Björklund, A. (1978). Organization of catecholamine neurons in the rat central nervous system. In *Handbook of psychopharmacology, vol. 9* (eds. L. L. Iversen, S. D. Iversen, and S. H. Snyder), pp. 139–231. Plenum Press, New York.

Llinas, R. and Sugimori, M. (1980). Electrophysiological properties of *in vitro* Purkinje cell dendrites in mammalian cerebellar slices. *J. Physiol.* **305**, pp. 197–213.

Llinas, R., Nicholson, C., and Precht, W. (1969). Preferred centripetal conduction of dendritic spikes in alligator Purkinje cells. *Science* **163**, pp. 184–7.

Lux, H. D., Shubert, P., and Kreutzberg, G. W. (1970). Direct matching of morphological and electrophysiological data in cat spinal motoneurons. In *Excitatory synaptic mechanisms* (eds. P. Anderson and J. K. S. Jansen), pp. 189–98. Scandinavian University Books, Oslo.

Maeda, T., Tohyama, M., and Shimizu, N. (1974). Modification of postnatal development of neocortex in rat brain with experimental deprivation of locus coeruleus. *Brain Res.* **70**, pp. 515–20.

Mannen, H. (1968). Neuronal stereophotogrammetry. *Med. Biol. Illus.* **18**, pp. 96–102.

Mariani, J. (1982). Extent of multiple innervation of Purkinje cells by climbing fibres in the olivocerebellar system of weaver, reeler and staggerer mutant mice. *J. Neurobiol.* **13**, pp. 119–26.

Mariani, J., Crepel, F., Mikoshiba, K., Changeux, J. P., and Sotelo, C. (1977). Anatomical, physiological and biochemical studies of the cerebellum from reeler mutant mouse. *Phil. Trans. R. Soc. Lond. B.* **281**, pp. 1–28.

Meininger, V. and Baudrimont, M. (1981). Postnatal modifications of the dendritic tree of cells in the inferior colliculus of the cat. A quantitative Golgi analysis. *J. Comp. Neurol.* **200**, pp. 339–55.

Mikoshiba, K., Nagaike, K., Kohsaka, K., Takamatsu, K., Aoki, E., and Tsukada, Y. (1984). Developmental studies on the cerebellum from reeler mutant mouse *in vivo* and *in vitro*. *Dev. Biol.* **79**, pp. 64–80.

Morest, D. K. (1969*a*). Differentiation of cerebral dendrites. A study of the post-migratory neuroblast in the medial nucleus of the trapezoid body. *Z. Anat. Entwickl-Gesch.* **128,** pp. 271–89.

Morest, D. K. (1969b). The growth of dendrites in the mammalian brain. *Z. Anat. Entwickl-Gesch.* **128,** pp. 290–317.

Mouren-Mathieu, A. M. and Colonnier, M. (1969). The molecular layer of the adult cat cerebellar cortex after lesion of the parallel fibres. An optic and electron microscopic study. *Brain Res.* **16,** pp. 307–23.

Mugnaini, E. (1969). Ultrastructural studies on cerebellar histogenesis. II. Maturation of nerve cell populations and establishment of synaptic connections in the cerebellar cortex of the chick. In *Neurobiology of cerebellar evolution and development* (ed. R. Llinas), pp. 749–82. American Medical Association, Chicago, IL.

Mugnaini, E. (1983). The length of cerebellar parallel fibres in chickens and rhesus monkey. *J. Comp. Neurol.* **220,** pp. 7–15.

Mugnaini, E. and Dahl, A. -L. (1975). Mode of distribution of aminergic fibres in the cerebellar cortex of the chicken. *J. Comp. Neurol.* **162,** pp. 417–32.

Overdijk, J., Uylings, H. B. M., Kuypers, K., and Kamstra, A. W. (1978). An economical, semi-automatic system for measuring cellular tree structures in three dimensions, with special emphasis on Golgi-impregnated neurons. *J. Microsc.* **114,** pp. 271–84.

Paldino, A. M. and Purpura, D. P. (1979). Quantitative analysis of the spatial distribution of axonal and dendritic terminals of hippocampal pyramidal neurons in immature human brain. *Exp. Neurol.* **64,** pp. 620–31.

Pappas, G. D. and Purpura, D. P. (1961). Fine structure of dendrites in the superficial neocortical neuropil. *Exp. Neurol.* **4,** pp. 507–30.

Parnavelas, J. G. and Uylings, H. B. M. (1980). The growth of non-pyramidal neurons in the visual cortex of the rat: a morphometric study. *Brain Res.* **193,** pp. 373–82.

Pasternak, J. F. and Woolsey, T. A. (1975). On the 'selectivity' of the Golgi-Cox Method. *J. Comp. Neurol.* **160,** pp. 307–12.

Pellionisz, A. and Llinas, R. (1977). A computer model of cerebellar Purkinje cells. *Neuroscience* **2,** pp. 37–48.

Perkel, D. H. (1983). Functional role of dendritic spines. *J. Physiol. (Paris.)* **78,** pp. 695–9.

Pettigrew, J. D. and Kasamatsu, T. (1978). Local perfusion of noradrenaline maintains visual cortical plasticity. *Nature* **271,** pp. 761–6.

Pfenninger, K. H. and Bunge, R. P. (1974). Freeze-fracturing of nerve growth cones and young fibres. A study of developing plasma membrane, *J. Cell Biol.* **63,** pp. 180–96.

Pongracz, F. (1985). The function of dendritic spines: a theoretical study. *Neuroscience.* **15,** pp. 933–46.

Puro, D. G. and Woodward, D. J. (1977). The climbing fibre system in the weaver mutant. *Brain Res.* **129,** pp. 141–6.

Purves, D. and Hadley, R. D. (1985). Changes in the dendritic branching of adult neurons revealed by repeated imaging *in situ. Nature* **315,** pp. 404–6.

Purves, D., Hadley, R. D., and Voyvodic, J. T. (1986). Dynamic changes in the dendritic geometry of individual neurons visualised over periods of up to three months in the superior cervical ganglion of living mice. *J. Neurosci.* **6,** pp. 1051–60.

Pysh, J. J. and Weiss, G. M. (1979). Exercise during development induces an increase in Purkinje cell dendritic tree size. *Science* **206,** pp. 230–1.

Rakic, P. (1976). Synaptic specificity in the cerebellar cortex: study of anomalous circuits induced by single gene mutations in mice. *Cold Spring Harb. Symp. Quant. Biol.* **40**, pp. 333–46.

Rakic, P. and Sidman, R. L. (1973a). Sequence of developmental abnormalities leading to granule cell deficit in cerebellar cortex of weaver mutant mice. *J. Comp. Neurol.* **152**, pp. 103–32.

Rakic, P. and Sidman, R. L. (1973b). Organisation of cerebellar cortex secondary to deficit of granule cells in weaver mutant mice. *J. Comp. Neurol.* **152**, pp. 133–62.

Rall, W. (1959). Branching dendritic trees and motoneuron membrane resistivity. *Exp. Neurol.* **1**, pp. 491–527.

Rall, W. (1962). Theory of physiological properties of dendrites. *Ann. N.Y. Acad. Sci.* **96**, pp. 1071–92.

Rall, W. (1964). Theoretical significance of dendritic trees for neuronal input–output relations. In *Neural theory and modelling* (ed. R. F. Reiss), pp 73–97. Stanford University Press, Stanford, CA.

Rall, W. (1970). Cable properties of dendrites and effects of synaptic location. In *Excitatory synaptic mechanisms* (eds. P. Anderson and J. K. S. Jansen), pp. 175–89. Scandinavian University Books, Oslo.

Rees, R. P., Bunge, M. B., and Bunge, R. P. (1976). Morphological changes in the neuritic growth cone and target neuron during synaptic junction development in culture. *J. Cell Biol.* **68**, pp. 240–63.

Rutledge, L. T., Wright, C., and Duncan, J. (1974). Morphological changes in the pyramidal cells of mammalian neocortex associated with increased use. *Exp. Neurol.* **44**, pp. 209–28.

Sadler, M. and Berry, M. (1983a). Vertex analysis of the growth of Purkinje cell dendritic fields of the mouse. *Acta. Stereol.* **2**, pp. 63–71.

Sadler, M. and Berry, M. (1983b). Morphometric study of the development of Purkinje cell dendritic trees in the mouse using vertex analysis. *J. Microsc.* **131**, pp. 341–54.

Sadler, M. and Berry, M. (1984). Remodelling during development of the Purkinje cell dendritic tree in the mouse. *Proc. R. Soc. Lond. B.* **221**, pp. 349–68.

Schlumpf, M., Shoemaker, W. J., and Bloom, F. E. (1977). The development of catecholamine fibres in the prenatal cerebellar cortex of the rat. *Neurosci. Abstr.* **3**, p. 361.

Sholl, D. A. (1953). Dendritic organization in the neurons of the visual and motor cortices of the cat. *J. Anat.* **87**, pp. 387–407.

Sholl, D.A. (1955). The organization of the visual cortex in the cat. *J. Anat.* **89**, pp. 33–46.

Sholl, D. A. (1956). *Organization of the cerebral cortex.* Methuen, Andover, Hants.

Sievers, J., Berry, M., and Baumgarten, H. G. (1981). The role of noradrenergic fibres in the control of post-natal cerebellar development. *Brain Res.* **207**, pp. 200–8.

Sievers, J., Klemm, H. P., Jenner, S., Baumgarten, H. G., and Berry, M. (1980). Neuronal and extraneuronal effects of intracisternally administered 6-OHDA on the developing rat brain. *J. Neurochem.* **34**, pp. 765–73.

Siggins, G. R., Hoffer, B. J., and Bloom, F. E. (1971). Studies on norepinephrine-containing afferents to Purkinje cells of rat cerebellum. III. Evidence for mediation of norepinephrine effects by cyclic 3, 5-adenine monophosphate. *Brain Res.* **25**, pp. 535–53.

Smit, G. J. and Colon, E. J. (1969). Quantitative analysis of the cerebral cortex. I. Aselectivity of the Golgi-Cox staining technique. *Brain Res.* **13**, pp. 485–510.

Sotelo, C. (1975). Anatomical, physiological and biochemical studies of the cerebellum from mutant mice. II. Morphological study of cerebellar cortical neurons and circuits in the weaver mouse. *Brain Res.* **94,** pp. 19–44.

Sotelo, C., Hillman, D. E., Zamora, A. K., and Llinas, R. (1975). Climbing fibre deafferentation, its action on Purkinje cell dendritic spines. *Brain Res.* **98,** pp. 574–81.

Spinelli, D. N., Jensen, F. E., and Viana Di Prisco, G. (1980). Early experience effect on dendritic branching in normally reared kittens. *Exp. Neurol.* **68,** pp. 1–11.

Stirling, R. V. (1986). Video techniques in neurobiology. *Trends Neurosci.* **9,** pp. 145–7.

Uylings, H. B. M., Kuypers, K., Diamond, M. C., and Veltman, W. A. M. (1978). Effects of differential environments on plasticity of dendrites of cortical pyramidal neurons in adult rats. *Exp. Neurol.* **62,** pp. 658–77.

Volkmar, F. R. and Greenough, W. T. (1972). Rearing complexity affects branching of dendrites in the visual cortex of the rat. *Science* **176,** pp. 1445–7.

Weber, A. and Schachner, M. (1984). Maintenance of immunocytologically identified Purkinje cells from mouse cerebellum in monolayer culture. *Brain Res.* **311,** pp. 119–30.

Weiss, G. M. and Pysh, J. J. (1978). Evidence for loss of Purkinje cell dendrites during late development: a morphometric Golgi analysis in the mouse. *Brain Res.* **154,** pp. 219–30.

West, M. J. and del Cerro, M. (1976). Early formation of synapses in the molecular layer of the foetal rat cerebellum. *J. Comp. Neurol.* **165,** pp. 137–60.

Wilson, L., Sotelo, C., and Caviness, V. S., Jr. (1981). Heterologous synapses upon Purkinje cells in the cerebellum of the reeler mutant mouse: an experimental light and electron microscopic study. *Brain Res.* **213,** pp. 63–82.

Wyss, U. R. (1972). Analysis of dendrite patterns by use of an adaptive scan system. *J. Microsc.* **95,** pp. 269–75.

Yamamoto, T., Ishikawa, M., and Tanaka, C. (1977). Catecholaminergic terminals in the developing and adult rat cerebellum. *Brain Res.* **132,** pp. 355–61.

Suggested further reading

PART 1

Eisen, J. S., Myers, P. Z., and Westerfield, M. (1986). Pathway selection by growth cones of identified motoneurons in live zebrafish embryos. *Nature (Lond.)* **320**, pp. 269–71.

Gimlich, R. L. and Braun, J. (1985). Improved fluorescent compounds for tracing cell lineage. *Develop. Biol.* **109**, pp. 509–14.

Gimlich, R. L. and Cooke, J. (1983). Cell lineage and the induction of second nervous systems in amphibian development. Nature (Lond.) **306**, pp. 471–3.

Kimmel, C. B. and Warga, R. M. (1986). Tissue-specific cell lineages orginate in the gastrula of the zebrafish. *Science* **231**, pp. 365–8.

Lawrence, P. A. and Martinez-Arias, A. (1985). The cell lineage of segments and parasegments in *Drosophila. Phil. Trans. Roy. Soc. B.* **312**, pp. 83–90.

Myers, P. Z. (1985). Spinal motoneurons of the larval zebrafish. *J. Comp. Neurol.* **236**, pp. 555–61.

Slack, J. M. W. (1984). *From egg to embryo.* Cambridge University Press, Cambridge.

Winklbauer, R. and Hausen, P. (1983). Development of the lateral line system in *Xenopus laevis*. II. Cell multiplication and organ formation in the supraorbital system. *J. Embryol. exp. Morph.* **76**, pp. 283–96.

PART 2

Nakamura, O. and Toivonen, S. (eds.) (1978). *Organizer—a milestone of a half-century since Spemann.* Elsevier, Amsterdam.

Nüsslein-Volhardt, C. and Wieschaus, E. (1980). Mutants affecting segment number and polarity in *Drosophila. Nature (Lond.)* **287**, pp. 795–801.

Schofield, P. (1986). *Trends Neurosci.* (in press).

Scott, M. P. (1984). Homoeotic gene transcripts in the neural tissue of insects. *Trends Neurosci.* **7**, pp. 221–3.

Smith, J. C., Dale, L., and Slack, J. M. W. (1985). Cell lineage labels and region-specific markers in the analysis of inductive interactions. *J. Embryol. exp. Morph.* **89** (suppl.), pp. 317–31.

Spemann, H. and Mangold, H. (1964). Induction of embryonic primordia by implantation of organizers from a different species. In *Foundations of experimental embryology* (eds. B. H. Wilher and J. M. Oppenheimer), pp. 145–84. Macmillan, London.

Waddington, C. H. (1940). *Organisers and genes.* Cambridge University Press, Cambridge.

Waddington, C. H. (1952). *The epigenetics of birds.* Cambridge University Press, Cambridge.

PART 3

Bate, C. M. (1976). Pioneer neurones in an insect embryo. *Nature* **260**, pp. 54–6.

Bastiani, M. J., Doe, C. Q., Helfand, L., and Goodman, C. S. (1985). Neuronal specificity and growth cone guidance in grasshopper and *Drosophila* embryos. *Trends Neurosci.* **8**, pp. 257–66.

Eisen, J. S., Myers, P. Z., and Westerfield, M. (1986). Pathway selection by growth cones of identified motoneurones in live zebra fish embryos. *Nature (Lond.)* **320**, pp. 269–71.

Hollyday, M. P. (1981). Development of motor innervation in chick embryos with supernumerary limbs. *Prog. Clin. Biol. Res.* **110A**, pp. 183–93.

Horder, T. J. and Martin, K. A. C. (1977). Morphogenetics as an alternative to chemospecificity in the formation of nerve connections. In *Cell–Cell recognition. Symp. Soc. exp. Biol. vol. 32.* (ed. Curtis, A. S. G.), pp. 275–58. Cambridge University Press, Cambridge.

Lance-Jones, C. and Landmesser, L. (1981). Pathway selection by chick lumbosacral motoneurons in an experimentally altered environment. *Proc. Roy. Soc. Lond. B.* **214**, pp. 19–52.

Sperry, R. W. (1963). Chemoaffinity in the orderly growth of nerve fiber patterns and connections. *Proc. Natl. Acad. Sci. (N.Y.)* **50**, pp. 703–10.

Stent, G. S. (1981). Strength and weakness of the genetic approach to the development of the nervous system. In *Studies in developmental neurobiology* (ed. W. M. Cowan), pp. 288–321. Oxford University Press, Oxford.

Wigston, D. J. and Sanes, J. R. (1982). Selective reinnervation of adult mammalian muscle by axons from different segmental levels. *Nature (Lond.)* **299**, pp. 464–7.

PART 4

Clarke, P. G. H. (1985). Neuronal cell death in the development of the vertebrate nervous system. *Trends Neurosci.* **8**, pp. 120–5.

Keating, M. J. (1975). The time course of experience dependent synaptic switching of visual connections in *Xenopus laevis*. *Proc. Roy. Soc. Edinburgh B.* **189**, pp. 603–10.

Liestøl, K., Mahelen, J., and Njå, A. (1986). Selective synaptic connections: significance of recognition and competition in mature sympathetic ganglia. *Trends Neurosci.* **9**, pp. 21–4.

Oppenheim, R. W. (1981). Neuronal cell death and some related regressive phenomena during neurogenesis: a selective historical review and progress report. In *Studies in developmental neurobiology* (ed. W. M. Cowan), pp. 74–133. Oxford University Press, Oxford.

Rakic, P. (1986). Mechanisms of ocular dominance segregation in the lateral geniculate nucleus: competitive elimination hypothesis. *Trends Neurosci.* **9**, pp. 11–15.

PART 5

Black, I. B. and Patterson, P. H. (1980). Developmental regulation of neurotransmitter phenotype. *Curr. Top. Develop. Biol.* **15,** pp. 27–40.

Bray, D. and Gilbert, D. (1981). Cytoskeletal elements in neurons. *Ann. Rev. Neurosci.* **4,** pp. 505–23.

Burnside, B. (1971). Microtubules and microfilaments in newt neurulation. *Develop. Biol.* **26,** pp. 416–41.

Froehner, S. C. (1986). The role of the post-synaptic cytoskeleton in AChR organization. *Trends Neurosci.* **9,** pp. 37–41.

Patterson, P. H. (1978). Environmental determination of autonomic neurotransmitter functions. *Ann. Rev. Neurosci.* **1,** pp. 1–17.

Pollard, T. D. (1976). Cytoskeletal functions of cytoplasmic contractile proteins. *J. Supramolec. Struct.* **5,** pp. 317–34.

Index

A2B4 antibody 270, 271
ablation experiments in nematodes 15–17, 19, 58–9
acetylcholine neurons (ChAT positive)
in cortex of mammals 436, 447, 449, 450
in insects 264
acetylcholine receptors 342, 343
nicotinic (AChRn) 454, 455, 457, 463
see also muscarinic acetylcholine receptors (AChRm)
adhesive interactions 128–9, 169
dendritic growth and 494
neural crest migration and 113, 116, 123–4
see also cell surface molecules; cellular interactions and neural cell adhesion molecule ageing, changes at neuromuscular junctions and 344–5, 349
alpha-adrenergic receptors 463, 465
alpha-bungarotoxin 389
binding sites 455, 457, 459, 461
Amblyostoma embryos, see axolotl embryos
amphibians
analysis of neural induction 75–82
astrocytes in spinal cord 276–7, 278
neural crest migration in 107, 110, 111, 117
see also axolotl embryos; frogs and newts
Amphioxus, segmentation of spinal cord 93–4
anterior commissure 323
aspartate 435
astrocytes
fibrous 268, 275
functional significance of heterogeneity of 271–5, 277
neurotransmitter receptors on 457
in optic nerve 268–75
protoplasmic 268, 275
in spinal cord 275–7
auditory cortex, transitory projections to 322, 325
auditory map, tectal 391
auditory nerve, neural crest cell pathways and development of 287–92, 310
Aves, see birds
axolotl embryos 119, 199, 233, 293

axonal branching (arborization)
of cutaneous sensory neurons in leeches 44–6
elimination of excess 46–7, 326–9, 334–5, 343, 348, 387, 407
shape of 421
see also axonal overproduction and elimination
axonal guidance 103, 148–9, 248
by chemotropic factors 166–83
of cutaneous sensory fibres 182
by 'labelled' pioneer axons 188–99
limb muscle motor axons 91–2, 135–8, 142, 181, 232–43
by neural cell adhesion molecule (NCAM) 135–8, 142
theories of 282
through sclerotomes 85–7, 88, 89, 94–5, 108
axonal outgrowth
formation of sensory fields in leeches 40–6
neural cell adhesion molecule (NCAM) expression during 133, 134–5, 141–2
axonal overproduction and elimination (developmental exuberance) 319–35
in central nervous system 320–3
mechanisms of 326–9
reasons for 331–5
timing of 323–6
see also axonal branching, elimination of excess; cell death and regeneration, of retinotectal axons
axon boundaries 235, 282
role of glia in 283–7, 309–10
role of neural crest and crest-like cells 294–308, 309–10
axon pathways 103, 166–7, 282
followed by regeneration retinotectal axons 215–16, 217–21, 222–3
formed by pioneering axons 189–99
to limb buds 232–7
of normal retinal axons in goldfish 204–14
role of glia in 283–7, 309–10
role of neural crest and crest-like cells in 287–93, 309–10